ECONOMICS
FOR HEALTHCARE
MANAGERS

ECONOMICS
FOR HEALTHCARE
MANAGERS

THIRD EDITION

ROBERT H. LEE

AUPHA

Health Administration Press, Chicago, Illinois

Association of University Programs in Health Administration, Arlington, Virginia

19 18 17 16   5 4 3

Library of Congress Cataloging-in-Publication Data

Lee, Robert H., 1948– author.
  Economics for healthcare managers / Robert H. Lee. — Third edition.
    p. ; cm.
  "HAP/AUPHA."
  Includes bibliographical references and index.
  ISBN 978-1-56793-676-6 (alk. paper)
  I. Health Administration Press. II. Association of University Programs in Health Administration. III. Title.
  [DNLM: 1. Health Services Administration—economics—United States. 2. Costs and Cost Analysis—United States. 3. Economics, Medical—United States. W 84 AA1]
  RA427
    362.1068'1—dc23
                    2014014759

Acquisitions editor: Tulie O'Connor; Project manager: Andrew Baumann; Manuscript editor: Karin Horler; Cover designer: Mark Oberkrom; Layout: Cepheus Edmondson

Found an error or a typo? We want to know! Please e-mail it to hapbooks@ache.org, and put "Book Error" in the subject line.

For photocopying and copyright information, please contact Copyright Clearance Center at www.copyright.com or at (978) 750–8400.

Health Administration Press
A division of the Foundation of the American
  College of Healthcare Executives
One North Franklin Street, Suite 1700
Chicago, IL 60606–3529
(312) 424–2800

Association of University Programs
  in Health Administration
2000 North 14th Street
Suite 780
Arlington, VA 22201
(703) 894–0940

BRIEF CONTENTS

DETAILED CONTENTS

PREFACE TO THE THIRD EDITION

A third edition of *Economics for Healthcare Managers* is needed for two reasons. The main reason is the dramatic changes underway in healthcare. Health insurance has changed, partly because of the effects of the Affordable Care Act of 2010 and partly because of the increasing ability of insurers and sponsors to identify efficient and inefficient providers of care. Healthcare providers will have to respond to these changes in insurance; the exact nature of those responses is impossible to forecast. Nonetheless, change is in the wind, and everyone in healthcare must be prepared. The radical idea that success requires offering one's customers exceptional value is becoming more common in healthcare. While challenging, this classic prescription for managing turbulent times is one of the most useful ideas that economics has to offer.

Second, two new topics need to be covered. One topic is an overview of initiatives to improve population health, reduce the per-person costs of healthcare, and improve the patient experience of care. The second topic is behavioral economics. This idea—that individuals often take shortcuts in decision making and make poor decisions as a result—is especially relevant for managers. Managers sometimes use rules of thumb to make choices, and some of these rules of thumb can harm employees, patients, and organizations. Being forewarned may prevent some of these errors.

The third edition remains firmly focused on the economics that healthcare managers need to understand, but it updates the references and offers students a glimpse into contemporary research. Although many classic citations remain vital, economists have done a great deal of interesting work since the publication of the previous edition. The third edition shares some of this work with students.

This textbook and the accompanying online instructor resources are designed to facilitate discussion and learning. Study questions are included at the end of each chapter, and the instructor resources include answers to the study questions, a PowerPoint presentation for each chapter as a teaching aid, and a test bank. For access information, e-mail hapbooks@ache.org.

1

WHY HEALTH ECONOMICS?

Learning Objectives

After reading this chapter, students will be able to

- describe the value of economics for managers,
- identify major challenges for healthcare managers,
- find current information about healthcare outcomes, and
- distinguish between positive and normative economics.

Key Concepts

- Economics helps managers focus on key issues.
- Economics helps managers understand goal-oriented decision making.
- Economics helps managers understand strategic decision making.
- Economics gives managers a framework for understanding costs.
- Economics gives managers a framework for understanding market demand.
- Economics gives managers a framework for assessing profitability.
- Healthcare managers must deal effectively with risk and uncertainty.
- Healthcare managers must contend with the management problems that insurance presents.
- Information asymmetries create a number of problems for healthcare managers.
- Not-for-profit organizations create unique problems for managers.
- Rapid change in the healthcare system forces managers to lead their organizations into unfamiliar territory on a routine basis.

1.1 Why Health Economics?

Why should working healthcare managers study economics? This simple question is really two questions. Why is economics valuable for managers? What special challenges do healthcare managers face? These questions motivate this book.

Why is economics valuable for managers? There are six reasons. We will briefly touch on each of them to highlight the themes we will develop in later chapters.

1. Economics helps managers focus on key issues. Economics helps managers wade through the deluge of information they confront and identify the data they need.
2. Economics outlines strategies for realizing goals given the available resources. One of the primary tasks of economics is to explore carefully the implications of rational decision making.
3. Economics gives managers ground rules for strategic decision making. When rivals are not only competing against them but watching what they do, managers must be prepared to think strategically (i.e., be prepared to use the insights of game theory).

Cost
The value of a resource in its next best use

4. Economics gives managers a framework for making sense of **costs**. Managers need to understand costs because good decisions are unlikely without this understanding.
5. Economics gives managers a framework for thinking about value. The benefits of the goods and services successful organizations provide to customers exceed the costs of producing those goods and services. Good management decisions require an understanding of how customers perceive value.
6. Most important, economics sensitizes managers to fundamental ideas that affect the operations of every organization. Effective management begins with the recognition that consumers are sensitive to price differences, that organizations compete to advance the interests of their stakeholders, and that success comes from providing value to customers.

1.2 Economics as a Map for Decision Making

Economics provides a map for decision making. Maps do two things. They highlight key features and suppress unimportant features. To drive from Des Moines, Iowa, to Dallas, Texas, you need to know how the major highways connect. You do not want to know the name and location of each street in each town you pass through. Of course, what is important and what is unimportant depend on the task at hand. If you want to drive from West 116th Street and Ridgeview Road in Olathe, Kansas, to the Truman homestead in Independence, Missouri, a map that describes only the interstate highway system will be of limited value to you. You need to know which map is the right tool for your situation.

Using a map takes knowledge and skill. You need to know what information you need, or you may choose the wrong map and be swamped in extraneous data or lost without key facts. Having the right map is no guarantee that you can use it, however. You need to practice to be able to use a map quickly and effectively. In the same sense, economics is a map for decision making.

Like a map, economics highlights some issues and suppresses others. For example, economics tells managers to focus on **marginal** or **incremental costs**, which makes understanding and managing costs much simpler, but economics has little to say about the belief systems that motivate consumer behavior. If you are seeking to make therapeutic regimens easier to adhere to by making them more consistent with consumers' belief systems, economics is not a helpful map. If, on the other hand, you want to decide whether setting up an urgent care clinic is financially feasible, economics helps you focus on how your project will change revenues and costs.

Economics also gives managers a framework for understanding rational decision making. **Rational decision making** means making choices that further one's goals given the resources available. Whether those goals include maximizing profits, securing the health of the indigent, or other objectives, the framework is much the same. It entails looking at benefits and costs to

Marginal/ incremental
Involving a small change from the current situation

Marginal or incremental cost
The cost of producing an additional unit of output

Rational decision making
Choosing the course of action that gives you the best outcomes, given the constraints you face

---

CASE 1.1 An Upset Customer

I ran into one of my neighbors last night. He was really upset with us. He had a routine echocardiogram at his cardiologist's office and was shocked to learn that it cost $1,600. Six months ago he paid $400 for the same test in the same office. He called the doctor's office and asked why the fee went up so much. The office staff told him that the practice had been acquired by our hospital system, so there was now a facility fee plus the higher rate that our system had negotiated with his insurer. That did not make him happier. Nor did it increase our revenue for long. The next time he went to an independent imaging center and got the test done for $300. He has a high-deductible insurance plan, so he had to pay the entire higher fee. He is also thinking of finding a new cardiologist.

Discussion questions:
- Do negotiated fees really vary as much as this case suggests?
- Are hospitals buying increasing numbers of medical practices?
- Do prices typically go up when a hospital buys a practice?
- What is a high-deductible insurance plan?
- Are high-deductible plans becoming more common?
- Is buying medical practices a profitable strategy for hospitals?
- If you were this customer, how would you react?

realize the largest net benefit. (We will explore this question further in section 1.5.)

Managers must understand costs and be able to explain costs to others. Confusion about costs is common, so confusion in decision making is also common. Confusion about benefits is even more widespread than confusion about costs. As a result, management decisions in healthcare often leave much to be desired.

Economists typically speak about economics at a theoretical level, using "perfectly competitive markets" (which are, for the most part, mythical social structures) as a model, which makes application of economics difficult for managers competing in real-world markets. Yet, economics offers concrete guidance about pricing, contracting, and other quandaries that managers face. Economics also offers a framework for evaluating the strategic choices managers must make. Many healthcare organizations have rivals, so good decisions must take into account what the competition is doing. Will being the first to enter a market give your organization an advantage, or will it give your rivals a low-cost way of seeing what works and what does not? Will buying primary care practices bring you increased market share or buyer's remorse? Knowing economics will not make these choices easy, but it can give managers a plan for sorting through the issues.

1.3 Special Challenges for Healthcare Managers

What special challenges do healthcare managers face? Healthcare managers face five issues more often than other managers do:

1. The central roles of risk and uncertainty
2. The complexities created by insurance
3. The perils produced by information asymmetries
4. The problems posed by not-for-profit organizations
5. The rapid and confusing course of technical and institutional change

Let's look at each of these challenges in more depth.

1.3.1 Risk and Uncertainty

Risk and uncertainty are defining features of healthcare markets and healthcare organizations. Both the incidence of illness and the effectiveness of medical care should be described in terms of probabilities. For example, the right therapy, provided the right way, usually carries some risk of failure. A proportion of patients will experience harmful side effects, and a proportion of patients will not benefit. As a result, management of costs and quality presents difficult challenges. Has a provider produced bad outcomes because he was unlucky and had to treat an extremely sick panel of patients, or because he encountered a panel of patients for whom standard therapies were ineffective? Did his colleagues let him down? Or was he incompetent, sloppy, or lazy? The reason is not always evident.

1.3.2 Insurance

Because risk and uncertainty are inherent in healthcare, most consumers have medical insurance. As a result, healthcare organizations have to contend with the management problems insurance presents. First, insurance creates confusion about who the customer is. Customers use the products, but insurance plans often pay most of the bill. Moreover, most people with private medical insurance receive coverage through their employer (in large part because the tax system makes this arrangement advantageous). Although economists generally agree that employees ultimately pay for insurance via wage reductions, most employees do not know the costs of their insurance alternatives (and unless they are changing jobs, they have limited interest in finding out). As a result of the employer plan default, employees remain unaware of the true costs of care and are not eager to balance cost and value. If insurance is footing the bill, most patients choose the best, most expensive treatment—a choice they might not make if they were paying the full cost of care.

In addition, insurance makes even simple transactions complex. Most transactions involve at least three parties (the patient, the insurer, and the provider), and many involve more. To add to the confusion, most providers deal with a wide array of insurance plans and face blizzards of disparate claim forms and payment systems. Increasing numbers of insurance plans have negotiated individual payment systems and rates, so many healthcare providers look wistfully at industries that simply bill customers to obtain revenues. The complexity of insurance transactions also increases opportunity for error and fraud. In fact, both are fairly common.

Despite this bewildering array of insurance plans, many providers still rely on a select few plans for their revenue (a circumstance most managers seek to avoid). For example, most hospitals receive at least a third of their revenue from Medicare. As a result, changes in Medicare regulations or payment methods can profoundly alter a healthcare organization's prospects. Overnight, changes to reimbursement terms may transform a market that is profitable for everyone to one in which only the strongest, best-led, best-positioned organizations can survive.

1.3.3 Information Asymmetries

Information asymmetries are common in healthcare markets and create a number of problems. When an information asymmetry exists, the party with more information has an opportunity to take advantage of the party with

Information asymmetry
When one party in a transaction has less information than another

less information. Recognizing a disadvantage, the party with less information may become skeptical of the other party's motivation and decline a recommendation that would have been beneficial. For example, physicians and other healthcare providers usually understand patients' medical options better than patients do. Unaware of their choices, patients may accept recommendations for therapies that are not cost-effective or, recognizing their vulnerability to physicians' self-serving advice, may resist recommendations made in their best interests.

From a manager's perspective, asymmetric information means that providers have a great deal of autonomy in recommending therapies. Because providers' recommendations largely define the operations of insurance plans, hospitals, and group practices, managers need to ensure that providers do not have incentives to use their superior information to their advantage. Conversely, in certain situations, patients have the upper hand and are likely to forecast their healthcare use more accurately than insurers. Patients know whether they want to start a family, whether they seek medical attention whenever they feel ill, or whether they have symptoms that indicate a potential condition. As a result, health plans are vulnerable to **adverse selection**.

Adverse selection
High-risk consumers' willingness to pay more for insurance than low-risk consumers (Organizations that have difficulty distinguishing high-risk from low-risk consumers are unlikely to be profitable.)

1.3.4 Not-for-Profit Organizations

Most not-for-profit organizations have worthy goals that their managers take seriously, but these organizations can create problems for healthcare managers as well. For example, not-for-profit organizations usually have multiple stakeholders. Multiple stakeholders mean multiple goals, so organizations become much harder to manage, and managers' performance becomes harder to assess. The potential for managers to put their own needs before their stakeholders' needs exists in all organizations but is more difficult to detect in not-for-profit organizations because they do not have a simple bottom line. In addition, not-for-profit organizations may be harder to run well. They operate amid a web of regulations designed to prevent them from being used as tax avoidance schemes. These regulations make setting up incentive-based compensation systems for managers, employees, and contractors (the most important of whom are physicians) more difficult. Further, when a project is not successful, not-for-profit organizations have greater difficulty putting the resources invested in the failed idea to other uses. For example, the trustees of a not-for-profit organization may have to get approval from a court to sell or repurpose its assets. Because of these special circumstances, managers of not-for-profit organizations can always claim that substandard performance reflects their more complex environment.

1.3.5 Technological and Institutional Change

This fifth challenge makes the others pale in comparison. The healthcare system is in a state of flux. Virtually every part of the healthcare sector is reinventing itself,

CASE 1.2　Questions About Tax Exemptions

Pittsburgh mayor Luke Ravenstahl announced on March 20, 2013, that he was going to challenge the nonprofit status of the University of Pittsburgh Medical Center. The mayor's legal review concluded that the medical center provides too little charity care, has diversified overseas, and structures its operations to serve wealthy customers. The review also noted that the CEO had a $5.9 million salary; that the CEO's headquarters included a chef, a chauffeur, and a dining room; that more than 20 employees are paid more than $1 million; that the medical center owned a corporate jet; and that the medical center had profits of nearly $1 billion during the last several years. Most observers believe that the mayor is seeking a negotiated settlement that will result in payments in lieu of taxes (Hamill 2013).

Hospitals began as refuges for the poor, with clearly charitable missions. But the increasing use of hospitals by paying customers, the resulting expansion of the hospital sector, and higher tax rates necessitated clear standards for tax exemption. In 1956 the Internal Revenue Service published a statement requiring that a tax-exempt hospital "be operated to the extent of its financial ability for those not able to pay for the services rendered." In addition, a tax-exempt hospital could not "refuse to accept patients in need of hospital care who cannot pay for such services," nor was it dispensing charity if it operated "with the expectation of full payment" and incurred bad debt as a result of non-payment (US Internal Revenue Service 1956).

Thirteen years later, following the introduction of Medicare and Medicaid, the Internal Revenue Service substituted a broader "community benefit" standard, which expanded the definition of activities eligible for tax exemption. After lying dormant for a number of years, the issue resurfaced in the 1980s when local groups began complaining about hospitals' tax exemptions. In the 1990s, the conversion of not-for-profit hospitals to for-profit status seemed to have little effect on taxes (other than increases in local tax revenues), and concern spread. A study by the US Government Accountability Office found that the volume of charity care provided by not-for-profit hospitals was only marginally greater than the volume of charity care provided by for-profit hospitals (Walker 2005).

(continued)

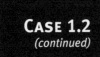

CASE 1.2
(continued)

The issue is not settled. Clearly, though, losing tax-exempt status can have a major impact on a hospital's finances. This issue is a major concern for any not-for-profit manager. Most economists are skeptical of a subsidy without a clear link to the desired outcome. At a minimum, the manager must be able to explain what taxpayers receive in return.

The Affordable Care Act (ACA) requires tax-exempt hospitals to conduct community needs assessments and address the needs that are found. Most tax-exempt hospitals were required to do so by the end of 2013. In addition, the ACA is intended to reduce the number of uninsured, hence the amount of charity care that hospitals must provide.

Discussion questions:
- What do hospitals have to do to qualify for tax-exempt status?
- How much charity care do hospitals provide on average?
- How much is tax-exempt status worth to hospitals?
- Should the University of Pittsburgh Medical Center be required to pay Pittsburgh taxes?

and no one seems to know where the healthcare system is headed. Leadership is difficult to provide if you don't know where you are going. Because change presents a pervasive test for healthcare managers, we will examine it in greater detail.

1.4 Turmoil in the Healthcare System

Why is the healthcare system of the United States in such turmoil? One explanation is common to the entire developed world: rapid technical change. The pace of medical research and development is breathtaking, and the public's desire for better therapies is manifest. These demands challenge healthcare managers to regularly lead their organizations into unmapped territory. To make matters worse, changes in technology or changes in insurance can quickly affect healthcare markets. In healthcare, as in every other sector of the economy, new technologies can create winners and losers. For example, between 2000 and 2007 Medicare payments to ambulatory surgery centers more than doubled. Medicare changed its policy, and growth slowed down (MedPac 2013). What appears profitable today may not be profitable tomorrow if technology, competition, rates, or regulations change significantly.

The ACA seems to have resulted in a wave of innovations by providers, insurers, employers, and governments. (See Chapter 6 for more detail.) Which of these innovations will succeed is not clear. In addition, some healthcare organizations will thrive in the new environment, and some will fail. The passage of the ACA appears to have been transformative, but its repeal might not undo the changes it led to.

1.4.1 The Pressure to Reduce Costs

The economics of high healthcare costs are far simpler than the politics of high healthcare costs. To reduce costs, managers must reallocate resources from low-productivity uses to high-productivity uses, increase productivity wherever feasible, and reduce prices paid to suppliers and sectors that have excess supply. They also must recognize that cost cutting is politically difficult. Reallocating resources and increasing productivity will cost some people their jobs. Reducing prices will lower some people's incomes. These steps are difficult for any government to take, and many of those who will be affected (physicians, nurses, and hospital employees) are politically well organized.

CASE 1.3   **Why Is the Pressure to Reduce Healthcare Costs So Strong?**

The United States spends far more on healthcare than other wealthy industrial countries do but, according to health indicators, fares worse than most of them. Spending per person is nearly double the spending per person in Germany, Canada, and France (see Exhibit 1.1). Differences this large should be reflected in the outcomes of care.

Country	2000	2011
Canada	$2,519	$4,522
France	$2,544	$4,118
Germany	$2,677	$4,495
Japan	$1,969	$3,213
United Kingdom	$1,827	$3,405
United States	$4,791	$8,508

EXHIBIT 1.1
Healthcare Spending per Person

Source: Data from OECD (2013b).
Note: Spending figures have been converted into US dollars.

(continued)

CASE 1.3
(continued)

As you can see in Exhibit 1.2, of the six countries listed, the United States has the shortest life expectancy at birth. In an analysis of potentially avoidable deaths, Nolte and McKee (2012) noted that the United States had a higher rate of potentially avoidable deaths and slower rates of improvement than France, Germany, or the United Kingdom. Greater spending should not produce these results.

EXHIBIT 1.2
Life Expectancy at Birth, 2011

Country	Males	Females
Canada[a]	78.7 years	83.3 years
France	78.7 years	85.7 years
Germany	78.4 years	83.2 years
Japan	79.4 years	85.9 years
United Kingdom	79.1 years	83.1 years
United States	76.3 years	81.1 years

Source: Data from OECD (2013b).
[a] Canadian data are for 2009.

Discussion questions:

- Why is spending so much more than other countries on healthcare a problem?
- What can Americans not buy because of high spending on healthcare?
- What factors other than healthcare affect population health?
- Does this evidence suggest that the American healthcare system is not efficient?

1.4.2 The Fragmentation of Healthcare Payments

The fragmentation of healthcare bills compounds the political problem. Most Americans see only a part of the cost of healthcare. A typical American pays his or her share of healthcare costs through a mixture of direct payments for care; payroll deductions for insurance premiums; lower wages; higher prices for goods and services; and federal, state, and local taxes. Because so much of the payment system is hidden, most Americans cannot track healthcare costs. The exceptions, notably employers who write checks for the entire cost of insurance policies and the trustees of the Medicare system, understand the need to reduce costs. Given that so few Americans recognize how much their healthcare system costs, the complex system of public regulations and subsidies will change slowly, at best.

1.5 What Does Economics Study?

What does economics study? Economics analyzes the allocation of **scarce resources**. Although this answer appears straightforward, several definitions are needed to make this sentence understandable. Resources include anything useful in consumption or production. From the perspective of a manager, resources include the flow of services from supplies or equipment the organization owns and the flow of services from employees, buildings, or other entities the organization hires. A resource is scarce if it has alternative uses, which might include another use within the organization or use by another person or organization. Most issues that managers deal with involve scarce resources, so economics is potentially useful for nearly all of them.

Scarce resources
Anything useful in consumption or production that has alternative uses

Economics focuses on rational behavior—that is, it focuses on individuals' efforts to best realize their goals, given their resources. Because time and energy spent in collecting and analyzing information are scarce resources (i.e., the time and energy have other uses), complete rationality is irrational. Everyone uses shortcuts and rules to make certain choices, and doing so is rational, even though better decisions are theoretically possible.

Much of economics is positive. **Positive economics** uses objective analysis and evidence to answer questions about individuals, organizations, and societies. Positive economics might describe the state of healthcare, for example, in terms of hospital occupancy rates over a certain period. Positive economics also proposes hypotheses and assesses how consistent the evidence is with them. For example, one might examine whether the evidence supports the conjecture that reductions in direct consumer payments for medical care (measured as a share of spending) have been a major contributing factor in the rapid growth of healthcare spending per person. Although values do not directly enter the realm of positive economics, they do shape the questions economists ask (or do not ask) and how they interpret the evidence.

Positive economics
Using objective analysis and evidence to answer questions about individuals, organizations, and societies

Normative economics often addresses public policy issues, but not always. The manager of a healthcare organization who can identify additional services or additional features that customers are willing to pay for is demonstrating normative economics. Likewise, the manager who can identify features or services that customers do not value is also demonstrating normative economics.

Normative economics
Using values to identify the best options

Normative economics takes two forms. In one, citizens use the tools of economics to answer public policy questions. Usually these questions

Why Does the United States Spend More on Medical Care Than Other Wealthy Countries Do?

Compared to that of other wealthy countries (those that are members of the Organisation for Economic Co-operation and Development [OECD]), healthcare spending in the United States is very high. In 2011 spending per person in the United States was $8,508. This figure was more than 50 percent higher than spending in Norway and Switzerland, which had the second and third highest spending per person (OECD 2013b). Average incomes are actually higher in Norway and Switzerland than in the United States, so income levels don't explain the difference.

The population of the United States is actually one of the youngest in the OECD (OECD 2013a). In addition, alcohol and tobacco use are lower than in most other wealthy countries. Obesity rates, however, are the highest in the OECD, but obesity doesn't lead to high rates of service use. Residents of the United States generally use *fewer* services than residents of other OECD countries.

For the most part, Americans use fewer medical services than other OECD residents but pay substantially higher prices. For example, compared to patients in other wealthy countries, American patients average 61 percent fewer physician visits and 24 percent fewer hospital stays (OECD 2013b). But prices are much higher in the United States. For example, at $1,634 the Medicare payment to a physician for hip replacement is 70 percent higher than the average amount paid by public programs in Australia, Canada, France, Germany, or the United Kingdom. The average private insurance payment is $3,996, which is more than double the Medicare payment and the average private insurance payment in Australia, France, or the United Kingdom (Laugesen and Glied 2011). Because private hospital and physician prices are higher in the United States, the total payments for a major procedure are much higher. In 2012, for example, average hospital and physician payments for a hip replacement were $40,364 in the United States versus $9,574 in Switzerland, $10,927 in France, $11,187 in the Netherlands, and $27,810 in Australia (International Federation of Health Plans 2013).

Americans also spend far more on hospital care, even though they are less likely to be admitted and usually have a shorter stay if they

(continued)

> *(continued)*
>
> are admitted. Some of the difference can be attributed to prices, but higher levels of staffing and equipment in American hospitals are also factors. Sorting out how much of the difference in the cost per hospitalization is attributable to price differences and how much is attributable to higher levels of staffing and equipment is an example of positive economics. Sorting out whether higher levels of staffing and equipment are worth the extra cost takes us into the realm of normative economics.

involve ethical and value judgments (which economics cannot supply) as well as factual judgments (which economics can support or refute). A question like "Should the Medicare program provide coverage for prescription drugs?" involves balancing benefits and harms. Economic analysis can help assess the facts that underlie the benefits and harms but cannot provide an answer. The second form of normative economics is the basis for this book's content. This form tells us how to analyze what we *should* do, given the circumstances that we face. In this part of normative analysis, market transactions indicate value. For example, we may believe that a drug is overpriced, but we must treat that price as a part of the environment and react appropriately if no one will sell it for less. Most managers find themselves in such an environment.

To best realize our goals within the constraints we face, we can use the explicit guidance economics gives us:

1. First, identify plausible alternatives. Breakthroughs usually occur when someone realizes there is an alternative to the way things have always been done.
2. Second, consider modifying the standard choice (e.g., charging a slightly higher price or using a little more of a nurse practitioner's time).
3. Next, pick the best choice by determining the level at which its *marginal benefit* equals its *marginal cost*. (We will explain these terms shortly.)
4. Finally, examine whether the total benefits of this activity exceed the total cost.

Skilled managers routinely perform this sort of analysis. For example, a profit-seeking organization might conclude that a clinic's profits would be as large as possible if it hired three physicians and two nurse practitioners, but that the clinic's profits would still be unacceptably low if it did. Profits would fall even further if it increased or decreased the number of physicians and nurse practitioners, so the profit-seeking organization would choose to close the clinic.

Let's back up and define some terms to make this discussion clearer. *Cost*, as noted previously, is the value of a resource in its next best use. For example, the cost of a plot of land for a medical office would be the most another user would pay for it, not what it sold for 20 years ago. The next best use of that land might be for housing, for a park, for a store, or for some other use. Usually the next best use of a resource is someone else's use of it, so a resource's cost is the price we must pay for it. If 30 Lipitor tablets are worth $80 to another consumer, that will be our cost for it. *Benefit* is the value we place on a desired outcome. We describe this value in terms of our willingness to trade one desired outcome for another. Often, but not always, our willingness to pay money for an outcome is a convenient measure of value. A *marginal* or an *incremental* amount is the increased cost we incur from using more of a resource or the increased benefit we realize from a greater outcome. So, if a 16-ounce soda costs 89 cents and a 24-ounce soda costs 99 cents, the incremental cost of the larger size is $(99 - 89) \div (24 - 16)$, or 1.25 cents per ounce. A rational consumer might conclude that

1. the incremental benefit of the larger soda exceeds its incremental cost and buy the larger size;
2. the incremental cost of the larger soda exceeds its incremental benefit and buy the smaller size; or
3. the total benefit of both sizes was less than their total cost and buy neither.

Remember, however, that rational decisions are defined by the goals that underpin them. A consumer with a train to catch might buy an expensive small soda at the station to save time.

1.6 Conclusion

Why should healthcare managers study economics? To be better managers. Economics offers a framework that can simplify and improve management decisions. This framework is valuable to all managers. It is especially valuable to clinicians who assume leadership roles in healthcare organizations.

Managers are routinely overwhelmed with information, yet lack the key facts that they need to make good decisions. Economics offers a map that makes focusing on essential information easier.

Exercises

1.1 Why is the idea that value depends on consumers' preferences radical?

1.2 Mechanics usually have better information about how to fix automobiles than their customers do. What problems does this advantage create? Do mechanics or their customers do anything to limit these problems?

1.3 A mandatory health insurance plan costs $4,000. One worker earns $24,500 in employment income and $500 in investment income. Another worker earns $48,000 in employment income and $2,000 in investment income. A third worker earns $68,000 in employment income and $7,000 in investment income. A premium-based system would cost each worker $4,000. A wage tax–based system would cost each worker 8.5 percent of wages. An income tax–based system would cost each worker 8 percent of income. For each worker, calculate the cost of the insurance as a share of total income.

	Worker 1	Worker 2	Worker 3
E = Employment income	$24,500	$48,000	$68,000
I = Investment income	$500	$2,000	$7,000
P = Premium cost of insurance	$4,000	$4,000	$4,000
Premium as a percentage of income = P/(E + I)			
W = Wage tax cost of insurance = 0.085 × E			
Wage tax cost as a percentage of income = W/(E + I)			
T = Income tax cost of insurance = 0.080 × (E + I)			
Income tax cost as a percentage of income = T/(E + I)			

1.4 Which of the payment systems in Exercise 1.3 would impose the larger burden on those with incomes under $25,000: a plan financed via premiums, via the income tax, or via a payroll tax?

1.5 Which of the plans in Exercise 1.3 would be fairer?

1.6 Which of the preceding questions can you answer using positive economics? For which of the preceding questions must you use normative economics?

1.7 The following table shows data for Australia, Canada, and the United States.

   a. How did female life expectancy at birth change between 2000 and 2010?

   b. How did expenditure per person change between 2000 and 2010?

c. What conclusions do you draw from these data?

d. If you were the "manager" of the healthcare system in the United States, what would be a sensible response to data like these?

	Life Expectancy (years)		Expenditure per Person	
	2000	2010	2000	2010
Australia	82.0	84.0	$2,861	$3,800
Canada	81.7	83.3[a]	$3,190	$3,965
United States	79.3	81.1	$6,067	$8,508

Source: Data from OECD (2013b).
Notes: Life expectancy is female life expectancy at birth. Expenditure per person has been translated into US dollars and adjusted for inflation.
[a] Data from 2009.

References

Hamill, S. D. 2013. "UPMC, Pittsburgh Stake Positions for Court Fight on Non-profit Status." *Pittsburgh Post-Gazette*, March 22.

International Federation of Health Plans. 2013. *2012 Comparative Price Report.* Accessed July 2, 2014. www.ifhp.com.

Laugesen, M. J., and S. A. Glied. 2011. "Higher Fees Paid to US Physicians Drive Higher Spending for Physician Services Compared to Other Countries." *Health Affairs* 30 (9): 1647–56.

Medicare Payment Advisory Commission (MedPAC). 2013. *A Data Book: Health Care Spending and the Medicare Program.* Published June. www.medpac.gov/documents/Jun13DataBookEntireReport.pdf.

Nolte, E., and C. M. McKee. 2012. "In Amenable Mortality—Deaths Avoidable Through Health Care—Progress in the US Lags That of Three European Countries." *Health Affairs* 31 (9): 2114–22.

Organisation for Economic Co-operation and Development (OECD). 2013a. *OECD Factbook 2013: Economic, Environmental and Social Statistics.* Published January 9. www.oecd-ilibrary.org/content/book/factbook-2013-en.

———. 2013b. "OECD Health Data 2013." Accessed April 23, 2014. www.oecd.org/health/health-systems/oecdhealthdata.htm.

US Internal Revenue Service. 1956. Revenue Ruling 56-185. Accessed July 2, 2014. www.irs.gov/pub/irs-tege/rr56-185.pdf.

Walker, D. M. 2005. *Nonprofit, For-Profit, and Government Hospitals: Uncompensated Care and Other Community Benefits.* Washington, DC: US Government Accountability Office.

AN OVERVIEW OF THE US HEALTHCARE SYSTEM

Learning Objectives

After reading this chapter, students will be able to

- apply marginal analysis to a simple economic problem,
- articulate the input and output views of healthcare products,
- find current national and international information about healthcare,
- compare the US healthcare system to those in other countries, and
- identify major trends in healthcare.

Key Concepts

- Healthcare products are inputs into health.
- Healthcare products are also outputs of the healthcare sector.
- The usefulness of healthcare products varies widely.
- Marginal analysis helps managers focus on the right questions.
- Life expectancies have increased sharply in the United States in recent years.
- Other wealthy countries have seen larger health gains with smaller cost increases.
- The healthcare sector may change radically in response to technology and policy changes.

2.1 Input and Output Views of Healthcare

This chapter describes the healthcare system of the United States from an economic point of view and introduces tools of economic analysis. It looks at the healthcare system from two perspectives. The first perspective, called the *input view*, emphasizes healthcare's contribution to the public's well-being. The second perspective, called the *output view*, emphasizes the goods and services the healthcare sector produces. In the language of economics, an

Input
Goods and
services used in
production

Output
Goods and
services produced
by an organization

input is a good or service used in the production of another good or service, and an **output** is the good or service that emerges from a production process. Products (which include both goods and services) are commonly both inputs and outputs. For example, a surgical tool is an input into a surgery and an output of a surgical tool company. Similarly, the surgery itself can be considered an output of the surgical team or an input into the health of the patient.

2.1.1 The Input View

The input view of the healthcare system stresses the usefulness of healthcare products. From this perspective, healthcare products are neither good nor bad; they are simply tools used to improve and maintain health. The input view is important because it focuses our attention on alternative ways of achieving our goals, and healthcare products are only one of many inputs into health. Others, such as exercise, diet, and rest, are alternative ways to improve or maintain health. From this perspective, a switch from medical therapies for high blood pressure to meditation or exercise would be based on the following question: Which is the least expensive way to get the result I want? This apparently simple question can be very difficult to answer.

The input view stresses that the usefulness of any resource depends on the problem at hand and other available resources. Whether the health of a particular patient or population will improve as a result of using more healthcare products depends on a number of factors, including the quality and quantity of healthcare products already being used, the quality and quantity of other health inputs, and the general well-being of the patient or population. For example, the effect of a drug on an otherwise healthy 30-year-old is likely to be different from its effect on an 85-year-old who is taking 11 other medications. Or, increasing access to medical care is not likely to be the best way to reduce infant mortality in a population that is malnourished and lacks access to safe drinking water, given the powerful effects of better food and water on health outcomes. Likewise, consider the question, What is the best way to use our resources, given that most preventable mortality is a result of risky behavior? Sometimes, more medical care is not the answer. All of these examples illustrate that the usefulness of resources varies with the situation.

Marginal analysis
The assessment
of the effects of
small changes in a
decision variable
(such as price or
volume of output)
on outcomes (such
as costs, profits,
or probability of
recovery)

The economic perspective of **marginal analysis** challenges us to examine the effects of changes on what we do. Marginal analysis proposes questions such as these: How much healthier would this patient or population be if we increased use of this resource? How much unhealthier would this patient or population be if we reduced use of this resource? Most management decisions are made on the basis of marginal analysis, although the questions used to arrive at the decisions are often more concrete. For example, what costs would we incur if we increased the chicken pox immunization rate among three-year-olds from 78 to 85 percent, and how much would increased immunization reduce the incidence of chicken pox among preschoolers?

Reasonable answers to these questions tell us the cost per case of chicken pox avoided, and we can decide whether we want to use our resources for this proposition. Managers who focus on healthcare products as outputs of their organizations ask the same types of questions, although they frame them differently: How much will profits rise if we increase the number of skilled nursing beds from 12 to 18? What costs would we incur if we added a nurse midwife to the practice, and how would this addition change patient outcomes and revenues? In any setting, marginal analysis helps managers focus on the right questions.

Using estimates from an article on the cost-effectiveness of prevention (Tengs 1996), Exhibit 2.1 illustrates how variable the effects of medical interventions can be. It estimates how many life years would be saved by spending $1 million on a particular population. (A **life year** is one additional year of life. One person living for nine additional years, and nine persons living for one additional year, equally represent nine life years.) The data indicate that spending $1 million on screening black newborns for sickle cell disease would save more than 4,000 life years but that spending the same amount on screening nonblack newborns at high risk for sickle cell disease would save less than ten life years. Exhibit 2.1 also reminds us that our attitudes toward health are more complex than we sometimes admit. Spending $1 million on mandatory motorcycle helmet laws would save a few more life years than spending $1 million on vaccinating adults older than 65 years against pneumonia would save, yet the helmet law is controversial and these vaccinations are not.

We have to make some choices. Screening nonblack, low-risk newborns for sickle cell disease saves virtually no life years. On rare occasions, though, this screening identifies a nonblack, low-risk newborn with sickle

Life year
One additional year of life (A life year can equal one added year of life for an individual or an average of $1/n$th of a year of life for n people.)

Intervention	Life Years Saved
Sickle cell screens for black newborns	4,167
Defibrillators in emergency vehicles	2,564
Mandatory motorcycle helmet laws	500
Pneumonia vaccinations for those older than 65 years	476
Sickle cell screens for nonblack, high-risk newborns	9
Sickle cell screens for nonblack, low-risk newborns	0

EXHIBIT 2.1
How Many Life Years Will $1 Million Save?

Source: These calculations are based on estimates presented in Tengs (1996).

cell disease. We cannot avoid a decision about whether the benefits of this intervention are large enough to justify its substantial costs. In different ways, these illustrations remind us that the usefulness of healthcare products varies dramatically.

The input view also stresses that changes in technology or prices may affect the mix or amount of healthcare products citizens want to use. For example, lower surgery costs will increase the number of people who choose vision correction surgery rather than eyeglasses. Conversely, advances in pharmaceutical therapy for coronary artery disease might reduce the rate of bypass graft surgeries (and reduce the number of attendant hospital stays).

In the past, healthcare managers did not spend much time on the input view. They were charged with running healthcare organizations well, so products that their organizations did not produce were of little interest. This perception is changing. Our collective rethinking of the role of health insurance makes the input view practical. For example, if offering instruction on meditation reduces healthcare use enough, the chief executive of an insurance plan, the medical director of a **capitated** healthcare organization, or the benefits manager of a self-insured employer will find it an attractive option. Increasingly, healthcare managers must be prepared to evaluate a wide range of options.

Capitated
Payment is per person (The payment does not depend on the services provided.)

2.1.2 The Output View

New ways of thinking do not always invalidate former perspectives. The output view of the healthcare sector is more relevant than ever. The importance of producing goods and services efficiently has increased. Those struggling with the rising cost of healthcare are increasingly purchasing care from low-cost producers. At present, third parties (i.e., insurers, governments, and employers) have difficulty distinguishing between care that is inexpensive because it is of inferior quality and care that is inexpensive because it is produced efficiently, but their ability to make this distinction is improving.

To succeed, managers must lead their organizations to become efficient producers that attract customers. In many organizations, this task will be formidable.

2.2 Health Outcomes

Americans often celebrate their healthcare system as "the best in the world." While parts of the system are superb, the system as a whole needs improvement. As indicated in Chapter 1, the American healthcare system incurs high costs and produces mediocre outcomes. Although the United States spends far more on healthcare per person than does any other large, developed country, American life expectancy at birth ranks twenty-sixth among the 34 members of a group of industrialized nations called the Organisation for Economic Co-operation and Development (OECD). Only Chile, the Czech Republic, Poland, Estonia, the Slovak Republic, Hungary, Turkey, and Mexico trailed the United States (OECD 2013).

Given the political decision to subsidize healthcare resources for the elderly, life expectancy at 65 years might represent a fairer test. On this measure, the United States ranked twenty-fifth in 2011 (OECD 2013). Despite its many areas of excellence, it is hard to argue that the US healthcare system is the best in the world.

This caustic appraisal should not hide the fact that the health of the American public has improved dramatically. Between 1960 and 2004 the infant mortality rate fell by 77 percent in the United States, and the death rate among new mothers and mothers-to-be fell nearly as sharply (OECD 2013). All in all, Americans are living longer. Life expectancy at birth rose from 69.9 years in 1960 to 78.7 years in 2011, an increase of 8.8 years (OECD 2013).

From one perspective, this increase in life expectancy reflects impressive performance. From another, it does not compare well to the performance of other industrialized countries. For example, French life expectancy at birth rose from 70.3 years in 1960 to 82.2 years in 2011. Making the comparison look even less favorable, costs increased more than twice as much in the United States as in France (OECD 2013).

This conclusion rests on a simple marginal analysis in which we compare the change in spending to the change in life expectancy. What appears to be higher spending, however, might just be the effects of inflation. To avoid inaccuracies resulting from changes in the value of money, economists use two strategies. The simplest and most reliable strategy to report spending uses shares of national income, or *gross domestic product* (GDP). This examination of shares removes the effects of inflation (see Exhibits 2.2–2.4). When we need to compare dollar amounts, we adjust all the spending figures to a common basis. These inflation-adjusted spending levels are often called *real spending levels.* The price indexes that underlie these adjustments are imperfect, so the adjustments are as well. Consequently, economists are reluctant to make much of small changes in real spending.

To compare French and US spending, we also need to convert figures into a common currency. The OECD regularly publishes estimates of spending per person for a number of countries in US dollars, so we can use these data as a starting point. Converting these figures into inflation-adjusted US dollars, we find that real spending per person in the United States rose from $1,122 in 1960 to $8,508 in 2011. In contrast, real spending per person in France rose from $524 in 1960 to $4,118 in 2011. Therefore, annual inflation-adjusted spending per person rose by $7,386 in the United States and $3,594 in France. This simple marginal analysis does not tell us why costs rose more and life expectancy rose less in the United States, but spending nearly twice as much for a smaller payoff suggests we are not using our resources wisely.

Calculating Inflation-Adjusted Values

Per capita healthcare spending was $7,026 in 2006 and $8,915 in 2012. Did real spending go up? After all, prices generally increased during this period. The Consumer Price Index increased from 201.6 to 229.6, implying that prices rose by 14 percent from 2006 to 2012: 229.6 ÷ 201.6 = 114 percent. To express the 2006 spending figure in inflation-adjusted terms, we multiply it by the value of the Consumer Price Index for 2012 and divide it by the value of the Consumer Price Index in 2006 ($7,026 × 229.6) ÷ 201.6 = $8,002. We conclude that inflation-adjusted spending did go up.

2.3 Outputs of the Healthcare System

In 2012, Americans spent $2.8 trillion on healthcare, meaning that healthcare claimed 17.2 percent of the nation's output (see Exhibit 2.2). In 2000, healthcare spending totaled $1.4 trillion, or 13.4 percent of output. Why is how much we spend on healthcare interesting? Is there anything wrong with healthcare spending?

2.3.1 Why Is How Much We Spend on Healthcare Interesting?

How much we spend on healthcare is interesting for two reasons. First, although healthcare is claiming an increasing share of national income worldwide, other industrialized countries appear to be realizing larger health

EXHIBIT 2.2
US Health Expenditures as a Share of Gross Domestic Product

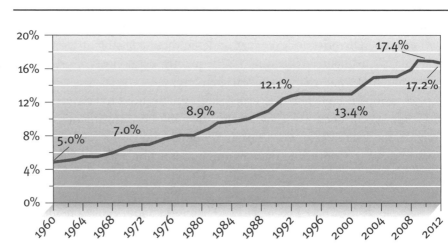

Source: Centers for Medicare & Medicaid Services (2013).

gains while spending less than the United States. Second, the rising share of national income claimed by healthcare has prompted most governments and employers to question whether the benefits of this increased spending warrant it. If not, there is something wrong with healthcare spending. If the benefits of healthcare spending are smaller than the benefits of using our resources in other ways, a shift would be in order. For example, would we be better off if we had spent less on educating new physicians and more on educating new teachers? The **opportunity cost** of producing a product consists of the other goods and services we cannot make instead. Stating that the benefits of healthcare are less than its costs does not imply that it is bad or worthless, only that it is worth less than some other use of our resources.

Opportunity cost
The value of a resource in its next best use (The opportunity cost of a product consists of the other goods and services we cannot have because we have chosen to produce the product in question.)

Comparing Health Outcomes in Utah and Nevada

In 1974, Victor Fuchs compared health outcomes for residents of Utah and Nevada, noting that, despite their many apparent similarities, inhabitants of the two states were at opposite ends of the health spectrum. Residents of Utah were among the healthiest in the nation; residents of Nevada were among the least healthy. Fuchs (1974, 53) argued that the explanation for these health differences "almost surely lies in the different life-styles of the residents of the two states."

Despite major changes in the populations of both states, large differentials persist. Focusing on death rates (the crudest but most accurate measures of health), Exhibit 2.3 shows that death rates for adults in Nevada remain much higher. Moreover, the differences are similar to those found by Fuchs.

Age	Males	Females
Under 1 year	12%	25%
1–14 years	12%	4%
15–44 years	23%	22%
45–64 years	45%	31%
65–84 years	21%	15%
85 years and older	–1%	–1%

Source: Centers for Disease Control and Prevention (2014b).

EXHIBIT 2.3
Excess Death Rates in Nevada over Utah, 1999–2010

(continued)

(continued)

One striking change has taken place: the two states' infant mortality rates have converged. In 1974, Fuchs found infant mortality rates more than 35 percent higher in Nevada, much more than the differential in Exhibit 2.3. This change likely reflects improvements in the treatment of low-birthweight (less than 2,500 grams) infants. Differences in infant mortality rates largely depend on the proportion of children with low birth weights, which is heavily influenced by what individuals do, and survival rates among children with low birth weights, which largely reflect effects of the healthcare system (Mac-Dorman and Mathews 2009). The proportion of children with low birth weights is about 18 percent higher in Nevada (Centers for Disease Control and Prevention 2014a), so the convergence of infant mortality rates appears to reflect improvements in the treatment of low-birthweight infants.

A significant portion of the excess mortality in Nevada can be traced to different patterns of alcohol and tobacco use (see Exhibit 2.4). Greater use leads to much larger age-adjusted death rates for malignant neoplasms of the respiratory system (an uncommon disease among nonsmokers) and for chronic liver disease (including cirrhosis).

EXHIBIT 2.4
Excess Age-Adjusted Death Rates in Nevada over Utah, 1999–2010

Cause of Death	Males	Females
Malignant neoplasms of the respiratory system	161%	203%
Chronic liver disease and cirrhosis	194%	136%

Source: Centers for Disease Control and Prevention (2014b).

The consequences of alcohol and tobacco abuse are purely medical issues, but finding ways to reduce the consequences of abuse is a classic problem for those taking the input view of healthcare.

These differences in health outcomes are unlikely to be attributable to differences in healthcare resources. What citizens do (e.g., smoke) and do not do (e.g., exercise) are much more likely to explain these differences. Spending more on healthcare is not the only way to improve outcomes.

Inefficiency is another concern. Seemingly, many healthcare outputs could be produced using fewer resources, and some health outcomes could be realized in ways that use fewer resources. The healthcare system may be wasting resources that have other, more valuable uses.

CASE 2.1 A Pain in the Back

Americans with back pain are using more pain-killers, having more surgeries, and undergoing more imaging studies (magnetic resonance imaging and computed tomography) than ever, yet they do not appear to be feeling better. In 2005, patients with back problems reported more limited functioning than patients did in 1997, even though inflation-adjusted spending was up more than 60 percent (Martin et al. 2008).

Neck and back pain are common, and a majority of adults have an episode during the course of a year. Neck and back pain are also common reasons for physician visits. During these visits, physicians usually (or should) reassure patients that most low back pain improves with conservative treatment (a combination of ice and nonprescription pain relievers, followed by moderate strengthening and stretching exercises that can be done at home without special equipment). Diagnostic imaging is being prescribed more frequently for patients with back and neck pain, even though the value of imaging appears to be limited (Carragee 2005). Few imaging studies yield a definitive diagnosis or a new treatment plan. Furthermore, Medicare data show that rates of back surgery have increased dramatically, even though there is little scientific evidence that surgery is superior to conservative treatment. The United States has the highest rates of back surgery in the world, even though back problems are no more common here than in other countries. In addition, surgery rates also vary greatly between cities. For example, in 2010, the back surgery rate for residents of Fort Myers, Florida, was 140 percent higher than the rate for residents of Miami (Dartmouth Atlas of Health Care 2014).

Discussion questions:
- If imaging followed by surgery is as effective as conservative therapy, what's wrong with letting physicians and patients do what they want?
- What explains this rise of imaging and surgery for back pain?

(continued)

CASE 2.1
(continued)
- Who makes decisions about surgery?
- Should insurers take action to reduce surgery rates? Should individuals?
- How do providers' revenues change if imaging and surgery rates rise?
- How do patients' costs change if imaging and surgery rates rise?
- How do current incentive systems affect physicians' and patients' decisions?

2.3.2 The Shifting Pattern of Healthcare Spending

The output of the healthcare sector has changed. New technologies and new insurance arrangements are altering what the public buys. In addition, the scope and pace of change will likely increase.

Hospitals' share of healthcare outputs has been falling since the early 1980s. Even though they have expanded into nontraditional markets and are earning more revenue, hospitals produced slightly less than a third of the output of the healthcare sector in 2011 (Centers for Medicare & Medicaid Services 2013). The number of inpatient days has been falling, however, and other healthcare sectors have been expanding rapidly (Exhibit 2.5). It seems likely that inpatient days will continue to fall.

Physicians' output share has risen only a little since 1960. This fact is attributable to the rapid growth in other healthcare sectors, not to slowing spending on physicians' services. Inflation-adjusted spending on physicians' services increased by 35 percent between 2000 and 2011 (Centers for Medicare & Medicaid Services 2013).

EXHIBIT 2.5
Age-Adjusted Days of Care per 10,000 Population

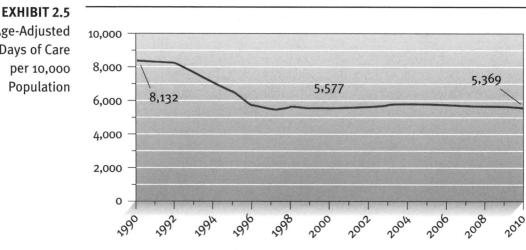

Source: National Center for Health Statistics (2013).

Nonetheless, many of the payment innovations that are described in Chapter 6 directly or indirectly focus on reducing the prices paid to physicians. One of the main reasons that healthcare costs are so high in the United States is that prices for physicians' services are much higher than in other countries. For example, Laugesen and Glied (2011) report that US private insurers paid an average of $3,996 to orthopedic surgeons for a hip replacement operation. The Medicare price averaged $1,634, and private insurance prices in other countries ranged from $1,340 to $2,160.

Prescription Drugs and the Consumer Price Index

The Consumer Price Index may overstate the rate of growth of prescription prices. The Bureau of Labor Statistics, which compiles the Consumer Price Index for prescription drugs, samples 300 retail outlets that are representative of the locations where Americans buy prescription drugs. The outlets include chain pharmacies, neighborhood pharmacies, discount stores, and mail-order firms. The Bureau of Labor Statistics tracks the prices of 20 representative drugs but faces four major problems in the rapidly changing pharmaceutical market: shifts in insurance coverage, the emergence of generics, the conversion from prescription to over-the-counter status, and the introduction of new drugs. These ongoing changes make constructing a good index of prices more difficult. For example, what should happen to the price index if the price of a branded drug remains $100 but a third of consumers switch to a generic version costing $40? Or what should happen to the price index if a third of consumers switch to a new drug that costs $120? Presumably this new drug represents a better value than the older, less expensive drug, and the index should reflect this difference. The Bureau of Labor Statistics has implemented changes to address these issues but is having difficulty keeping up with shifts in the pharmaceutical market.

2.4 Disruptive Change in the Healthcare System

For many years six trends were evident in the healthcare system of the United States. They were

- Rapid technological change;
- The shrinking share of direct consumer payments;
- The rapid growth of the healthcare sector;

- The rapid growth of the outpatient sector;
- The slower growth of the inpatient sector; and
- The steady increase in the number of uninsured Americans.

Only two of these trends continue unabated: rapid technological change and the shrinking share of direct consumer payments.

Exhibit 2.6 depicts the steady decline in the share of direct consumer payments for healthcare. This decline is primarily due to broader coverage among Americans with health insurance coverage, as the number of Americans without health insurance steadily increased through 2010. For example, in 2000 consumers directly paid 28 percent of pharmacy costs, but by 2011 that share had fallen to 17 percent (Centers for Medicare & Medicaid Services 2013). Consumers ultimately pay all healthcare bills. Increasingly, though, they are doing so indirectly via taxes and premiums.

The most surprising development of recent years has been the slowing growth of the healthcare sector. Rapid expansion of the healthcare sector has been a feature of American life for most of this century, but its pace has clearly slowed. As Exhibit 2.2 showed, healthcare spending in 1960 claimed only 5.0 percent of national income. By 2012, healthcare spending had risen to 17.2 percent of national income. However, in contrast to the rapid expansion of previous years, the share had fallen slightly from its peak in 2010.

Why spending grew more slowly is not clear. Job loss during the Great Recession and changes in health insurance benefits played a role, but these factors explained only part of the slowdown (Ryu et al. 2013). Forecasting

EXHIBIT 2.6
Direct Payments by Consumers as a Share of National Health Spending

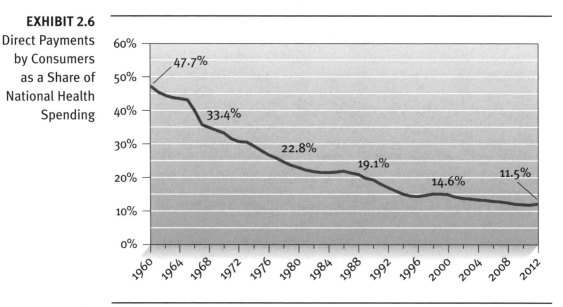

Source: Centers for Medicare & Medicaid Services (2013).

what will happen during the next several years is difficult because the health-care environment appears to have changed due to two major shocks: the implementation of the Affordable Care Act (ACA) and the transformation of the health insurance industry. Section 2.4.2 discusses the ACA, and Section 2.4.3 discusses the reconfiguration of the health insurance industry.

The ACA has already reduced the number of uninsured and promises to continue to do so. Many of these newly insured Americans have coverage that is similar to a catastrophic plan. For example, a fairly typical set of plans had deductibles that ranged from $500 to $5,000 and out-of-pocket limits that ranged from $2,500 to $7,000 (Blue Cross Blue Shield of Kansas City 2012). Use of health services will likely depend on the type of insurance that consumers choose (Fronstin 2010).

Many healthcare managers are maintaining an inpatient focus. They seek improved hospital operations (a worthy aim) for the purpose of increasing the census (an unlikely result). In most areas, the census of well-managed hospitals will drop more slowly than the census of hospitals that are less well managed. Similarly, in hopes of building the inpatient census, many managers want to start satellite clinics or acquire physician practices. Once the hospital has assumed management of these additions, however, they may not be profitable. The continuing drop in inpatient services will overwhelm the modest increase in referrals that ensues.

2.4.1 Rapid Technological Change

Rapid technological change is pervasive in healthcare. Technological change makes transformation of the healthcare system possible, and policy changes are apt to make transformation desirable. Only luck will rescue management decisions that ignore technological change.

Monitoring of implantable cardioverter defibrillators illustrates the interaction of technological and policy change. Patients with an implantable cardioverter defibrillator—a small device used to treat irregular heartbeats—require regular follow-up visits to monitor their health and whether their device is working properly. The stakes are high. An untreated arrhythmia may be life threatening, and more than 2 percent of the population experience some arrhythmia (Ball et al. 2013).

Although little scientific evidence exists, the professional consensus is that these patients should be seen two to four times per year even if no difficulties are evident. A recent evaluation of a remote monitoring system concluded that it offered more rapid detection of problems and had the potential to lower costs sharply by reducing office visits by up to 75 percent (Varma et al. 2010). In a **fee-for-service** environment, in which revenues depend on the volume of visits, physicians and healthcare organizations would have little interest in remote home monitoring. However, in a capitated environment, in which

Fee-for-service
A reimbursement model that pays providers on the basis of their charges for services

reducing visits reduces workload without reducing revenue, physicians, healthcare organizations, patients, and insurers have a common interest in expanding remote monitoring. (In a capitated insurance plan, a payment is made per member per month, and an extra visit generates no revenue.) For a variety of reasons, participation in capitated plans is rising quite rapidly. Enrollment in Medicare Advantage HMOs (private health insurance plans for Medicare beneficiaries) has grown very fast (Kaiser Family Foundation 2013). In addition, in response to recent policy changes, many states have moved aggressively to move beneficiaries who are eligible for Medicare and Medicaid into HMOs.

Other innovations could prove even more disruptive. For example, pharmacogenomics—the science of predicting differing responses to drugs based on genetic variations—could have profound effects on the healthcare system. Even after adjusting for individual factors such as age, weight, race, sex, diet, and other medications, patients can respond very differently to a drug. One patient may have the desired relief of symptoms, another may have no apparent response, and a third may have a life-threatening reaction. Obviously this difference matters a great deal to patients and practitioners. It also matters to managers. An adverse drug reaction is the fourth leading cause of death in the United States, and genetic testing to ensure that patients get safe, effective pharmaceuticals could reduce hospitalization rates by up to 30 percent (Karczewski, Daneshjou, and Altman 2012; Ventola 2013). Even a much smaller reduction in hospitalization rates would have profound effects on the healthcare sector.

Like every sector of society, healthcare illustrates the struggle to take advantage of the information revolution and demonstrates the paradox of technological change. The essence of the information revolution is that the cost of performing a single calculation has dropped precipitously. As a result, many more calculations are possible, and spending on some types of information processing (e.g., computer games) has increased sharply as spending on other types of information processing (e.g., inventory management) has plummeted. Technological advances almost always make a process less expensive, yet spending may rise because volume increases dramatically.

The challenges of the information revolution are even greater in healthcare than in most sectors. Much of the output of the healthcare sector involves information processing, yet relatively few healthcare workers are highly skilled users of computerized information. In addition, healthcare organizations have lagged behind other service organizations in investing in computer hardware, software, and personnel.

The rapid pace of change in other areas further intensifies these challenges. Healthcare's diagnostic and therapeutic outputs are changing even faster than the organizational structure of the sector, which itself is changing rapidly. In some areas (most notably imaging and laboratory services), technological change is tightly linked to the information processing revolution. In other areas, the links are much looser. For example, advances in information processing speed the development and assessment of new drugs, yet because pharmaceutical innovations can be extremely profitable, a powerful incentive for pharmaceutical innovation exists regardless of these advances.

2.4.2 Major Features of the Affordable Care Act

The ACA is a complex law with multiple provisions. This section briefly sketches some of its major provisions, focusing on ones that have the potential to reshape the healthcare sector.

1. The ACA incorporates several mechanisms for *expanding insurance coverage*. These include new regulations, state and federal insurance marketplaces, subsidies for those with low incomes, and the option for states to expand Medicaid coverage for those with the lowest incomes.
2. The ACA incorporates several mechanisms for *reducing Medicare spending*. These include penalties for higher-than-expected readmission rates, reductions in Medicare payments to hospitals with large numbers of uninsured patients, reductions in payments to Medicare Advantage plans, incentive payments for care of high quality and for significant improvements in quality, and the establishment of the Independent Payment Advisory Board to identify opportunities for Medicare savings.
3. The ACA authorizes a number of *payment reform demonstrations*. These include trials of accountable care organizations, bundled payments, medical homes, and **managed care** for beneficiaries who are eligible for Medicare and Medicaid.

Managed care
A loosely defined term that includes all plans except open-ended fee-for-service, sometimes used to describe the techniques insurance companies use

Many years will pass before the full effects of the ACA are understood. This section briefly notes some ACA provisions that have the capacity to change incentives and about which there is some evidence. Chapter 6 will explore these issues in more detail.

    Narrow networks are common in ACA marketplace plans (McKinsey & Company 2013). These plans may be limited to a single healthcare system or may exclude just a few providers. The main motivation for narrow networks is that some healthcare systems have traditionally been able to negotiate very high prices—sometimes four or five times Medicare rates—with private insurers (Ginsburg 2010). The benefit to marketplace insurance customers is sharply lower premiums, often 15 to 20 percent lower. The true effect of narrow networks is likely to be seen in the years to come because they are likely to become common in the much bigger employer-sponsored health insurance and Medicare Advantage markets.

Narrow network
A limited group of providers who have contracted with an insurance company (Patients will usually pay more if they get care from a provider not in the network. The network is usually restricted to providers with good quality who will accept low payments.)

Medicare penalties for higher-than-expected readmission rates clearly give hospitals an incentive to reduce readmissions. A 2 percent reduction in Medicare payments would have a significant effect on most hospitals' revenues, so reducing readmissions will be a priority for most hospitals. Note that reducing readmissions will reduce hospital volumes. For 2007 through 2011, the Medicare 30-day readmission rate averaged 19 percent, so bringing down the readmission rate will also bring down inpatient volumes (Gerhardt et al. 2013). Although commonly interpreted as a measure of the quality of hospital care, readmissions are clearly influenced by the quality of postdischarge care (Lin, Barnato, and Degenholtz 2011).

Bundled payment
A single payment, also called a *bundled episode payment*, that covers all services delivered during a given episode of care (Examples of an episode of care include hip replacement, a year of diabetes care, or pregnancy.)

Bundled payments already have been tested, but the ACA dramatically expands testing of this concept. As a part of the ACA, Medicare has launched bundled payment trials in more than 450 healthcare organizations. Termed the Bundled Payments for Care Improvement Initiative, these trials will explore whether paying lump sums for episodes of care will reduce healthcare costs without harming care. One model, which is being tested only in New Jersey, lets hospitals give physicians bonuses if they help the hospital reduce costs and improve quality. A second model puts hospital and posthospital services in a common bundle. A third model pays a flat fee for all posthospital care (skilled nursing, inpatient rehabilitation, long-term care hospital or home health services). A fourth model covers all services provided during a hospital stay (hospital, physician, and other). The common denominator in all of these bundled payment trials is that services are viewed as cost centers rather than revenue centers.

2.4.3 The Transformation of the Health Insurance Industry

The health insurance industry looks very different than it did a few years ago. To begin with, its revenues will grow. Deloitte Consulting forecasts that industry revenues will double by 2020, with most of the growth coming from Medicare Advantage, Medicaid, and ACA marketplace plans (Keckley, Copeland, and Scott 2013).

Second, the industry's customers look different. Until fairly recently, most purchasing decisions were made by firms or governments. Americans had coverage through work, Medicare, or Medicaid. Typically just one plan was offered. Increasingly, though, individuals are making their own choices. Millions of Americans have chosen Medicare Advantage plans already, and millions more have chosen marketplace plans. Both options seem likely to grow more, and insurers are planning to roll out private exchanges so that employees can choose their plans as well.

Third, the basis for competition seems likely to change. The ACA has made avoiding risk more difficult and, with other regulations, has made pricing and quality easier for consumers to discern. Starting in 2007, individuals seeking Medicare Advantage plans could use summary ratings based on clinical quality, the experience of patients, and customer service. Customers are using these ratings in choosing plans, and ratings systems seem likely to spread (Reid et al. 2013).

Fourth, the structure of the industry has changed. The industry has already consolidated, and this process is likely to continue. If, as many predict, profit margins will drop, additional mergers and acquisitions seem likely.

Fifth, the health insurance industry is increasingly using data to measure cost and quality. For the most part, insurers are using data from claims, which give at best an imprecise picture of clinical quality (Berenson, Pronovost, and Krumholz 2013). Increasingly, however, insurers are using claims data to estimate the cost of an entire episode of care, provide feedback to providers, and make judgments about which providers offer good value. Underlying insurers' increasing willingness to create narrow networks and designate preferred providers of care is the conclusion that cost and quality are not highly correlated, so steering patients to low-cost providers will be a winning strategy (Ho and Sandy 2013).

2.5 Conclusion

During the 1980s, a consensus emerged that the US healthcare system needed to be redirected despite its many triumphs. Underlying this consensus was the recognition that costs were the highest in the world even though outcomes were not the best in the world.

How the healthcare system should change is much less clear. Managing under such circumstances is stressful, but an awareness of the trends presented in this chapter should guide any organization's managers, and a number of strategies (such as striving to be the low-cost producer) make sense in almost any environment. These low-risk strategies, and ways to deal with risk and uncertainty, will be discussed in the next chapters.

Exercises

2.1 Identify a product that is one organization's output and another organization's input.

2.2 Can you think of any initiatives that reflect the input view of healthcare?

2.3 What's wrong with spending 17.2 percent of GDP on healthcare?

2.4 Americans spend more on smartphones than the citizens of other countries do, yet this type of spending is seldom described as a problem. Why is spending more on healthcare different?

2.5   US national health expenditure was $7,026 per person in 2006 and $4,790 in 2000. The Consumer Price Index had a value of 201.6 in 2006 and a value of 172.2 in 2000. Adjusted for inflation, how much was spending in 2000?

2.6   US national health expenditure was $148 per person in 1960 and $4,790 in 2000. The Consumer Price Index had a value of 29.6 in 1960 and a value of 172.2 in 2000. In 1960 dollars, how much was spending in 2000?

2.7   How did the state and local government share of national health expenditures change between 2000 and last year? What accounts for this change? Go to the "Actuarial Studies" page on the website of the Centers for Medicare & Medicaid Services (www.cms.gov/Research-Statistics-Data-and-Systems/Research/ActuarialStudies/index.html) to get data.

2.8   When was the last year that GDP grew faster than national health expenditure? Go to the "Actuarial Studies" page on the website of the Centers for Medicare & Medicaid Services (www.cms.gov/Research-Statistics-Data-and-Systems/Research/ActuarialStudies/index.html) to get data.

2.9   Your accountants tell you that it costs $400 to set up an immunization program at a preschool and immunize one child against polio. It will cost $460 more to immunize 20 more children. What is the cost per child for the first child? What is the cost per child for these additional 20 children? What is the average cost per child? What concepts do these calculations illustrate?

2.10   A new treatment of cystic fibrosis costs $2 million. The life expectancy of 1,000 patients who were randomly assigned to the new treatment increased by 3.2 years. What is the cost per life year of the new treatment?

2.11   Setting up nurse practitioner clinics to serve 20,000 newborns in Georgia would cost $6 million. This program would increase life expectancy at birth from 75.1 years to 75.3 years. How many life years would be gained? What is the cost per life year? Should this program be started?

2.12   Why has the share of healthcare output produced by hospitals fallen? Will this trend continue? Can you think of a policy or technology change that would further reduce hospital use? Can you think of a policy or technology change that would increase hospital use? What implications do these changes have for the careers of healthcare managers?

References

Ball, J., M. J. Carrington, J. J. McMurray, and S. Stewart. 2013. "Atrial Fibrillation: Profile and Burden of an Evolving Epidemic in the 21st Century." *International Journal of Cardiology* 167 (5): 1807–24.

Berenson, R. A., P. J. Pronovost, and H. M. Krumholz. 2013. "Achieving the Potential of Health Care Performance Measures." *Timely Analysis of Immediate Health Policy Issues* May. Robert Wood Johnson Foundation and Urban Institute. www.rwjf.org/content/dam/farm/reports/reports/2013/rwjf406195.

Blue Cross Blue Shield of Kansas City. 2012. "Preferred-Care Blue Premium Benefits." Published November. www.bluekc.com/Content/themes/base/PDF/2013Plan/PCB_Premium_PPO_ProductBenefits.pdf.

Carragee, E. J. 2005. "Clinical Practice: Persistent Low Back Pain." *New England Journal of Medicine* 352 (18): 1891–98.

Centers for Disease Control and Prevention. 2014a. "Linked Birth/Infant Death Records 2007–2010." CDC WONDER Online Database. Accessed March 8. http://wonder.cdc.gov/lbd-current.html.

———. 2014b. "Underlying Cause of Death 1999–2010." CDC WONDER Online Database. Accessed April 23. http://wonder.cdc.gov/ucd-icd10.html.

Centers for Medicare & Medicaid Services. 2013. "National Health Expenditure Data." Accessed July 2, 2014. www.cms.gov/Research-Statistics-Data-and-Systems/Statistics-Trends-and-Reports/NationalHealthExpendData/NationalHealthAccountsHistorical.html.

Dartmouth Atlas of Health Care. 2014. "Inpatient Back Surgery per 1,000 Medicare Enrollees." Accessed March 8. www.dartmouthatlas.org/data/region/.

Fronstin, P. 2010. *What Do We Really Know About Consumer-Driven Health Plans?* Employee Benefit Research Institute. Issue Brief No. 345. Published August. www.ebri.org/pdf/briefspdf/EBRI_IB_08-2010_No345_CDHP.pdf.

Fuchs, V. R. 1974. *Who Shall Live? Health, Economics, and Social Choice.* New York: Basic Books.

Gerhardt, G., A. Yemane, P. Hickman, A. Oelschlaeger, E. Rollins, and N. Brennan. 2013. "Medicare Readmission Rates Showed Meaningful Decline in 2012." *Medicare & Medicaid Research Review* 3 (2): E1–E12.

Ginsburg, P. B. 2010. *Wide Variation in Hospital and Physician Payment Rates Evidence of Provider Market Power.* Center for Studying Health System Change Research Brief No. 16. Published November. www.hschange.com/CONTENT/1162/.

Ho, S., and L. G. Sandy. 2013. "Getting Value from Health Spending: Going Beyond Payment Reform." *Journal of General Internal Medicine.* Published online November 6. doi:10.1007/s11606-013-2687-7.

Kaiser Family Foundation. 2013. "Medicare Advantage Fact Sheet." Accessed April 23, 2014. http://kff.org/medicare/fact-sheet/medicare-advantage-fact-sheet/.

Karczewski, K. J., R. Daneshjou, and R. B. Altman. 2012. "Chapter 7: Pharmacogenomics." *PLOS Computational Biology* 8 (12): e1002817.

Keckley, P., B. Copeland, and G. Scott. 2013. "The Future of Health Care Insurance: What's Ahead?" *Deloitte Review* 13: 117–31.

Laugesen, M. J., and S. A. Glied. 2011. "Higher Fees Paid to US Physicians Drive Higher Spending for Physician Services Compared to Other Countries." *Health Affairs* 30 (9): 1647–56.

Lin, C. Y., A. E. Barnato, and H. B. Degenholtz. 2011. "Physician Follow-up Visits After Acute Care Hospitalization for Elderly Medicare Beneficiaries Discharged to Noninstitutional Settings." *Journal of the American Geriatrics Society* 59 (10): 1947–54.

MacDorman, M. F., and T. J. Mathews. 2009. "The Challenge of Infant Mortality: Have We Reached a Plateau?" *Public Health Reports* 124 (5): 670–81.

Martin, B. I., R. A. Deyo, S. K. Mirza, J. A. Turner, B. A. Comstock, W. Hollingworth, and S. D. Sullivan. 2008. "Expenditures and Health Status Among Adults with Back and Neck Problems." *Journal of the American Medical Association* 299 (6): 656–64.

McKinsey & Company. 2013. "Hospital Networks: Configurations on the Exchanges and Their Impact on Premiums." Updated December 14. www.mckinsey.com/client_service/healthcare_systems_and_services/center_for_us_health_system_reform.

National Center for Health Statistics. 2013. *Health, United States, 2012: With Special Feature on Emergency Care.* Hyattsville, MD: National Center for Health Statistics.

Organisation for Economic Co-operation and Development (OECD). 2013. "OECD Health Data 2013." Accessed April 23, 2014. www.oecd.org/health/health-systems/oecdhealthdata.htm.

Reid, R. O., P. Deb, B. L. Howell, and W. H. Shrank. 2013. "Association Between Medicare Advantage Plan Star Ratings and Enrollment." *Journal of the American Medical Association* 309 (3): 267–74.

Ryu, A. J., T. B. Gibson, M. R. McKellar, and M. E. Chernew. 2013. "The Slowdown in Health Care Spending in 2009–11 Reflected Factors Other Than the Weak Economy and Thus May Persist." *Health Affairs* 32 (5): 835–40.

Tengs, T. O. 1996. "Enormous Variation in the Cost-Effectiveness of Prevention: Implications for Public Policy." *Current Issues in Public Health* 2: 13–17.

Varma, N., A. E. Epstein, A. Irimpen, R. Schweikert, and C. Love. 2010. "Efficacy and Safety of Automatic Remote Monitoring for Implantable Cardioverter-Defibrillator Follow-up: The Lumos-T Safely Reduces Routine Office Device Follow-up (TRUST) Trial." *Circulation* 122 (4): 325–32.

Ventola, C. L. 2013. "Role of Pharmacogenomic Biomarkers in Predicting and Improving Drug Response: Part 1. The Clinical Significance of Pharmacogenetic Variants." *Pharmacy & Therapeutics* 38 (9): 545–60.

AN OVERVIEW OF THE HEALTHCARE FINANCING SYSTEM

Learning Objectives

After reading this chapter, students will be able to

- use standard health insurance terminology,
- identify major trends in health insurance,
- describe why health insurance is common,
- describe the major problems faced by the current insurance system, and
- find current information about health insurance.

Key Concepts

- Consumers pay for most medical care indirectly, through taxes and insurance premiums.
- Direct payments for healthcare are often called out-of-pocket payments.
- Insurance pools the risks of high healthcare costs.
- Moral hazard and adverse selection complicate risk pooling.
- About 85 percent of the US population has medical insurance.
- Most consumers obtain coverage through an employer- or government-sponsored plan.
- Receiving insurance as a benefit of employment has significant tax benefits.
- Managed care has largely replaced traditional insurance.
- Managed care plans differ widely.

3.1 Introduction

3.1.1 Paying for Medical Care

Consumers pay for most medical care indirectly, through taxes and insurance premiums. Healthcare managers must understand the structure of private and social insurance programs because much of their organizations' revenues will be shaped by these programs. Managers must also be aware that consumers ultimately pay for healthcare products, a key fact obscured by the complex structure of the US healthcare financing system. A prudent manager will anticipate a reaction when healthcare spending invokes higher premiums or taxes, thereby forcing consumers to spend less on other goods and services. Some consumers may drop coverage, some employers may reduce benefits, and some plans may reduce payments. This reaction need not occur if a consensus has emerged in support of increased spending, but even then managers should be wary of the profound effects that changes to insurance plans can mean for them. Finally, managers must consider more than the amount subsidized by insurance. Even though the bulk of healthcare firms' revenue comes from payments for products covered by insurance plans, consumers do pay directly for some products. Consumers directly spent more than $328 billion on healthcare products in 2012 (Centers for Medicare & Medicaid Services 2013b). No firm should ignore this huge market.

Out-of-pocket payment
Total amount that a consumer spends directly for healthcare

Coinsurance
A form of cost sharing in which a patient pays a share of the bill rather than a set fee

3.1.2 Indirect Spending

Despite the large amount, direct consumer spending accounts for only a fraction of total healthcare spending. Exhibit 3.1 depicts a healthcare market in general terms—consumers directly pay the full cost of some services and part of the costs of other services. These direct payments are often called **out-of-pocket payments**. For example, a consumer's payment for the full cost of a pharmaceutical product, her 20 percent **coinsurance** payment to her dentist,

EXHIBIT 3.1
The Flow of Funds in Healthcare Markets

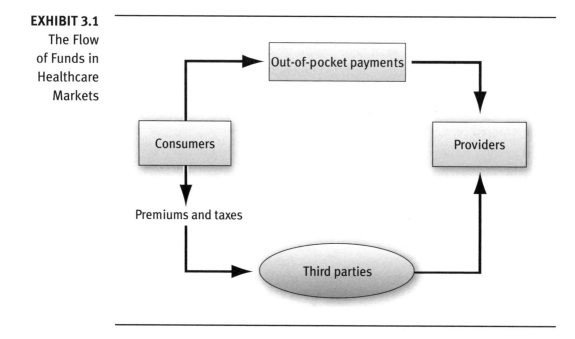

and her $25 **copayment** to her son's pediatrician are all considered out-of-pocket payments. Insurance beneficiaries make some out-of-pocket payments for services that are not covered, for services in excess of their policy's coverage limits, or for **deductibles** (amounts consumers are required to spend before their plan pays anything). Another name for out-of-pocket payments is **cost sharing**. Economics teaches us that a well-designed insurance plan usually incorporates some cost sharing. We will explore this concept in detail in the discussion of demand in Chapter 7.

Insurance payments continue to be the largest source of revenue for most healthcare providers. In 2011, they represented 97 percent of payments to hospitals, 81 percent of payments to physicians, and 67 percent of payments to nursing homes (Centers for Medicare & Medicaid Services 2013b). Because indirect payments are a factor in most healthcare purchases, their structure has a profound influence on the healthcare system and healthcare organizations.

Copayment
A fee the patient must pay in addition to the amount paid by insurance

Deductible
Amount a consumer must pay before insurance covers any healthcare costs

Cost sharing
The general term for direct payments to providers by insurance beneficiaries (Deductibles, copayments, and coinsurance are forms of cost sharing.)

Medicare
An insurance program for the elderly and disabled that is run by the Centers for Medicare & Medicaid Services

Boom and Bust in Home Care

The history of home care in the 1990s should be a warning to any manager whose business model relies on a single payer. **Medicare** home care spending grew rapidly between 1989 and 1997. Visits per user nearly doubled, and the number of users increased sharply (Spector, Cohen, and Pesis-Katz 2004). This boom had several causes. The introduction of the prospective payment system encouraged hospitals to discharge patients quickly to other settings, such as home care. Legal action in 1989 resulted in more generous eligibility and coverage, and new technology increased the number of patients who could receive adequate care at home. Some of the increased spending was for services of questionable value, and some was for services that were never delivered.

In 1997, however, the home care boom halted abruptly. Exploding spending and stories of fraud prodded the government to act. The Balanced Budget Act of 1997 reduced payments and eligibility for home care and reduced incentives for hospitals to discharge patients to home care. In addition, Medicare took steps to reduce fraud and abuse. The number of Medicare beneficiaries using home care fell by 20 percent, and visits per beneficiary fell by 40 percent. Home care spending fell sharply, and more than 10 percent of home care agencies

(continued)

(continued)

went out of business. The boom was too good to be true, and a prudent manager would have anticipated a response by Medicare.

A new version of this story seems to be in the works. As a part of the Affordable Care Act (ACA), the Centers for Medicare & Medicaid Services has launched 65 trials of Medicare bundled payments that include post-acute care, of which home health care is one part (Centers for Medicare & Medicaid Services 2013a). These trials almost certainly indicate that the Centers for Medicare & Medicaid Services believes that opportunities exist to reduce spending in this sector.

The extent of indirect payment in the healthcare market distinguishes it from most other markets. Indirect payment has three important effects on patients:

- It protects them against high healthcare expenses, which is one goal of insurance.
- It encourages them to use more healthcare services, which is a side effect of insurance.
- It limits their autonomy in healthcare decision making, which is not a goal of insurance.

Nonetheless, the advantages of indirect payment continue to exceed its disadvantages. As discussed in Chapter 2, the share of direct payments for healthcare has steadily fallen during the past 50 years.

3.1.3 The Uninsured

For many years the share of the population without medical insurance rose steadily, even as insurance payments rose as a share of total spending. Since the enactment of the ACA, the percentage of the population without health insurance has edged down.

Uninsured consumers enter healthcare markets with two significant disadvantages. First, they must finance their needs from their own resources or the resources of family, friends, and well-wishers. If these funds are not adequate, they must do without care or rely on charity care. The uninsured do not have access to the vast resources of modern insurance companies when large healthcare bills arrive. Second, unlike most insured consumers, uninsured consumers may be expected to pay list prices for services. The majority of insured consumers are covered by plans that have secured discounts from providers. For example, none of the major government insurance plans and few private insurance plans pay list prices for care. Although, in principle, uninsured patients could negotiate discounts, this practice is not routine.

The uninsured tend to have low incomes. In 2012, 16 percent of Americans lacked health insurance. A quarter of those with annual household incomes below $25,000 did not have health insurance, compared with only 8 percent of those with annual household incomes above $75,000 (DeNavas-Walt, Proctor, and Smith 2013).

The combination of low income and no insurance often creates access problems. For example, in 2012, 60 percent of uninsured adults reported not filling a prescription; skipping a recommended medical test, treatment, or follow-up; not seeing a specialist when recommended; or not making a clinic visit when they had a medical problem (Collins et al. 2013). This percentage was more than double the rate for well-insured adults. Delaying or forgoing care can lead to worse health outcomes.

3.2 What Is Insurance, and Why Is It So Prevalent?

3.2.1 What Insurance Does

Insurance pools the risks of healthcare costs, which have a skewed distribution. Most consumers have modest healthcare costs, but a few incur crushing sums. Insurance addresses this problem. Suppose that one person in a hundred has the misfortune to run up $20,000 in healthcare bills. For simplicity, let's say no one else will have any healthcare bills. Consumers cannot predict if they will be lucky or unlucky, so they may buy insurance. If a private firm offers insurance for an annual premium of $240, many consumers would gladly buy insurance to eliminate a 1 percent chance of a $20,000 bill. (The insurer gets $4,000 extra per 100 people to cover its selling costs, claims processing costs, and profits.)

3.2.2 Adverse Selection and Moral Hazard

Alas, the world is more complex than the preceding scenario, and such a simple plan probably would not work. To begin with, insurance tends to change the purchasing decisions of consumers. Insured consumers are more likely to use services, and providers no longer feel compelled to limit their diagnosis and treatment recommendations to amounts that individual consumers can afford. The increase in spending that occurs as a result of insurance coverage is known as **moral hazard**. Moral hazard can be substantially reduced if consumers face cost-sharing requirements, and most contemporary plans have this provision.

Moral hazard
The incentive to use additional care that having insurance creates

Another, less tractable problem remains. Some consumers, notably older people with chronic illnesses, are much more likely than average to face large bills. Such consumers would be especially eager to buy insurance. On the other hand, some consumers, notably younger people with healthy ancestors and no chronic illnesses, are much less likely than average to face large bills. Such consumers would not be especially eager to buy insurance. This situation illustrates **adverse selection**: people with high risk are apt to be eager to buy insurance, but people with low risk may not be. Wary of this phenomenon, insurance firms have tried to assess the risks that individual consumers pose and base their premiums on those risks, a process known as **underwriting**. Of course underwriting drives up costs, making coverage more expensive. In the worst case, no private firm would be willing to offer insurance to the general public.

In the United States, three mechanisms reduce the effects of adverse selection: employment-sponsored medical insurance, government-sponsored medical insurance, and medical insurance subsidies. In 2012, 85 percent of the population had medical insurance. About 32 percent had government-sponsored medical insurance, and 57 percent had private medical insurance. Virtually all Americans 65 years or older have health insurance coverage through Medicare, a government insurance program. About 83 percent of those under 65 years have coverage, and most of them have private coverage (DeNavas-Walt, Proctor, and Smith 2013). More than 95 percent of privately insured consumers under 65 years obtained their coverage through their own or their spouse's employer.

Why is the link between employment and medical insurance so strong? To begin with, insurers are able to offer lower prices on employment-based insurance because they have cut their sales costs and their adverse selection risks by selling to groups. Selling a policy to a group of 1,000 people costs only a little more than selling a policy to an individual; thus the sales cost is much lower. And because few people take jobs or stay in them just because of the medical insurance benefits, adverse selection rarely occurs (i.e., all of the employees get the insurance, whether or not they think they'll need it soon). Medical insurance can also benefit employers. If coverage improves the health of employees or their dependents, workers will be more productive, thereby improving profits for the company. Companies also benefit because workers with employment-based medical insurance are less likely to quit. The costs of hiring and training employees are high, so firms do not want to lose employees unnecessarily.

The most salient factor in the link between employment and medical insurance is the substantial tax savings that employment-based medical insurance provides. Medical insurance provided as a benefit is excluded from Social Security taxes, Medicare taxes, federal income taxes, and most state and local income taxes. Earning $5,000 in cash instead of a $5,000 medical insurance benefit could easily increase an employee's tax bill by $2,500.

This system is clearly advantageous from the perspective of insurers, employers, and employees. From the perspective of society as a whole,

Adverse selection
High-risk consumers' willingness to pay more for insurance than low-risk consumers (Organizations that have difficulty distinguishing high-risk from low-risk consumers are unlikely to be profitable.)

Underwriting
The process of assessing the risks associated with an insurance policy and setting the premium accordingly

however, its desirability is less clear. The subsidies built into the tax code tend to force tax rates higher, may encourage insurance for costs such as eyeglasses and routine dental checkups, and give employees an unrealistic sense of how much insurance costs.

Another disadvantage is found in the way most employers frame health insurance benefits. In 2013, less than 15 percent of private employers allowed employees to choose between plans (Kaiser Family Foundation and Health Research & Educational Trust 2013). Larger employers were more likely to offer a choice of plans. In addition, most employers pay more when an employee selects a more expensive plan, which encourages employees to choose one. Few employers share information about the quality of care offered through different plans or other aspects of plan performance. Without this information, employees are unlikely to be able to identify plans with better provider networks or better customer service.

Understanding Health Risks and Insurance

Adverse selection is one reason for governments to intervene in health insurance markets. A persistent fear is that people with low risks will not buy insurance, pushing up premiums for people with higher risks. Once premiums go up, additional people with low risks will drop out. This sequence is called a *death spiral* because it will ultimately result in no one buying insurance. To prevent this, governments subsidize insurance or mandate that it be bought.

Little evidence suggests that people understand their health risks very well, and evidence shows that some consumers poorly understand health insurance plans. A study of the Medicare supplementary insurance market found that those with supplementary coverage spend an average of $4,000 less than those without. One factor explaining this advantageous selection was cognitive ability (Fang, Keane, and Silverman 2008). People who did not buy coverage may not have understood the risks they were running or the benefits of having supplementary coverage. A recent survey of Americans who might seek insurance through the ACA marketplace found that many struggled with such basic concepts as a premium, a provider network, or covered services (Long et al. 2014).

A person under 65 years has a 10 percent chance of having medical bills of $30,000 or more (Bernard 2013). Because such bills are not part of their experience, some people tend to underestimate the financial and health risks of not having insurance.

3.2.3 Medicare as an Example of Complexity

The health insurance system in the United States is so complex that only a few specialists understand it. Exhibit 3.2 illustrates the complexity of healthcare financing, even in simple cases. To demonstrate this complexity, we will examine the flow of funds in Medicare, starting with Medicare beneficiaries. Many pay premiums for Medigap policies that cover deductibles, coinsurance, and other expenses that Medicare does not cover. Like many insurers, Medicare requires a deductible. In 2014, the **Medicare Part A** deductible was $1,216 per year and the **Medicare Part B** deductible was $147. The most common coinsurance payments spring from the 20 percent of allowed fees Medicare beneficiaries must pay for most Part B services. To keep Exhibit 3.2 simple, we have focused on Medigap policies that reimburse beneficiaries rather than pay providers directly. Beneficiaries with these sorts of policies (and many without Medigap coverage) must make required out-of-pocket payments directly to

Medicare Part A
Coverage for inpatient hospital, skilled nursing, hospice, and home health care services

Medicare Part B
Coverage for outpatient services and medical equipment

EXHIBIT 3.2
The Flow of Funds in Medicare

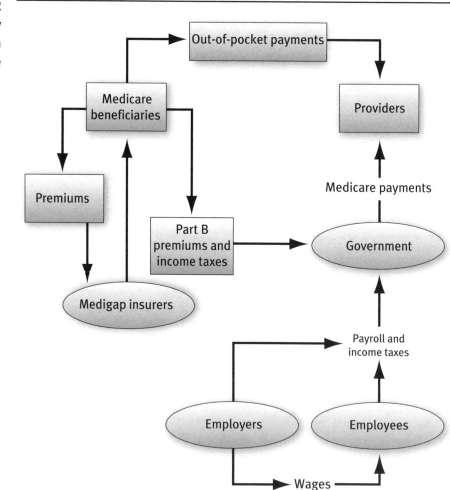

providers. Beneficiaries must also pay the Part B premiums that fund 25 percent of this Medicare component. Like other taxpayers, beneficiaries must also pay income taxes that cover the other 75 percent of Part B costs.

Employers and employees also pay taxes to fund the Medicare system. The most visible of these taxes is the Medicare payroll tax, which is levied on wages to fund Part A (which covers hospital, home health, skilled nursing, and hospice services). In addition, corporation and individual income taxes help fund the 75 percent of Part B costs that premiums do not cover. The Centers for Medicare & Medicaid Services, the federal agency that operates Medicare, combines these tax and premium funds to pay providers. Not surprisingly, few taxpayers, beneficiaries, or public officials understand how Medicare is financed.

3.3 The Changing Nature of Health Insurance

Traditional, open-ended **fee-for-service** (FFS) plans (of which pre-1984 Medicare was a classic example) have three basic problems. First, they encourage providers and consumers to use covered services as long as the direct cost to consumers is less than the direct benefit. Because the actual total cost of care is much greater than the amount consumers pay, some consumers may use services that are not worth as much as they actually cost. In addition, open-ended FFS plans discourage consumers from using services that are not covered, even highly effective ones. Finally, much of the system is unplanned, in that the prices paid by consumers and the prices received by providers do not reflect actual provider costs or consumer valuations.

Given the origins of traditional medical insurance, this inattention to efficiency makes sense. Medical insurance was started by providers, largely in response to consumers' inability to afford expensive services and the unwillingness of some consumers to pay their bills once services had been rendered. The goal was to cover the costs of services, not to provide care in the most efficient manner possible and not to improve the health of the covered population.

Managed care is a varied collection of insurance plans with only one common denominator: they are different from FFS insurance plans. FFS plans covered all services if they were included in the contract and if a provider, typically a physician, was willing to certify that they were medically necessary. No FFS features tried to influence the decisions of patients or physicians (aside from the effects of subsidizing higher spending).

At present, insurance takes five basic forms: FFS plans, **PPOs (preferred provider organizations)**, **HMOs (health maintenance organizations)**, **point-of-service (POS) plans**, and high-deductible plans. We will briefly describe each of the alternatives to FFS plans.

Fee-for-service
A reimbursement model that pays providers on the basis of their charges for services

PPO (preferred provider organization)
An insurance plan that contracts with a network of providers (Network providers may be chosen for a variety of reasons, but a willingness to discount fees is usually required.)

HMO (health maintenance organization)
A firm that provides comprehensive healthcare benefits to enrollees in exchange for a premium (Originally, HMOs were distinct from other insurance firms because providers were not paid on a fee-for-service basis and because enrollees faced no cost-sharing requirements.)

Point-of-service (POS) plan
Plan that allows members to see any physician but increases cost sharing for physicians outside the plan's network (This arrangement has become so common that POS plans may not be labeled as such.)

Medicaid
A collection of state-run programs that meet standards set by the Centers for Medicare & Medicaid Services (Medicaid serves those with incomes low enough to qualify for their state's program.)

CASE 3.1   Federal Employees Health Benefits Program as the Model for Marketplace Plans

Many Americans have little choice about health insurance. For the majority, the choices are to accept the plan offered by their employer, by their state **Medicaid** agency, or by Medicare, or to do without. Even Americans who have a choice lack the information needed to choose wisely. In many respects, the Federal Employees Health Benefits Program is superior. Its structure reflects the concept of managed competition first advocated by a Stanford University economist (Enthoven 1984):

- Each year employees choose one of several private insurance plans in an online exchange.
- Employees pay the marginal cost of choosing more expensive coverage.
- Insurance providers must accept everyone and must charge everyone the same premium.

How has this program worked? Compared to private employer plan premiums, federal plan premiums have risen more slowly in some years and have risen more rapidly in others (Liu and Jin 2013). The overall pattern, however, is similar to the patterns of other private insurer plan premiums.

Although the Federal Employees Health Benefits Program served as model for ACA marketplace plans, it differs from those plans in several ways. The most important difference is that federal employees are typically well-paid professionals. Nearly two-thirds of federal employee households have incomes that are at least four times the federal poverty level; only 11 percent of uninsured households do (Bovbjerg 2009). Not surprisingly, given that their customers are apt to be very sensitive to insurance premiums, ACA marketplace plans have been aggressive in taking steps to keep premiums low. Many excluded high-priced providers from their 2014 networks, and they appear poised to implement additional steps to bring down costs.

Discussion questions:
- One plan costs $8,000. The government will pay $6,500. How much would a $10,000 plan cost the employee?

(continued)

CASE 3.1
(continued)

- Is equal government payment important, regardless of the plan the employee chooses?
- How does equal payment affect employees' choices?
- Would varying premiums (such as premiums based on age) work better, so that older employees would be attractive risks for insurers?
- What problems would varying premiums cause?
- Why didn't insurers for the Federal Employees Health Benefits Program take aggressive steps (like creating narrow networks) to bring down premiums?
- Why do the high incomes of federal employees affect their choices?

PPOs are the most common form of managed care organization. All PPOs negotiate discounts with a panel of hospitals, physicians, and other providers, but their similarities end there. Some PPOs have small panels; others have large panels. Some PPOs require that care be approved by a primary care physician; some do not.

PPOs are far less diverse than HMOs, however. Some HMOs are structured around large medical group practices and are called **group model HMOs**. Group model HMOs typically make a flat payment per consumer enrolled with the group. This practice is called **capitation**. Other HMOs, called **staff model HMOs**, employ physicians directly and pay them salaries. Both staff and group model HMOs still exist, but they are expensive to set up and make sense only for large numbers of enrollees.

HMO expansion largely has been fueled by the growth of **independent practice association (IPA) HMOs**. These plans contract with large groups of physicians, small groups of physicians, and solo practice physicians. These contracts assume many forms. Physicians can be paid per service (as PPOs usually operate) or per enrollee (as group model HMOs usually operate). IPAs also pay hospitals and other providers in different ways.

The POS plan is another form of HMO. These plans are a combination of PPO and IPA. Unlike an IPA, they cover nonemergency services provided by nonnetwork providers, but copayments are higher. Unlike a PPO, they pay some providers using methods other than discounted FFS.

A high-deductible (HD) plan typically has a deductible of more than $1,000 for an individual. These plans are also sometimes called *consumer-directed health plans*. Many HD plans also incorporate health savings accounts, in which funds deposited by the worker or the employer can earn interest if not spent.

Group model HMO
HMO that contracts with a physician group to provide services

Capitation
Payment per person (The payment does not depend on the services provided.)

Staff model HMO
HMO that directly employs staff physicians to provide services

Independent practice association (IPA) HMO
HMO that contracts with an independent practice association, which in turn contracts with physician groups

EXHIBIT 3.3
Enrollment
Patterns in
Employer-
Sponsored
Insurance

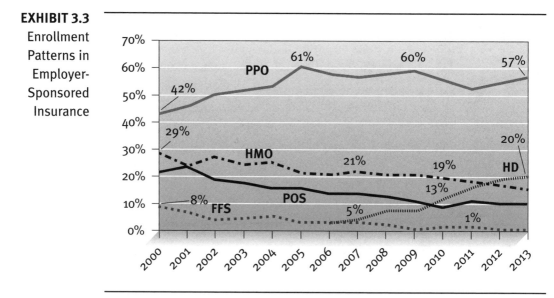

Source: Kaiser Family Foundation and Health Research & Educational Trust (2013).

Health insurance continues to evolve in a disorderly fashion. Where this development will lead is not clear. The belief that managed care is in retreat is widespread, but Exhibit 3.3 indicates otherwise. FFS plans have all but disappeared, and the market share of PPO plans has risen. HMOs and POS plans have lost market share, likely because of the fact that PPO plans do not cost much more, are easier to operate, and have been better accepted by consumers. HD plans (which were not even tracked separately until 2006) claimed 20 percent of the market in 2013.

Complicating this already complex picture are recent developments in Medicare, Medicaid, and ACA marketplace plans. A series of changes in these plans could have widespread effects.

Medicare has launched a series of demonstration projects and major changes in Medicare Advantage. The demonstration projects include trials of accountable care organizations, trials of bundled payments, trials of primary care innovations, and initiatives to improve the speed of innovation (Centers for Medicare & Medicaid Services 2013a). Accountable care organizations include doctors, hospitals, and other providers who assume the risk for the quality of care and the cost of care delivered to Medicare beneficiaries. When an accountable care organization succeeds, it gets paid more. A 2012 evaluation of one of the first accountable care organizations found that it met quality targets and realized modest savings (Colla et al. 2012). As of early 2014, no results were available from any of the bundled payment trials, but earlier models did show cost and quality gains (Cromwell, Dayhoff, and Thoumaian 1997). A bundled payment creates incentives for clinicians to streamline and standardize care. Medicare's primary care initiative emphasizes paying bonuses to primary care doctors who take steps to improve coordination of care. In essence, Medicare's primary care initiative is testing medical homes. The evidence suggests that some medical homes improve care and reduce cost, but some do not (Peikes et al. 2012). As of early 2014, no results were available for the initiatives to speed innovation.

The changes to Medicare Advantage appear to have been successful. The main driver appears to have been the creation of a rating system that summarizes the performance of an insurance plan (and its network of providers) using a rating of one to five stars. This system appears to have improved outcomes for Medicare Advantage customers and has increased enrollment significantly (Ayanian et al. 2013; Landon et al. 2012; Reid et al. 2013). Given the complexities of making health insurance decisions, this innovation might prove useful in other health insurance sectors.

Changes in Medicaid have taken place since the passage of the ACA in 2010. Most of these changes entail creation of managed care plans for beneficiaries who are also eligible for Medicare. These dually eligible beneficiaries typically face grave health problems and have very low incomes. No general results are available, although a trial of accountable care organizations for dually eligible Medicare beneficiaries showed improvements in cost and quality (Colla et al. 2012).

ACA marketplace plans are new, but most have used narrow provider networks to keep premiums down. About 70 percent of these plans have very small networks, and plans with broader networks have significantly higher premiums (McKinsey & Company 2013). Some of these innovations will likely work well, and some of them will be incorporated into standard insurance plans. However, it is too soon to tell which ones will become routine.

CASE 3.2   Group Health Cooperative's Patient-Centered Medical Home

Group Health Cooperative is a nonprofit, consumer-governed healthcare system that provides healthcare and health insurance coverage to residents of Idaho and Washington. Originally a staff model HMO that employed physicians, Group Health became a **network HMO**, meaning that it contracted with a large multispecialty medical group and with independent physicians.

Group Health had traditionally stressed primary care. But as it transitioned away from being a staff model HMO, its primary care practices began showing signs of strain. Primary care patient panels kept getting larger, referrals to specialists increased, hospitalization costs rose, emergency department use mounted, evidence of workforce burnout

Network HMO
HMO that has a variety of contracts (including contracts with physician groups, IPAs, and individual physicians)

(continued)

CASE 3.2
(continued)

increased, and recruiting primary care physicians kept getting harder.

In response, Group Health began turning one of its locations into a patient-centered medical home. Doing so entailed using its electronic health record system to recognize patient care needs, expanding use of phone and e-mail communication to reduce patient visits, and increasing the time physicians spent per patient visit. This process involved adding a medical assistant for each physician. It also involved adding a nurse practitioner to handle same-day visits, adding one clinical pharmacist per 10,000 panel members, and adding two licensed practical nurses per 10,000 panel members.

The practice that became a patient-centered medical home improved in patient satisfaction and clinical quality more than comparable Group Health practices (Reid et al. 2010). Cost per member per month also rose more slowly than in other practices, primarily because hospitalization rates did not rise in the patient-centered medical home. At 21 months, admission rates were 6 percent lower in the patient-centered medical home practice, and use of emergency and urgent care was 29 percent lower.

Discussion questions:
- Why would it make sense to become a network model HMO?
- Would you like to get your primary care at a patient-centered medical home?
- Did it make sense for Group Health to support the patient-centered medical home transition?
- Could an independent practice afford to become a patient-centered medical home?
- Why is Medicare sponsoring patient-centered medical home demonstrations?
- How would a 6 percent reduction in hospitalization rates affect hospitals?

3.4 Payment Systems

In the past, most healthcare providers were paid on a simple FFS basis. Today, managed care plans have begun to experiment with alternative payment arrangements. Different payment systems are important because they create different incentive systems for providers. Differences in financial incentives lead to different patterns of care, so the power of changing incentives should not be underestimated. In contracting with insurers or providers, managers need to recognize the strengths and weaknesses of different systems. The four basic payment methods—salary, FFS, case-based, and capitation—can be modified by the addition of incentive payments, increasing the number of possible payment methods.

A **salary** is fixed compensation paid per defined period. As such, it is not directly linked to output. Typically, physicians are paid a salary when their productivity is difficult to measure (e.g., in the case of academic physicians) or when the incentives created by FFS payments are seen as undesirable (e.g., an incentive to overtreat increases costs). As stated earlier, most physicians in the United States have traditionally been paid on a fee-for-service basis, meaning that each physician has a schedule of fees and expects to be paid that amount for each unit of service provided.

Case-based payments make single payments for all covered services associated with an episode of care. Medicare's **diagnosis-related group (DRG)** system is a case-based system for hospital care, although it does not include physicians' services or posthospital care. In essence, case-based payments are FFS payments for a wider range of services. Bundled payments are a form of case-based payments. Capitation is compensation paid per beneficiary enrolled with a physician or an organization. Capitation is similar to a salary but varies according to the number of customers.

Each of the four basic payment methods has advantages and disadvantages. Salaries are straightforward and incorporate no incentives to provide more care than necessary, but they do not encourage outstanding effort or exemplary service. In addition, salaries give providers incentives to use resources other than their time and effort to meet their customers' needs. In the absence of incentives not to refer patients to other providers, salaried providers may well seek to refer substantial numbers of patients to specialists, urgent care clinics, or other sources of care.

Capitation incorporates many of the same incentives as a salary, with two important differences. One is that capitation payments drop if customers leave the practice, so physicians have more incentive to serve patients well. The other is that capitation arrangements often generate extra costs. Profits rise if these extra costs fall, so capitation encourages greater efficiency, referral to other providers, or insufficient treatment.

In contrast, FFS payments create powerful incentives to provide superior service, so much that overtreatment of insured consumers often results. Services that are more costly than beneficial can be profitable in this system, as long as the benefits exceed the consumer's out-of-pocket cost. These incentives can complicate efforts to control costs. For example, attempts to

Salary
Fixed compensation paid per period

Case-based payment
A single payment for an episode of care (The payment does not change if fewer services or more services are provided.)

Diagnosis-related groups (DRGs)
Case groups that underlie Medicare's case-based payment system for hospitals

impose or negotiate lower rates are likely to provoke providers to "unbundle" care by billing separately for procedures or tests that had been combined as one service.

The case-based method combines features of the FFS and capitation methods. Like FFS, it creates strong incentives to provide exceptional service, as well as an additional incentive to increase profits by reducing costs included in the case rate. Costs can be reduced by improving efficiency, shifting responsibility for therapy to "free" sources (such as the health department), and narrowing the definition of a case. The challenge is to keep providers focused on improving efficiency, not on duping the system.

Any of these four basic methods can be modified by including bonuses and penalties. A base salary plus a bonus for reducing inpatient days in selected cases is not a straight salary contract. Similarly, a capitation plan with bonuses or penalties for exceeding or not meeting customer service standards (e.g., a bonus for returning more than 75 percent of after-hours calls within 15 minutes) would not generate the same incentives a plain capitation plan would.

Capitation was previously expected to become the dominant method of payment. Experience with capitation suggests, however, that few providers (or insurers, for that matter) have the administrative skills or data that capitation demands. In addition, the financial risks of capitation can be substantial. Few providers have enough capitated patients for variations in average costs to cease being worrisome, and capitation payments are seldom risk-adjusted (i.e., increased when spending can be expected to be higher than average). These considerations have dampened most providers' enthusiasm for capitation. Insurers also have realized that capitation is not a panacea, recognizing that providers have ways other than becoming more efficient to reduce their costs. At present, FFS payments to providers remain the norm, even in most HMOs, but incentive payments for quality are proliferating. What compensation arrangements will look like in ten years remains to be seen.

3.5 Conclusion

The days of traditional, open-ended insurance plans are over. Despite the ubiquity of managed care, most consumers are enrolled in plans that are minimally managed, such as PPOs or POS plans that pay providers in familiar ways, and most providers are not part of an organized delivery system. This situation may change.

The central challenge of cost remains. In 2012 the median household income for a family of four was $66,000. This statistic means that half of the households in the country made less than $66,000. The Milliman Medical Index, which tracks all healthcare costs, shows that an average family of four spent $20,728 on healthcare in 2012 (Milliman 2013). Many families simply cannot afford this level of spending.

The process of change substantially increases the risks healthcare managers must face. The next chapter will introduce the basics of how to manage these risks.

Exercises

3.1 Why is health insurance necessary?

3.2 Explain how adverse selection and moral hazard are different, and give an example of each.

3.3 "The United States is the land of the overinsured, the underinsured, and the uninsured." What do you think these concepts mean? Why might this comment be true?

3.4 Private health insurers have been slow to develop and adopt proven cost containment innovations (e.g., case rates or disease management programs). Why do you think this is the case?

3.5 A radiology firm charges $2,000 per exam. Uninsured patients are expected to pay list price. How much do they pay?

3.6 A radiology firm charges $2,000 per exam. An insurer's allowed fee is 80 percent of charges. Its beneficiaries pay 25 percent of the allowed fee. How much does the insurer pay? How much does the beneficiary pay?

3.7 If the radiology firm raised its charge to $3,000, how much would the insurer pay? How much would the beneficiary pay?

3.8 A surgeon charges $2,400 for hernia surgery. He contracts with an insurer that allows a fee of $800. Patients pay 20 percent of the allowed fee. How much does the insurer pay? How much does the patient pay?

3.9 You have incurred a medical bill of $10,000. Your plan has a deductible of $1,000 and coinsurance of 20 percent. How much of this bill will you have to pay directly?

3.10 Why do employers provide health insurance coverage to their employees?

3.11 Your firm offers only a PPO with a large deductible, high coinsurance, and a limited network. You pay $400 per month for single coverage. Some of your employees have been urging you to offer a more generous plan. Who would you expect to choose the more generous plan and pay any extra premium?

3.12 What are the fundamental differences between HMO and PPO plans?

3.13 Suppose that your employer offered you $4,000 in cash instead of health insurance coverage. Health insurance is excluded from state income taxes and federal income taxes. (To keep the problem simple, we will ignore Social Security and Medicare taxes.) The cash would be subject to state income taxes (8 percent) and federal income taxes (28 percent). How much would your after-tax income go up if you took the cash rather than the insurance?

3.14 How different would this calculation look for a worker who earned $500,000 and lived in Vermont? This worker would face a state income tax rate of 9.5 percent and a federal income tax rate of 35 percent.

References

Ayanian, J. Z., B. E. Landon, A. M. Zaslavsky, R. C. Saunders, L. G. Pawlson, and J. P. Newhouse. 2013. "Medicare Beneficiaries More Likely to Receive Appropriate Ambulatory Services in HMOs Than in Traditional Medicare." *Health Affairs* 32 (7): 1228–35.

Bernard, T. S. 2013. "Weighing the Risks of Going Without Health Insurance." *New York Times*, November 19.

Bovbjerg, R. R. 2009. "Lessons for Health Reform from the Federal Employees Health Benefits Program." *Timely Analysis of Immediate Health Policy Issues* August. Robert Wood Johnson Foundation and the Urban Institute. www.urban.org/UploadedPDF/411940_lessons_for_health_reform.pdf.

Centers for Medicare & Medicaid Services. 2013a. "Innovation Models." http://innovation.cms.gov/.

———. 2013b. "National Health Expenditure Data." www.cms.gov/Research-Statistics-Data-and-Systems/Statistics-Trends-and-Reports/NationalHealth ExpendData/NationalHealthAccountsHistorical.html.

Colla, C. H., D. E. Wennberg, E. Meara, J. S. Skinner, D. Gottlieb, V. A. Lewis, C. M. Snyder, and E. S. Fisher. 2012. "Spending Differences Associated with the Medicare Physician Group Practice Demonstration." *Journal of the American Medical Association* 308 (10): 1015–23.

Collins, S. R., R. Robertson, T. Garber, and M. M. Doty. 2013. *Insuring the Future: Current Trends in Health Coverage and the Effects of Implementing the Affordable Care Act*. New York: The Commonwealth Fund.

Cromwell, J., D. A. Dayhoff, and A. H. Thoumaian. 1997. "Cost Savings and Physician Responses to Global Bundled Payments for Medicare Heart Bypass Surgery." *Health Care Financing Review* 19 (1): 41–57.

DeNavas-Walt, C., B. D. Proctor, and J. C. Smith. 2013. *Income, Poverty, and Health Insurance Coverage in the United States: 2012*. Washington, DC: US Government Printing Office.

Enthoven, A. C. 1984. "A New Proposal to Reform the Tax Treatment of Health Insurance." *Health Affairs* 3 (1): 21–39.

Fang, H., M. P. Keane, and D. Silverman. 2008. "Sources of Advantageous Selection: Evidence from the Medigap Insurance Market." *Journal of Political Economy* 116 (2): 303–50.

Kaiser Family Foundation and Health Research & Educational Trust. 2013. *2013 Employer Health Benefits Survey.* Menlo Park, CA: Kaiser Family Foundation and Chicago: Health Research & Educational Trust.

Landon, B. E., A. M. Zaslavsky, R. C. Saunders, L. G. Pawlson, J. P. Newhouse, and J. Z. Ayanian. 2012. "Analysis of Medicare Advantage HMOs Compared with Traditional Medicare Shows Lower Use of Many Services During 2003–09." *Health Affairs* 31 (12): 2609–17.

Liu, Y., and G. Z. Jin. 2013. *Employer Contribution and Premium Growth in Health Insurance.* National Bureau of Economic Research. Working Paper 19760. Published December. www.nber.org/papers/w19760.

Long, S. K., G. M. Kenney, S. Zuckerman, D. E. Goin, D. Wissoker, F. Blavin, L. J. Blumberg, L. Clemans-Cope, J. Holahan, and K. Hempstead. 2014. "The Health Reform Monitoring Survey: Addressing Data Gaps to Provide Timely Insights into the Affordable Care Act." *Health Affairs* 33 (1): 161–67.

McKinsey & Company. 2013. "Hospital Networks: Configurations on the Exchanges and Their Impact on Premiums." Updated December 14. www.mckinsey.com/client_service/healthcare_systems_and_services/center_for_us_health_system_reform.

Milliman. 2013. *2013 Milliman Medical Index.* Published May. www.milliman.com/uploadedFiles/insight/Periodicals/mmi/pdfs/mmi-2013.pdf.

Peikes, D., A. Zutshi, J. L. Genevro, M. L. Parchman, and D. S. Meyers. 2012. "Early Evaluations of the Medical Home: Building on a Promising Start." *American Journal of Managed Care* 18 (2): 105–16.

Reid, R. J., K. Coleman, E. A. Johnson, P. A. Fishman, C. Hsu, M. P. Soman, C. E. Trescott, M. Erikson, and E. B. Larson. 2010. "The Group Health Medical Home at Year Two: Cost Savings, Higher Patient Satisfaction, and Less Burnout for Providers." *Health Affairs* 29 (5): 835–43.

Reid, R. O., P. Deb, B. L. Howell, and W. H. Shrank. 2013. "Association Between Medicare Advantage Plan Star Ratings and Enrollment." *Journal of the American Medical Association* 309 (3): 267–74.

Spector, W. D., J. W. Cohen, and I. Pesis-Katz. 2004. "Home Care Before and After the Balanced Budget Act of 1997: Shifts in Financing and Services." *Gerontologist* 44 (1): 39–47.

DESCRIBING, EVALUATING, AND MANAGING RISK

After reading this chapter, students will be able to

- calculate an expected value and standard deviation,
- describe the key features of a risky outcome,
- construct and use a decision tree to frame a choice, and
- discuss common approaches to managing risk.

- Clinical and managerial decisions typically entail uncertainty about what will happen.
- Decision makers often have imprecise estimates of the probabilities of various outcomes.
- Decision making about risk involves describing, evaluating, and managing potential outcomes.
- Insurance and diversification are two ways to manage risk.

4.1 Introduction

Clinical and managerial decisions typically entail risk. Important information is often incomplete or missing when the time to make a decision arrives. At best, one is aware of potential outcomes and the probability of each outcome's occurrence. At worst, one has little to no information about outcomes and their probabilities. The challenge for managers is to identify risks that are worth analyzing, risks that are worth taking, and the best strategies for dealing with them.

When outcomes are uncertain, decision making has three components: describing, evaluating, and managing potential outcomes. Because uncertainty is central to many areas of healthcare, the same techniques (e.g., hedging bets and monitoring uncertain situations aggressively) are recommended for describing and evaluating potential outcomes regarding real investments (e.g., buildings, equipment, and training), financial investments (e.g., stocks, bonds, and insurance), and clinical decisions (e.g., testing and therapy).

4.2 Describing Potential Outcomes

The first step in any decision is to describe what could happen, including the probabilities and value of possible outcomes, and calculate descriptive statistics about the possible outcomes.

Objective probability
An estimate of probability based on observed frequencies

Description begins with an assessment of the probabilities of the possible outcomes. Ideally, the assessment should generate an **objective probability**—an estimate based on evidence about the frequencies of different outcomes. For example, if 250 of 1,000 patients reported nausea after taking a medication, a good estimate of the probability of nausea would be 0.25 (250 divided by 1,000). More often, though, description assesses the **subjective probability**—the decision maker's perception of how likely an outcome is to occur.

Subjective probability
An individual's judgment about how likely a particular event is to occur

In some cases, decision makers have incomplete data. In other cases, the data do not fit the situation. For example, if a careful study of a drug in a population of men older than 18 years finds that the probability of nausea is 0.25, what value should we use for a sample of women older than 65 years? In still other cases, individuals may feel that population frequencies do not apply to them. Someone who claims to have a cast-iron stomach may believe that his probability of nausea is much less than 0.25. The decision maker with a cast-iron stomach may be correct in thinking that the population frequency does not apply to him, or he may just be overly optimistic.

In practice, decision makers predominantly use subjective probabilities. Unfortunately, these subjective probabilities are often inaccurate, even when the estimates are made by highly trained clinicians or experienced managers. Studies have found that physicians overestimate the probability of skull fractures, cancer, pneumonia, and streptococcal infections, and managers are notorious for being overenthusiastic in their forecasts of how well new projects will be run and how well they will be received. For a variety of reasons, humans generally are poor probability calculators. Examining data about population frequencies can significantly improve decision makers' choices. For example, even if you believe that your hospital is less likely than average to lose money on the primary care practices it has just purchased, knowing that the majority of hospitals have lost money tells you that your hospital is still prone to loss. Moreover, in many cases, an honest assessment of the probabilities results in broad generalizations, not a point estimate of probabilities. A manager may be able to say only that he or she thinks one scenario is more likely than another. This information is still useful; general impressions can often clarify the situation and help managers make the best decision.

CASE 4.1   Betting on Medicare Advantage

Aetna announced on August 19, 2012, that it would buy Coventry Health Care for nearly $6 billion (de la Merced 2012). The acquisition represents a strategy to expand its Medicaid managed care, Medicare Advantage, and health insurance marketplace lines of business. Most analysts anticipate rapid growth in these markets.

These markets do present major risks, however. First, much of the growth in Medicaid managed care will be due to expanded coverage of aged or disabled beneficiaries. These new enrollees tend to have multiple, complex health problems, meaning that prior experience with Medicaid managed care plans may be of little help. Prior to the passage of the Affordable Care Act in 2010, Medicaid managed care enrollees were largely children, pregnant women, and parents. Second, profitability in Medicaid managed care and Medicare Advantage depends on government rates. Medicare Advantage rates are scheduled to be gradually cut to bring them in line with costs in traditional Medicare, and no one can really forecast what will happen to rates for Medicaid managed care or marketplace products. Third, no one knows what will happen to Medicare Advantage enrollment if the structure or payment systems of traditional Medicare are changed. Fourth, some time will be needed to sort out who will sign up for coverage via health insurance marketplaces. If too few low-risk individuals sign up, insurers could lose substantial amounts of money.

Risk is intrinsic to the health insurance business. Insurers take on risk by selling coverage for consumers' variable medical expenditures. When you average risk over the spending patterns of tens of thousands of consumers, however, the risk becomes less uncertain—in most cases. In 2008, Humana nearly halved its profit forecast because claims for its Medicare prescription drug plan ran much higher than anticipated (Donley and Britt 2008). Apparently, its emphasis on

(continued)

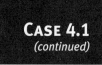

CASE 4.1
(continued)

covering well-known, branded pharmaceuticals attracted a large number of customers with above-average utilization patterns. (This situation is an example of adverse selection.)

But the main perils do not come from the operational issues mentioned previously. The real risks spring from strategic decisions that could go wrong if an insurer misjudges the market. For example, Humana's decision to serve Medicare Advantage customers in 2007 was a major gamble, but it appears to have paid off. Humana has gained nearly 2.5 million new customers (Gold et al. 2013). That result does not guarantee that Aetna's similar bet will work out as well.

Discussion questions:
- What has happened to Medicare Advantage enrollment since 2012?
- What has happened to Medicaid managed care enrollment since 2012?
- Have any insurers pulled out of Medicaid managed care markets during the past year?
- Medicare Advantage contracts last a year. What is Aetna risking by betting that Medicare Advantage will be an attractive opportunity?
- Is Medicare Advantage riskier than other forms of private health insurance?
- What other healthcare firms also face risks due to changes in government policy?

4.3 Evaluating Outcomes

The next step is to evaluate possible outcomes. This chapter focuses on financial outcomes, typically profits. Financial outcomes are usually difficult to project. Skilled analysts commonly arrive at different answers when asked to calculate how much a therapy will cost under well-defined circumstances. Attempts at forecasting costs and revenues for a new project result in an even greater range of plausible outcomes because of all the uncertainties inherent in such an undertaking. Analysts may have ways of improving their forecasts, but in general, forecasts will never be more than educated guesses.

The problems mount when no simple measurement system, like profits, exists. How valuable is a new surgical procedure that reduces the chance of abdominal scarring from 0.12 to 0.08 but reduces the chance that the operation will succeed from 0.68 to 0.66? Any time a scenario involves opposing probabilities, evaluation becomes a challenge. Even though scholars have made progress in evaluating complex outcomes, considerable uncertainty remains. Chapter 14 will tackle this problem in more detail.

Calculating descriptive statistics is the final step in the process of evaluating outcomes. The most common statistic is the **expected value**. To calculate an expected value, multiply the value of each outcome by its probability of occurrence and then add the resulting products. For example, suppose your organization is contemplating buying a skilled nursing facility that currently has profits of $20,000. The price of the nursing home is $1 million, meaning that the return on investment would be only 2 percent, which is too low from your organization's point of view. (Return on investment equals annual profit divided by your investment.) One of your managers, however, has identified a number of operational improvements that she forecasts will boost profits to $120,000. Although this manager's improvements are reasonable, a consultant points out that, in his experience, ambitious proposals to increase profits fail about 40 percent of the time. So, the consultant estimates that the expected profit is $80,000 = (0.6 × $120,000) + (0.4 × $20,000).

This level of precision (e.g., "about 40 percent of the time") is representative of the reliability of managerial forecasts—they are inexact at best. Despite imprecise forecasts, managers must make a choice. In many cases, calculating the expected profit and then conducting a **sensitivity analysis** will help managers avoid bad decisions.

Formally, an expected value equals $P_1X_1 + P_2X_2 + \ldots + P_nX_n$, where P_i represents the probability that an outcome will occur and X_i represents the value of that outcome. An expected value differs from an average because the probabilities of some outcomes will be higher than the probabilities of others, so they get more weight. For example, the average of $120,000 and $20,000—the two estimates from our example above—is $70,000. But the expected value is $80,000 because the probability of earning $120,000 is larger than the probability of earning $20,000.

Does buying the skilled nursing home make sense? It might. The expected return on investment is 8 percent. Given that the worst-case scenario is a 2 percent return on investment, this gamble will seem reasonable to many firms, depending on the alternative investments the firm is considering.

Good decisions usually require more information than just an expected value because typically the expected value is not the outcome that occurs. Most decision makers find that a list of the best and worst outcomes is valuable. A list of the most likely outcomes can also be useful. Graphs, too, can help decision makers understand their choices. Many people find a well-designed graph more valuable than a calculation. Finally, remember that estimates are estimates; writing them down does not make them more reliable. The less mathematically sophisticated your target audience is, the more you need to emphasize that forecasts are imprecise.

Expected value
The sum of the probability of each possible outcome multiplied by the value of the outcome

Sensitivity analysis
The process of varying the assumptions in an analysis over a reasonable range and observing how the outcome changes

Decision tree
A visual decision support tool that depicts the values and probabilities of the outcomes of a choice

This simple example can be illustrated with a **decision tree**, which is a way of presenting information about a choice. A decision tree visually links a decision maker's choices with the outcomes that are likely to result. It is called a tree because the possible outcomes branch from a choice. For the analyst, much of the value lies in the process of constructing the decision tree because it highlights his or her perception of what will happen and where the information is weakest. In addition, many people find that examining a decision tree helps them understand the issues involved because it lays out their best estimates of the cost or payoff and the probability associated with each possible outcome. As you can see in Exhibit 4.1, the worst-case forecast is a profit of $20,000, which is less than ideal but not a catastrophe. Similarly, the best-case forecast is a profit of $120,000, which is good but not superb. As is usually the case, laying out the decision tree helps clarify the situation by making the probability and profit estimates explicit. It does not tell managers what decision to make. Alternatives have not yet been laid out, so a sensible decision cannot be made.

Calculating the expected values of alternatives is sometimes called *rolling back* a decision tree. Rolling back a decision tree means calculating its expected value. In Exhibit 4.1, the expected return is $80,000.

Decision trees probably don't need to be drawn for scenarios as simple as this example, but a little more complexity can make construction of a tree worthwhile (see Exhibit 4.2). The consultant might have noted that there is one chance in four that the state will reduce nursing home payments. If payments are reduced, profits will be $100,000 if the improvements succeed or $0 if they fail. The chance of rate cuts reduces expected profits to $75,000. The updated decision tree also displays the profit available from an alternative investment, in this case a short-term bond that returns $40,000. Most profit-oriented decision makers would prefer to invest in the nursing home

EXHIBIT 4.1
A Nursing Home Decision Tree

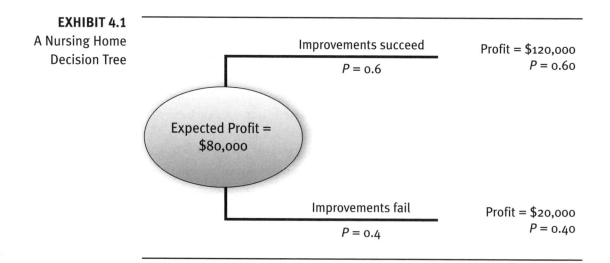

because its expected profit is higher and its outcomes with low profits do not entail losses.

To make sure that you understand Exhibit 4.2, answer the following questions.

- Why does the probability that the improvements fail and rates are cut equal 0.10?
- Why does profit equal $0 if the improvements fail and rates are cut?
- Why is expected profit less in Exhibit 4.2 than in Exhibit 4.1?

Range
The difference between the largest and smallest values of a variable

Estimates of the variability of outcomes can be useful for making comparisons. Variability is typically measured by listing the **range** of possible values or by listing the **standard deviation** (which is the square root of the **variance**). If you are not comparing outcomes, the standard deviation is not helpful. In contrast, the range can convey useful information even if you are not comparing outcomes. The range helps you see the best- and worst-case scenarios. To know whether a risk is worth taking, you need to know the size of the risk and the potential payoff. Few people will want to take a risk

Standard deviation
The square root of a variance

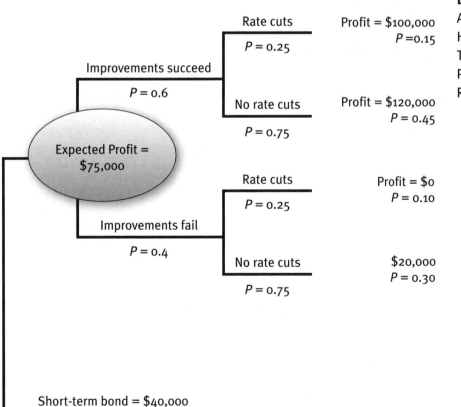

EXHIBIT 4.2
A Nursing Home Decision Tree with the Possibility of Rate Cuts

Variance
The squared deviation of a random variable from its expected value (If a variable takes the value 3 with a probability of 0.2, the value 6 with a probability of 0.3, and the value 9 with a probability of 0.5, its expected value is 6.9. Its variance is 5.49, which is $0.2 \times [3 - 6.9]^2 + 0.3 \times [6 - 6.9]^2 + 0.5 \times [9 - 6.9]^2$.)

if the best possible payoff is small or if the worst payoff is disastrous. On the other hand, if the best payoff is large, some people will be willing to accept significant risks.

To calculate variance, multiply the squared difference between the value of each outcome and the expected value by its probability of occurrence and then add the resulting products. (Find the appropriate probability of occurrence by multiplying the probability on the "branch" of the outcome by the probability on the preceding branch.) So, in our example, the variance equals $0.15 \times (\$100,000 - \$75,000)^2 + 0.45 \times (\$120,000 - \$75,000)^2 + 0.10 \times (\$0 - \$75,000)^2 + 0.3 \times (\$20,000 - \$75,000)^2$, or $\$2,475,000,000$. The standard deviation is the square root of $\$2,475,000,000$, which is $\$49,749$.

A standard deviation or variance has meaning only when you are comparing options. If two choices have similar expected values, the one with the higher standard deviation carries a higher risk because a larger standard deviation means that the bad outcomes are either more likely or much worse. For example, a project that has an 85 percent chance of earning $0 and a 15 percent chance of earning $500,000 also has an expected profit of $75,000. The standard deviation for this project is $178,536, confirming its higher risk.

CASE 4.2   Investing in Cardiology Services

"It's time for us to commit to building a center of excellence in cardiac care," said Shea, the hospital's chief financial officer. "Mercy and Central did it three years ago, and they are doing extremely well. Medicare pays well, and the private insurers pay even better. We cannot afford to miss this opportunity."

"Perhaps," said Emerson, the hospital's chief medical officer. "Let me lay out a couple of issues that we need to consider. First, there's no guarantee that the insurers will keep on paying so well for cardiology services. Most observers think that prices are higher than they need to be, and Medicare is facing a financial crisis. I think that Medicare will move to a bundled payment for many cardiology services before too long. The cardiologists will continue to do nicely, but they will have powerful incentives to cut back on imaging, to cut back on catheterizations, and to switch to less invasive interventions. The net effect will be to slash hospital revenues. Second, there's no guarantee that we will be able to attract a team of top-notch cardiologists. Those guys are in short supply these days. Without a really superb team, we will not get this off the ground."

(continued)

CASE 4.2
(continued)

"OK," said Shea. "Here is what the planning team has forecast. We will need a 24-bed unit, office space for three cardiologists, a 64-slice CT scanner, and a cardiac catheterization lab. We estimate that this setup will cost us $10 million. We estimate that this change will increase inpatient days by 1,500, resulting in profits of $2 million. We also estimate that we will have 1,000 new outpatient procedures, which will generate $500,000 in profits. That represents a very nice return on our investment and leaves us some room for error in our cost and revenue forecasts. Personally, I do not think that Medicare will make any changes fast. The ability of the federal government to avoid taking action is unsurpassed. And I am confident that we will be able to recruit cardiologists."

Discussion questions:
- How likely is a change in Medicare payment? What probability should you assign to it?
- What will happen to hospital profits if Medicare does switch to bundled payments?
- How likely is a failure to recruit three excellent cardiologists? What probability should you assign to this endeavor? What will happen to profits if you are able to recruit only two excellent cardiologists?
- If you set up this scenario as a decision tree, which of your assumptions become clear to other decision makers?
- What are the advantages of making your assumptions clear? What are the disadvantages?

Remember, though, the point of these calculations is to improve your analysis. The analysis should include an understanding of the size of the risk, how likely it is to occur, and whether it is worth taking. If your target audience, which might include members of the board or nonfinancial managers, is puzzled by your analysis and does not really understand the issues, you have failed to present it effectively. Your audience will not be able to offer useful feedback, and the decision to take or not take the risk will be all yours. Managers *could* be terminated for taking risks that the board and other managers understood and approved. Managers *will* be terminated for taking risks that the board and other managers did not understand.

4.3.1 Risk Preferences

Risk preferences may influence choices. A risk-seeking person prefers more variability. Someone who gambles in a casino must be a **risk seeker** because

Risk seeker
A decision maker who prefers more risk to less (A risk seeker would prefer a gamble with a 50 percent chance of getting nothing and a 50 percent chance of getting $10 to getting $5 for sure.)

the expected payoff from a dollar bet will always be less than a dollar because of taxes and the casino's take. Likewise, a patient who can expect to live 18 months if he undergoes standard therapy may be a risk seeker. He may prefer a therapy that gives him an expected life span of only 13 months if it increases his chances of significant recovery. The manager of a nearly bankrupt business is likely also a risk seeker. Taking chances, even chances with low expected payoffs, may be the only way to survive.

A **risk-neutral** person does not care about variability and will always choose the outcome with the highest expected value. Large organizations with substantial reserves can afford to be risk neutral. For example, a firm with $400 million in cash reserves will probably not buy fire insurance for a $200,000 clinic. If the expected loss is $4,000 per year (a 2 percent chance of a $200,000 loss), the organization's fire insurance will cost at least $4,400 because of processing costs and insurer profits. On average, the firm will have higher profits if it does not insure this risk, and it can afford not to. Spending $200,000 for a new clinic will not put much of a dent in the organization's reserves.

A risk-averse person avoids variability and will sometimes choose strategies with smaller expected values to avoid risk. An individual who buys health insurance is likely to demonstrate **risk aversion** because the expected value of his or her covered expenses will usually be less than the premium. Insurance premiums must cover the insurer's expected payout, its cost of operation, and some return on invested capital. Unless a beneficiary's expected benefits (the insurer's expected payouts) have been incorrectly estimated, the insurer's costs and profits will push insurance premiums above expected losses. By definition, someone who will pay an insurance premium is risk averse.

4.3.2 Decision Analysis

Formal decision analysis has three steps, and only one of them is difficult (Hammond, Keeney, and Raiffa 1998). The steps are setting up a decision tree, identifying the alternative with the largest expected value, and using sensitivity analysis to assess the robustness of the analysis. Setting up a decision tree is the hardest and most important part of decision analysis. Most insights are gained, but also most mistakes are made, in this step. Six steps are involved in setting up a decision tree.

1. Carefully define the problem. Often this task is harder than it sounds.
2. Identify the alternative courses of action. Serious mistakes are often made here.
3. Identify the outcomes associated with each alternative.
4. Identify the sequence of events leading to final outcomes. This sequence may include choices and chance events.

Risk neutral
Indifferent to risk in decision making (A risk-neutral person would think that getting $5 for sure is as good as a gamble with a 50 percent chance of getting nothing and a 50 percent chance of getting $10.)

Risk aversion
The reluctance of a decision maker to accept an outcome with an uncertain payoff rather than a smaller, more certain outcome (A risk-averse person would prefer getting $5 for sure to a gamble with a 50 percent chance of getting nothing and a 50 percent chance of getting $10.)

5. Calculate the probability of each outcome.

6. Calculate the value of each outcome.

Each of these steps is more difficult than it sounds, so often the first decision is whether to do a decision analysis at all.

4.3.3 Sensitivity Analysis

Any time setting up and solving a decision tree are worthwhile, performing a sensitivity analysis is equally worthwhile. A sensitivity analysis substitutes different, but plausible, values for the values in a decision tree. Gauging the effects of minor data changes on the results is always helpful. The data are never perfect, and using them as if they were would not make sense.

The decision tree for the nursing facility purchase tells us that the key issue is whether its manager can realize the operational improvements and product line changes that she is contemplating. If she can, the return on equity will be no less than 8.3 percent, no matter what Medicare does. A sensitivity analysis tells us that if she can realize about 70 percent of her projected gains, she can expect a 7 percent return on equity, no matter what Medicare does. What could she do to increase the odds of full improvement? The sensitivity analysis indicates that we can fall somewhat short of the manager's prediction and still hit the target rate of return.

4.4 Managing Risk

Risk sharing and diversification are the only two strategies for managing risk. Buying an insurance policy is the obvious way to share risk, although joint ventures or options can serve the same function. For insurance, consumers pay a fee to induce another organization to share risks; joint ventures or options share costs and profits with partners. Diversification can take a number of forms. Horizontal integration (creating an organization that can offer the full spectrum of healthcare services) is one diversification strategy because some aspects of healthcare are likely to be profitable no matter what the environment. All of these strategies limit potential losses, but they also limit potential profitability.

4.4.1 Risk Sharing

Joint ventures and options are common risk-sharing methods in the biotechnology and pharmaceutical fields. For example, in 2012 Pfizer and Zhejiang Hisun Pharmaceutical Company launched a joint venture to offer products for cardiovascular disease, infectious disease, oncology, and mental health in China (Khan 2012). This venture will be a full-service pharmaceutical company with manufacturing, marketing, and research capabilities. Likewise, Pfenex and

Agila Biotech announced a joint venture in 2013 to develop, manufacture, and commercialize an initial group of six products for the global market (Pfenex 2013). The two firms will share product development and marketing decisions. In 2013 Novartis purchased an option to buy Sideris Pharmaceuticals (Carroll 2013). Sideris, which got initial funding from a number of venture capital firms, was working on a drug that flushes iron from the body. Novartis has the option to complete the purchase if clinical trials confirm the drug's safety and efficacy. As a result, Novartis and the current owners share the risk that the drug will not be commercially viable. In a very different type of joint venture, Microsoft joined with General Electric to connect software applications with healthcare hardware. The objective was to offer a performance management suite that supports decision support and analysis (Tu 2012).

This example illustrates another facet of risk sharing. Often the cost that an organization seeks to share is the enormous cost of acquiring a key competency. Working with a knowledgeable partner allows the organization to gain experience. A lot of time and money is needed to build expertise, and joint ventures can reduce the risk of expending these resources needlessly. Of course, the organization must also assess what the gains are for the partner, such as expertise and profits.

4.4.2 Diversification
Diversification consists of identifying a portfolio of projects or therapies that are not highly positively correlated. Exhibit 4.3 compares investing in a clinic, investing in a trauma unit, and investing in a portfolio of 50 percent shares of each. Forecasts of return on investment for the projects depend on whether the growth of an HMO is rapid, moderate, or slow. The clinic is a better investment than the trauma unit (higher expected profits and lower standard

EXHIBIT 4.3
Diversification and Risk Reduction

| | HMO Growth | | | | |
	Rapid	Moderate	Slow		
Growth probabilities	0.160	0.700	0.140		

Profits				Expected	Standard Deviation
Clinic profits	10.0%	4.0%	−1.0%	4.3%	3.0%
Trauma unit profits	−3.0%	2.0%	13.0%	2.7%	4.5%
Portfolio profits (50% of each)	3.5%	3.0%	6.0%	3.5%	1.0%

deviation of profits). The portfolio is also a better investment than the trauma unit (higher expected profits and lower standard deviation of profits). The portfolio might be a better investment than the clinic for a risk-averse investor (lower expected profits but a lower standard deviation of profits).

Joint ventures can make diversification less risky, as Case 4.3 illustrates.

CASE 4.3   Diversification by Joint Venture

As of 2013 the University of Pittsburgh Medical Center (UPMC) had international operations in seven countries. It operates cancer centers and a full-service hospital in Ireland; transplantation, radiotherapy, and biotechnology centers in Italy; information technology and cancer centers in the United Kingdom; cancer center consults in Kazakhstan; transplantation in Singapore; pathology consulting in China; and educational training in primary care in Japan. UPMC is exploring expansion in Cyprus and Qatar. Most of these represent joint ventures with local partners (UPMC 2013).

In addition to its international operations, UPMC launched a domestic joint venture in 2011 with the Advisory Board, a consulting firm (Kliff 2013). Each partner invested $20 million in Evolent Health, which provides consulting services to other healthcare organizations. In addition, the Advisory Board brought consulting experience and a list of potential customers. UPMC brought years of experience in operating its own insurance plan, clinical expertise, and the infrastructure to coordinate care. Evolent Health supports the development strategies to reduce readmissions, to start medical homes, to create accountable care organizations, and even to form HMOs.

UPMC is headquartered in Pittsburgh, where it has a commanding presence. The largest employer in western Pennsylvania, with more than 50,000 employees and nearly $8 billion in revenue, UPMC owns 20 hospitals, 400 outpatient sites, a large insurance plan, and a number of other healthcare ventures (UPMC 2013).

Discussion questions:
- Why is expansion outside the United States an attractive form of diversification?
- What are the pitfalls of international expansion?
- What are the potential pitfalls of other diversification efforts?
- What are the main risks that UPMC faces in its Pittsburgh operations?

4.5 Conclusion

The goal of describing, evaluating, and managing risk is improving choices, not identifying perfect choices. Even when the evidence available to a decision maker is good and he or she makes a good decision, bad outcomes can result. More often, though, medical and managerial decisions are made with inadequate information. For example, managers often must make investment decisions long before they know how well technology will work, what volumes will be, and what rivals will do. Even when a manager has access to good information (which will never be the case with innovative choices), the possible consequences of his or her choices remain uncertain.

Good management, however, can reduce risk and reduce the consequences of risk. Some risks need not be taken because the payoff would not be adequate. Some risks can be shared via joint ventures or insurance. Some risks can be hedged via diversification. A balanced portfolio of projects and lines of business can be profitable in any market environment. Reducing variations in costs (so that risks are lower in capitated environments) or reducing fixed costs (so that sales slumps have fewer negative effects) can cut risk sharply. Finally, there's nothing like a high margin to reduce risk. If possible outcomes are a 15 percent return on equity or an 11 percent return on equity, most managers will sleep well.

Exercises

4.1 Five of ten people earn $0, four earn $100, and one loses $100. What is the expected payoff? What is the variance of the payoff?

4.2 There is a 50 percent chance of making $0, a 40 percent chance of making $100, and a 10 percent chance of losing $100. Calculate the expected value and variance of the payoff. How does your estimate compare to the previous problem?

4.3 There is a 1 percent chance that you will have healthcare bills of $100,000, a 19 percent chance that you will have healthcare bills of $10,000, a 60 percent chance that you will have healthcare bills of $500, and a 20 percent chance that you will have healthcare bills of $0. What is your expected healthcare spending?

4.4 There is a 1 percent chance that you will have healthcare bills of $100,000, a 19 percent chance that you will have healthcare bills of $10,000, a 60 percent chance that you will have healthcare bills of $500, and a 20 percent chance that you will have healthcare bills of $0. What will your expected insurance benefits be? Would you be willing to buy complete insurance coverage if it cost $3,712? Explain.

4.5 Instead of complete insurance as in Exercise 4.4, you have a policy with a $5,000 deductible. What will your expected out-of-pocket spending be? What will your expected insurance benefits be? Assuming that the premium equals 116 percent of expected insurance benefits, do you prefer the policy with a $5,000 deductible or complete coverage? Explain.

4.6 Your firm, which operates a nationwide system of cancer clinics, has annual profits of $800 million and cash reserves of $500 million. Your clinics have a replacement value of $200 million, and fire insurance for them would cost $5 million per year. Actuarial data show that your expected losses due to fire are $4 million. Should you buy insurance?

4.7 Your firm rents a supply management system to hospitals. You have received a buyout offer of $5 million. You forecast a 25 percent chance that you will have profits of $10 million, a 35 percent chance that you will have profits of $6 million, and a 40 percent chance that you will have profits of $2 million. Should you accept the offer? Explain.

4.8 You were given a lottery ticket. The drawing will be held in 5 minutes. You have a 0.1 percent chance of winning $10,000. You refuse an offer of $11 for your ticket. Are you risk averse? Explain.

4.9 Your house is worth $200,000. Your risk of a catastrophic flood is 0.5 percent. Such a flood would destroy your house and would not be covered by homeowner's insurance. Although you grumble, you buy flood coverage for $1,200. Are you risk averse or risk seeking?

4.10 Your firm faces considerable revenue uncertainty because you have to negotiate contracts with several customers. You forecast a 20 percent chance that your revenues will be $200,000, a 30 percent chance that your revenues will be $300,000, and a 50 percent chance that your revenues will be $500,000. Your costs are also uncertain because the prices of your supplies fluctuate considerably. You forecast a 40 percent chance that your costs will be $400,000 and a 60 percent chance that your costs will be $250,000. Use Excel to set up a decision tree for your profit forecast (it does not matter whether costs or revenues come first). How many possible profit outcomes do you have? What is your expected profit?

4.11 Your firm has been sued for $3 million by a supplier for breach of contract. Your lawyers believe that there are three possible outcomes if the suit goes to trial. One, which the lawyers term highly improbable, is that your supplier will win the lawsuit and be awarded $3 million. Another, which the lawyers term unlikely, is that your supplier will win the lawsuit and be awarded $500,000.

The third, which the lawyers term likely, is that your supplier will lose the lawsuit and be awarded $0. You have to decide whether to try to settle the case. To do so you need to assign probabilities to "highly improbable," "unlikely," and "likely." What probabilities correspond to these statements? Going to trial will cost you $100,000 in legal fees. One of your lawyers believes that your supplier will settle for $100,000 (and you will have legal fees of $25,000). Should you settle?

References

Carroll, J. 2013. "Novartis Grabs an Option to Buy Biotech Startup for Up to $300M." *FierceBiotech*. Published October 22. www.fiercebiotech.com/story/novartis-grabs-option-buy-biotech-startup-300m/2013-10-22.

de la Merced, M. J. 2012. "Aetna Agrees to Buy Coventry in $5.7 Billion Deal." *New York Times*, August 12.

Donley, M., and R. Britt. 2008. "Humana Slides Again on Profit Warning." *Market-Watch*. Published March 12. www.marketwatch.com/story/humana-warns-on-profit-shares-slide-for-second-day.

Gold, M., G. Jacobson, A. Damico, and T. Neuman. 2013. *Medicare Advantage 2013 Spotlight: Enrollment Market Update.* Kaiser Family Foundation Issue Brief. Published June. http://kaiserfamilyfoundation.files.wordpress.com/2013/06/8448.pdf.

Hammond, J. S., R. L. Keeney, and H. Raiffa. 1998. *Smart Choices: A Practical Guide to Making Better Decisions.* Boston: Harvard Business Review Press.

Khan, N. 2012. "Hisun-Pfizer Pharmaceutical to Hire 600 China Staff by Year-End." *Bloomberg*. Published September 13. www.bloomberg.com/news/2012-09-13/hisun-pfizer-pharmaceutical-to-hire-600-china-staff-by-year-end.html.

Kliff, S. 2013. "Is This the End of Health Insurers?" *Washington Post*, July 5.

Pfenex. 2013. "Pfenex Inc. and Agila Biotech Private Limited Announce Joint Venture to Develop Biosimilar Products for the Global Market." Published April 16. www.pfenex.com/news/details/31.

Tu, J. I. 2012. "Microsoft, GE Uniting to Create Better Health-Care Data Systems." *Seattle Times*. Published September 26. http://seattletimes.com/html/businesstechnology/2019270995_microsoftcaradigmxml.html.

University of Pittsburgh Medical Center (UPMC). 2013. "Business Ventures." Accessed July 2, 2014. www.upmc.com/about/partners/ventures/Pages/default.aspx.

UNDERSTANDING COSTS

Learning Objectives

After reading this chapter, students will be able to

- calculate average and marginal costs,
- articulate why efficiency is important,
- identify opportunity costs,
- forecast how changes in technology and prices will change costs, and
- discuss the relationship between cost and quality.

Key Concepts

- Costs depend on perspective.
- Costs can be hard to measure.
- Good managers have an accurate understanding of costs.
- Goods and services an organization produces are called *outputs*.
- Goods and services an organization uses in production are called *inputs*.
- *Incremental cost* equals the change in cost resulting from a change in output.
- *Average cost* equals the total cost of a process divided by the total output of a process.
- Large firms have a cost advantage if there are *economies of scale*.
- Multiproduct firms have a cost advantage if there are *economies of scope*.
- Higher quality should mean higher costs. If not, the organization is inefficient.
- Higher input prices mean higher costs.
- Costs depend on outputs, technology, input prices, and efficiency.
- *Opportunity cost* is the value of a resource in its best alternative use.
- *Sunk costs*, which are costs you cannot change, should be ignored.

5.1 Introduction

Efficient
Producing the most valuable output possible, given the inputs used (Viewed differently, an efficient organization uses the least expensive inputs possible, given the quality and quantity of output it produces.)

Output
Goods and services produced by an organization

Input
Goods and services used in production

Opportunity cost
The value of a resource in its next best use (The opportunity cost of a product consists of the other goods and services we cannot have because we have chosen to produce the product in question.)

Understanding and managing costs are core managerial tasks. Whatever the mission of the organization, cost control must be a priority. As evidence mounts that many healthcare firms are inefficient, cost control in the healthcare industry is becoming increasingly important. A firm is inefficient when its costs are higher than the quality of its service warrants, when the quality of a firm's products is lower than the cost of its service warrants, or when the quality of a firm's products is lower and its costs are higher than the quality and costs of comparable competitors.

An efficient producer of a good or service has a competitive advantage. For example, a pharmacy that can accurately dispense a product more cheaply than its competitors has an advantage. The **efficient** producer can win more contracts, enjoy higher profit margins, or more easily weather a slump. In healthcare, the bar has been raised as increased attention to the outcomes of care challenges us to think about health, not just medical care. Healthcare organizations are being challenged to work with customers to produce health efficiently, not just to produce goods and services efficiently.

Nonetheless, the pressure to become more efficient has grown considerably. As Chapter 6 details, public and private insurers have taken steps to steer patients to providers with lower costs. If your organization is a high-cost producer, there may not be much time to become more efficient.

This chapter focuses on what is necessary to turn an organization into an efficient producer. The starting point is to understand costs, which are defined by a combination of two definitions. First, the goods or services an organization uses in producing its **outputs** are called **inputs**. Second, **opportunity cost** equals the value of an input in its best alternative use. From this production-oriented perspective, costs equal the opportunity cost per unit of input multiplied by the volume of inputs the organization uses. Reducing the cost per unit that the organization pays for inputs reduces total costs, but real savings result from reducing the volume of inputs the organization uses. To reduce input volume, managers must lead efficiency improvement efforts or outsource the production of goods and services.

CASE 5.1   **Virginia Mason Medical Center**

In 2001, Virginia Mason Medical Center was under pressure to improve its financial performance. Its processes of care were overrun with waste and rework, increasing costs and putting patients at risk.

(continued)

CASE 5.1
(continued)
Virginia Mason used weeklong rapid process improvement workshops to examine processes, measure wasted resources, and identify activities that did not add value for customers. Workshop participants included leaders and frontline staff, supported by executive sponsors and performance improvement experts. After identifying areas for improvement, workshop participants discussed ways to standardize and optimize the work that would need to be done. Preliminary data collection (including observations of how care was delivered) started weeks before the workshops, and follow-up continued for months.

In 2005, an eight-person team (including a patient) participated in a workshop focused on a 27-bed telemetry unit that was experiencing numerous problems. Nurses were assigned patients with no consideration of how sick the patients were or where they were located, resulting in varied workloads and unnecessary travel between rooms. Supplies and equipment were not kept where they were needed. The work of nurses and technicians was poorly coordinated; some tasks were done twice, and some were not done at all. Communication was poor, patient status changes were missed too often, and nurses felt pressured to skip breaks and lunches. Furthermore, the unit's financial performance was unsatisfactory because it was consistently staffing over budget.

The workshop team made simple changes that dramatically streamlined care. First, they changed staff assignments so that nurses cared for patients in contiguous rooms, reducing travel by 85 percent. Second, they moved supplies to where they were needed and simplified ordering, reducing the time spent retrieving supplies by 85 percent. Third, they standardized and streamlined morning rounds, shortening them by 48 percent. As a result of these changes, costs and overtime hours dropped, patient falls and pressure ulcers decreased, patient satisfaction improved, and call light use fell (Nelson-Peterson and Leppa 2007).

Nonetheless, nurses' initial response to these changes was not positive. They wanted to focus on caring for patients rather than on improving financial performance. In addition, they were not happy with the standardization of their work and resisted some of the proposed changes. That resistance has largely faded. Now nurses spend almost 90 percent of their time on direct patient care, a major change from the less than 40 percent when the process started (Virginia Mason Institute 2012).

(continued)

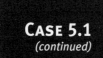

CASE 5.1
(continued)

Today other organizations can study at the Virginia Mason Institute, Virginia Mason's malpractice premiums have dropped by more than 50 percent, and Gary Kaplan, Virginia Mason's CEO, believes that its costs are much lower than those of comparable hospitals. Dr. Kaplan also argues that "there is still a lot of opportunity to get better" (Sloane 2012).

Discussion questions:
- Did standardizing care reduce quality? Did standardizing care reduce costs? What evidence supports your conclusions?
- How would reducing travel time between rooms reduce costs?
- Does including a patient in the rapid process improvement workshop make sense? Why?
- Was Virginia Mason efficient before it made these changes? Who is responsible for ensuring that care is efficient?
- Why did the nurses resist the changes? Would you expect to encounter resistance in other departments?

5.2 Cost Perspectives

Cost is a complex concept because it is difficult to measure and depends on the perspective of the beholder. For example, consumers will characterize the cost of a prescription in terms of their out-of-pocket spending and ancillary costs, such as the value of time spent filling a prescription. Pharmacists will focus on the spending required to obtain, store, and dispense the drug. Insurers will focus on their payments to the pharmacist for the prescription and their spending on claim management. Each of these perspectives on costs is valid. Exhibit 5.1 describes what costs look like from four perspectives.

A pharmacist acquires a prescription drug for $10 and incurs $5 in processing, storing, and billing costs. The pharmacist should recognize that reasonable returns on her time and on her investment in the pharmacy represent opportunity costs because both could be used in other ways.

The consumer is uninterested in the pharmacist's costs. What matters to him are his out-of-pocket costs and the $4 in travel expense he incurs when he drives to the pharmacy. When the consumer does not have insurance, as shown in the left half of Exhibit 5.1, the consumer's perspective on costs mirrors society's perspective. Both will say that the drug costs $20, although the two calculations are different. The consumer will focus on the price he pays and his travel costs. Society will ignore the price the consumer pays and focus on the underlying resource use by the pharmacist and the

EXHIBIT 5.1
Prescription Costs from Four Perspectives

	Without Insurance			With Insurance			
	Pharmacy	**Consumer**	**Society**	**Pharmacy**	**Consumer**	**Insurer**	**Society**
Wholesale price	$10	$0	$10	$10	$0	$0	$10
Travel	$0	$4	$4	$0	$4	$0	$4
Processing	$5	$0	$5	$5	$0	$9	$14
Return on assets	$1	$0	$1	$1	$0	$1	$2
Retail price	($16)	$16	$0	($16)	$5	$11	$0
Total	$0	$20	$20	$0	$9	$21	$30

consumer. The payment is an accounting entry, not a real use of resources (because it equals the amount the pharmacist receives).

The right side of Exhibit 5.1 lists cost perspectives when the prescription is covered by insurance. Three things change as a result of coverage. First, the additional perspective of the insurer must be considered. Second, the insurer incurs expense by processing the claim. Third, the consumer's perspective on costs differs from society's perspective.

The insurer focuses on its share of the retail price and its cost of paying the bill. Again, the insurer should factor in the opportunity cost of using its investment to provide pharmacy insurance benefits but will probably express this figure in terms of a required return on investment. From the perspective of the insurer, covering the prescription adds $21 in costs. From the perspective of the consumer, insurance coverage reduces costs by $11. Note also that society's perspective on costs differs from the perspective of any of the participants when insurance plays a role.

The concept of cost cannot be fully understood without stating a cost perspective. The part of cost that matters depends on your point of view. Your revenues are someone else's costs, and your costs are someone else's revenues.

Most people want to focus on costs from the perspective of the organization in which they work, but shifting costs to customers or suppliers seldom represents a good business strategy. Long-term business success rests on selling products that offer your customers excellent value and offer your suppliers adequate profits.

As stated earlier, the difficulty of measuring cost components also complicates the concept of costs. For example, opportunity costs are sometimes hard to measure. Managers sometimes become confused when calculating the opportunity cost of resources that have changed in value. For example, land that your organization bought a few years ago may be more valuable if rents in the area have risen or less valuable if rents have fallen. In most cases, though, an input's opportunity cost is simply its market price.

Linking the use of a resource to the organization's output also poses problems. A focus on incremental costs (i.e., the cost of the additional resources you use when you increase output by a small amount) often simplifies this task. "How much more of a hospital's information system does its intensive care unit use when it cares for an additional patient?" is an example of a way to reframe the relationship between resource use and output and facilitate its measurement.

5.3 Vocabulary

Average cost
Total cost divided by total output

Marginal or incremental cost
The cost of producing an additional unit of output

Fixed costs
Costs that do not vary according to output

Variable costs
Costs that change as output changes

To talk sensibly about costs, we need a clear vocabulary. At the core of that vocabulary are the concepts of average cost and incremental cost. **Average cost** equals the total cost of a process divided by the total output of a process. In Exhibit 5.2, when total cost equals $10,500 and output equals 300, average cost equals $35. **Incremental cost**, also called **marginal cost**, equals the change in a process's total cost that is associated with a change in the process's total output. In Exhibit 5.2, total cost rises from $8,000 to $10,500 as output rises from 200 to 300, so incremental cost equals ($10,500 – $8,000) ÷ (300 – 200), or $25 per unit of output.

In Exhibit 5.2, average cost is significantly larger than incremental cost. This difference is common because many processes require resources (such as equipment or key personnel) that do not change as output varies. For example, to open a pharmacy, a pharmacist has to rent a building and commit her own time. If sales fall short of expectations, the rent will not change. Rent is an example of a **fixed cost**, a component of total cost. In contrast, some labor costs and the cost of restocking the pharmacy will vary with sales. Average cost includes fixed and **variable costs**, but incremental cost includes only variable costs. The fact that average cost often exceeds

EXHIBIT 5.2
Total, Average, and Incremental Costs

Output	Total Cost	Average Cost	Incremental Cost
0	$3,000		
100	$5,500	$55	$25
200	$8,000	$40	$25
300	$10,500	$10,500/300 = $35	$2,500/100 = $25

incremental cost is important because management decisions often hinge on knowing how much increasing or decreasing production of a good or service will cost. Your willingness to negotiate with an insurer that offers $300 per service is likely to depend on whether you believe an additional service will cost you $440 (the average cost) or $120 (the incremental cost).

Average and incremental cost are both important concepts, although economists emphasize incremental values. Most management decisions concern incremental changes. Should we increase hours in the pediatric clinic? Should we reduce evening pharmacy staff? Should we accept patients needing skilled nursing care? These decisions demand data on incremental costs.

In addition to being the most relevant concept for managers, incremental cost is easier to calculate than average cost. Average cost calculations always involve difficult questions (e.g., How much of the cost incurred by the chief financial officer should we allocate to the pediatrics department?). In contrast, incremental cost calculations involve more straightforward questions and can be performed by most clinicians and frontline managers (e.g., What additional resources will we need to keep the pediatric clinic open until 8 p.m. on Wednesdays, and what are the opportunity costs of those resources?). To decide whether to start or stop a service, a manager needs to compare average revenue and average cost. For example, a telemedicine program that has average revenue of $84 and average cost of $98 is unprofitable. To decide whether to expand or contract a service, a manager needs to compare how revenue and costs will change. To make this comparison, information about incremental costs is essential. Usually confusion about cost arises because one person is talking about average cost and another is talking about incremental cost (or because one person is talking about costs to society and the other is talking about costs to the organization).

5.4 Factors That Influence Costs

Producer costs depend on what is produced (the outputs), the prices of inputs, how outputs are produced (the technology), and how efficiently inputs are used. We will explore each of these factors.

5.4.1 Outputs

Differences in outputs can profoundly affect costs. Firms that produce large volumes of a good or service may have lower costs than firms that produce small volumes. Large firms that have a cost advantage have **economies of scale**. Firms that produce several different kinds of goods or services may have lower costs than firms that produce just one. Multiproduct firms that have a cost advantage have **economies of scope**. Economies of scale and scope result from sharing resources.

Economies of scale
When larger organizations have lower average costs

Economies of scope
When multiproduct organizations have lower average costs

An example of economies of scale might be a large pharmacy's use of automated dispensing equipment. In a larger pharmacy the fixed costs of the equipment could be shared by a larger number of prescriptions, so the cost per prescription could be lower. An example of economies of scope might be a nursing home that expands to offer skilled care as well as intermediate care. Fixed costs (such as the cost of the director of nursing) would be shared by additional patients, so average costs for intermediate care could be lower.

Differences in the quality of outputs can affect costs as well. For an efficient firm, higher-quality products cost more. For an inefficient firm, higher-quality products may not.

What is higher quality? Economists define *quality* from the perspective of consumers, not from the clinical perspective common in healthcare. In economics, a good or service is of higher quality when it is more valuable to a well-informed customer than comparable goods or services. Consumers usually find greater value in goods or services that produce better clinical outcomes. Economists also define quality in terms of nonclinical factors. Well-informed consumers may attribute higher quality to a product that is easier to use, a service for which the wait is shorter, an insurance plan with less confusing referral requirements, a provider who bills more accurately, or a more cordial staff.

If higher quality does not cost more, failure to provide it demonstrates inefficiency. The many opportunities available to improve quality in healthcare without increasing costs reflect how inefficient most healthcare organizations are. Once an organization has become efficient, though, higher quality (better service, improved reliability, greater accuracy, less pain, and other enhancements) will cost more to produce.

CASE 5.2   Improving Performance

Atul Gawande is an employee of an academic, non-profit health system called Partners HealthCare, which owns a number of hospitals and is associated with dozens of practices in Massachusetts. As Dr. Gawande sees it, in today's environment Partners has very clear incentives: "This year, my employer's new contracts with Medicare, BlueCross BlueShield, and others link financial reward to clinical performance. The more the hospital exceeds its cost-reduction and quality-improvement targets, the more money it can keep" (Gawande 2012). In short, Partners is taking part in multiple accountable care organizations.

(continued)

CASE 5.2
(continued)

When Dr. Gawande's mother needed a knee replacement, he steered her to a team at the Brigham and Women's Hospital, his own hospital. He knew that this team (which included surgeons, anesthesiologists, physical therapists, and nurses) had worked together for several years to choose one best way of doing knee replacements. They looked at the medical literature and at what the best orthopedic teams were doing, and then made multiple changes in the whole knee replacement process. They changed how anesthesia and postoperative care were given, which reduced costs and got patients up and around faster. They also settled on a few standard prostheses, which reduced inventory costs and reduced prosthesis costs (by choosing cost-effective models and improving the hospital's bargaining position).

In addition to reducing costs, this redesign has led to vastly better outcomes. Patients leave the hospital sooner, with more mobility and less pain.

Discussion questions:
- Could limiting the number of prostheses improve the quality of care?
- Why was a team needed to choose the best way of doing knee replacements?
- Is standardization like this common? Should it be?
- Some of your staff object to standardizing care, calling it "cookbook nursing." How do you respond?
- What would happen to your organization if insurers started steering patients to the most efficient providers and you were not one of them?
- Was Brigham and Women's Hospital efficient before it made the changes described in this case?

5.4.2 Input Costs

Higher input prices mean higher costs. Shifting to a different combination of inputs will only partially offset the effects of higher input prices. The only times this rule does not hold are when a firm is inefficient or when a perfect, lower-priced substitute for the higher-priced input is available. An inefficient firm might be able to limit the effects of a cost increase by shifting to a more efficient production process. For example, even if the wages of pharmacy technicians increase, the cost of dispensing a prescription might not increase if the pharmacy switches to the automated system it should have been using before the wage increase. A firm also can avoid higher costs by switching to a perfect substitute. For example, if an Internet access provider tried to raise its monthly rates, firms could switch to rival Internet access providers and costs would not go up. Unfortunately, firms are unlikely to find such a replacement.

5.4.3 Technology

Advances in technology always reduce the cost of an activity. Adopting a new technology would be pointless if it increased the costs of a process. For example, installing an automated laboratory system would be absurd if it increased cost per analysis. An automated laboratory system that reduces cost per analysis, however, does not guarantee that laboratory costs will go down. Lower costs per analysis may prompt physicians to request more analyses, and the greater volume cancels the cost savings and might even drive up costs.

5.4.4 Efficiency

Increases in efficiency always reduce the cost of an activity. Production of almost every healthcare good or service can be made more efficient. Few production processes in healthcare have been examined carefully, and most healthcare workers have little or no training in process improvement. Consequently, mistakes, delays, coordination failures, unwise input choices, and excess capacity are routine. Techniques for improving production (total quality management, continuous quality improvement, and continuous process improvement) are just beginning to be applied in healthcare.

Even though greater efficiency reduces costs, not everyone is in favor of it. Greater efficiency often means that fewer workers will be needed. Workers whose jobs are in jeopardy may not want to help improve efficiency. (Commitment to a policy of no layoffs is usually one of the core terms of efficiency improvements.) Others have limited incentive to participate in efforts to improve efficiency. Physicians must help change clinical processes, yet many physicians have little to gain from these efforts. The gains produced by the changes will accrue to the healthcare organization, but the resulting billing reductions will be problematic for physicians and other healthcare workers not employed by the organization. A major challenge lies in devising incentives that will encourage workers and contractors to help improve efficiency.

5.5 Variable and Fixed Costs

Managing costs requires an understanding of opportunity costs and triggers that change costs. As stated earlier, opportunity costs usually are easy to assess. The opportunity cost of using $220 in supplies is $220. The opportunity cost of using an hour of legal time billed at $150 per hour is $150. Other cases demand more study. For example, the opportunity cost of a vacant wing of a hospital depends on its future use. If the wing will be reopened for acute care in response to a rising hospital census, the opportunity cost of the wing will depend on its value as an acute care unit. If the wing will be reopened because the hospital needs a skilled nursing unit, the opportunity cost of the wing will be determined by its value in that role.

Sunk costs should be ignored. A **sunk cost** is a cost you cannot change. A computer's purchase price is a sunk cost, as is money spent to train employees to operate the computer. If your current needs do not require the use of a computer, you should not fret about its initial cost. The opportunity cost of the computer will depend on its value in some other use (including its resale value).

Sunk costs
Costs that have been incurred and cannot be recouped

In the long run, all costs are variable. Buildings and equipment can be changed or built. The way work is done can be changed. Additional personnel can be hired. The entire organization could shut down, and its assets could be sold.

In the short run, some costs are fixed. An existing lease may not be negotiable, even if the building or equipment no longer suits your needs. Ignore fixed costs in the short run. They are sunk costs.

When fixed costs are substantial, average costs typically fall as output increases because the fixed costs are spread over a growing volume of output. As long as average variable costs are stable, this drop in average fixed costs will cause a reduction in average total costs. *Average total costs* equal average fixed costs plus average variable costs. As Exhibit 5.3 illustrates, average fixed cost drops from $30 to $15 as output rises from 100 to 200. If variable costs rise quickly enough, average total costs may rise despite the fall in average fixed costs. In Exhibit 5.3, variable costs rise by $10,000 as output increases from 200 to 300. As a result, average total cost rises to $60 even though average fixed cost continues to fall.

EXHIBIT 5.3
Fixed and Variable Costs

Output	Total Cost	Fixed Cost	Average Total Cost	Average Fixed Cost	Average Variable Cost
0	$3,000	$3,000			
100	$5,500	$3,000	$55	$30	$25
200	$8,000	$3,000	$40	$15	$25
300	$18,000	$3,000	$18,000/300 = $60	$3,000/300 = $10	$15,000/300 = $50

Fixed and variable costs are important concepts for day-to-day management of healthcare organizations. For example, an advantage of growth is that fixed costs can be spread over a larger volume of output. The idea is that lower average fixed costs result in lower average total costs, so profit margins can be larger. As Exhibit 5.3 illustrates, growth should not result in increases in average variable costs large enough to offset any reduction in average fixed costs. Otherwise, growth will be unprofitable.

Misclassification of costs can result in odd incentives. For example, fixed overhead costs are often allocated on the basis of some measure of output, which can make growth appear less profitable than it is because the overhead costs allocated to a unit increase as it grows. So that unit managers are not discouraged from expanding, allocated fixed costs should not vary with output.

CASE 5.3   The Costs of Nonurgent Care in the Emergency Department

"Obviously," said Kelly, director of patient accounts, "it costs more to see a patient in the emergency department than in a physician's office. We've got to channel these folks back to their primary care physicians. Plus, I'm sure they are money losers for us."

Cameron, director of emergency services, replied, "Actually, it's more complicated than that. Most patients seen in our emergency department have insurance, and it is not clear whether we are making money on them. There have been a couple of careful studies of costs in emergency departments, but they reach different conclusions. A study by Williams in 1996 concluded that the incremental cost of a patient visit for routine ambulatory care was not high and that these patients were quite profitable for hospitals. A subsequent study, by Bamezai and Melnick in 2006, found much higher costs. Emergency departments produce such a range of services, and there is so much overhead to allocate, that figuring out how much it costs to care for a child with an earache at 2 a.m. is a nightmare. We'd be happy to do a detailed cost analysis of the emergency department, but we have had other priorities up to now."

At that point, Morgan, chief executive, chimed in, "Let's think strategically here. First, I'll bet a month's pay that we could reduce costs in the emergency department and improve the experience of our patients, critically ill or not. Doing so will increase profits, whatever

(continued)

CASE 5.3
(continued)

our costs are. Second, our emergency department is overcrowded. We need to develop the capacity to see patients who are not critically ill more efficiently. Most of these patients do not need the sort of sophisticated care that our emergency department provides, and our emergency department was on diversion for eight days last month. That is not acceptable. In addition, we have made a commitment to have all of our primary care practices be recognized as patient-centered medical homes. To make that happen we need to create expanded after-hours options for patients. Cameron, I want you and Kelly to develop a menu of options for our next meeting."

Discussion questions:
- Why do patients who are not critically ill go to emergency departments?
- Why do the variety of services emergency departments produce and the amount of overhead to be allocated make cost finding difficult?
- Why was Morgan confident that costs could be reduced while quality could be improved? Is this conclusion supported in the literature?
- Thinking as a consumer, what would constitute higher quality in the emergency department?
- What options should the hospital consider? Why would you be confident that these options would incur lower costs than an emergency department? Do you think quality would be higher?
- If the hospital creates one or more urgent care clinics and adds evening and weekend hours to its primary care clinics, what will happen to emergency department volumes? What effect will that have on emergency department costs?

5.6 Conclusion

Cost management has become vital in healthcare. A more efficient producer always has an advantage. The increasingly competitive environment is forcing healthcare organizations to reduce costs and reassess product lines. More and more, healthcare organizations are seeking the cheapest production techniques and identifying core goods and services. This pressure has intensified as purchasers of goods and services have realized that high costs do not guarantee high quality and that high quality does not necessarily equate to high cost. Healthcare organizations are beginning to adopt cost-reducing technology, substitute low-cost production techniques for high-cost ones, purchase goods and services more conservatively, and rethink what they produce. Healthcare providers are also being challenged to improve the health of target populations in ways that are cost-effective—a task that is more difficult than the efficient production of healthcare products.

Exercises

5.1 Why is it important to distinguish between fixed and variable costs?

5.2 Explain how a decrease in input prices or an increase in efficiency would affect costs.

5.3 You spent $500,000 on staff training last year. Why should this cost be treated as a sunk cost? Why should this cost be ignored in making a decision whether to switch coding software?

5.4 Your president bought two acres of land for $200,000 ten years ago. Although it is zoned for commercial use, it currently holds eight small, single-family houses. A property management firm that wants to continue leasing the eight houses has offered you $400,000 for the property. A developer wants to build a 12-story apartment building on the site and has offered $600,000. What value should you assign to the property?

5.5 A community health center has assembled the following data on cost and volume. Calculate its average and marginal costs for volumes ranging from 25 to 40. What patterns do you see?

Visits	Total Cost
20	$2,200
25	$2,250
30	$2,300
35	$2,350
40	$2,400

5.6 Sweetwater Nursing Home has 150 beds. Its cost and volume data are as follows. Calculate its average and marginal costs for volumes ranging from 100 to 140. What patterns do you see?

Residents	Costs
80	$10,000
100	$11,000
120	$12,000
140	$13,200

5.7 It takes a phlebotomist 15 minutes to complete a blood draw. The supplies for each draw cost $4, and the phlebotomist earns $20 per hour. The phlebotomy lab is designed to accommodate 20,000 draws per year. Its rent is $80,000 per year. What are the average and incremental costs of a blood draw when the volume is 20,000? 10,000? What principle does your calculation illustrate?

5.8 How would the average and marginal costs change if the phlebotomist's wage rose to $24 per hour? What principle does your calculation illustrate?

5.9 A new computer lets a phlebotomist complete a blood draw in 10 minutes. The supplies for each draw cost $4, and the phlebotomist earns $20 per hour. The phlebotomy lab is designed to accommodate 20,000 draws per year. Its rent is $80,000 per year. What is the marginal cost of a blood draw? What principle does your calculation illustrate?

5.10 Use the data in Exercise 5.7. How would the average and marginal costs change if the rent rose to $100,000? What principle does your calculation illustrate?

5.11 A patient visits a clinic. She incurs $10 in travel costs and has a copayment of $20. The clinic's total charge is $60. The clinic spends $9 to bill the insurance company for the visit and uses resources worth $51 to produce the visit. The insurance company pays the clinic $40 and spends $11 to process the claim. Describe the cost of the visit from the perspective of the patient, the clinic, the insurer, and society.

5.12 A practice uses $40 worth of a dentist's time, $30 worth of a hygienist's time, $10 worth of supplies, and $15 worth of a billing clerk's time to produce a visit. The practice charges a patient $25 and charges her insurer $70. The insurer spends an additional $4 to process the claim. The patient incurs travel costs of $20. What are the costs of the visit from the perspective of society, the patient, the practice, and the insurer?

5.13   Kim and Pat underwrite insurance. Each underwrites 50 accounts per month. Each account takes four hours to underwrite. The value of their time is $40 per hour. Monthly costs for each are $1,500 for an office, $2,000 for a receptionist, and $2,400 for a secretary. Calculate the average and incremental cost per case for Kim and Pat.

5.14   If Kim and Pat merge their operations, they would need only one receptionist, and their rent for the joint office would be $2,800 per month. All other values stay the same. Calculate the average and incremental cost per case for the merged office. Are there economies of scale at 100 accounts per month? Should Kim and Pat merge their offices?

References

Bamezai, A., and G. Melnick. 2006. "Marginal Cost of Emergency Department Outpatient Visits: An Update Using California Data." *Medical Care* 44 (9): 835–41.

Gawande, A. 2012. "Big Med." *The New Yorker*. Published August 13. www.newyorker.com/reporting/2012/08/13/120813fa_fact_gawande.

Nelson-Peterson, D. L., and C. J. Leppa. 2007. "Creating an Environment for Caring Using Lean Principles of the Virginia Mason Production System." *Journal of Nursing Administration* 37 (6): 287–94.

Sloane, T. 2012. "The Learning Lab for Health Care Transformation." *Partners* September/October: 22–29.

Virginia Mason Institute. 2012. "Case Study: Adding Valuable Nursing Time at the Bedside." Accessed July 2, 2014. www.virginiamasoninstitute.org/workfiles/Virginia-Mason-Institute-Case-Study-Adding-Valuable-Nursing-Time-at-Bedside.pdf.

Williams, R. M. 1996. "The Costs of Visits to Emergency Departments." *New England Journal of Medicine* 334 (10): 642–46.

6

BENDING THE COST CURVE

Learning Objectives

After reading this chapter, students will be able to

- explain what the Triple Aim is,
- discuss several strategies for realizing the Triple Aim,
- describe several strategies for reducing services per patient, and
- identify several ways to reduce cost per service.

Key Concepts

- The Triple Aim includes improving the experience of care for patients, improving population health, and reducing healthcare costs per person.
- The Affordable Care Act (ACA) has changed incentives for insurers and providers in a number of ways.
- The ACA has already increased hospitals' incentives to reduce readmissions.
- Medicare Advantage HMOs are growing.
- Multiple trials of Medicare accountable care organizations (contracts with potential gains for providers if cost and quality goals are met) are underway.
- Private insurers are also testing accountable care organizations and simpler variants called *narrow networks*.
- The prices that private insurers pay for similar products vary a great deal.
- Private insurers are testing ways of steering patients to less expensive providers.
- Multiple trials of bundled payments (fixed payments for an episode of care) are underway.
- Multiple trials of medical homes are underway.
- A number of states are shifting Medicaid beneficiaries to HMOs.
- Some states have expanded Medicaid; some have not.

- Some evidence indicates that the ACA's initiatives have had positive effects.
- The full effects of the ACA's initiatives will not be known for years.

6.1 The Triple Aim

Berwick, Nolan, and Whittington (2008) argued that the United States should try to reach three aims simultaneously:

- improving the experience of care,
- improving population health, and
- reducing healthcare costs per person.

This chapter explores strategies for reducing costs while improving population health and customer satisfaction. Berwick, Nolan, and Whittington (2008, 768) noted that "the remaining barriers to integrated care are not technical; they are political."

In making this argument, Berwick, Nolan, and Whittington (2008) offered the example of congestive heart failure. Congestive heart failure is the most common reason that Medicare patients are hospitalized, and more than 25 percent are readmitted within 30 days of discharge (Ryan et al. 2013). Many of these readmissions can be prevented, and a number of interventions have succeeded in doing so (Takeda et al. 2012). These interventions typically involved enhancing the instruction about managing heart failure provided to patients and families during the hospitalization, scheduling a follow-up visit before discharge, and calling recently discharged patients to check on their health. An ongoing barrier to these steps was that hospitals had limited incentives to try to reduce readmission. Preventing readmissions took resources and reduced hospital profits.

The Affordable Care Act (ACA) changed hospitals' incentives. It reduced Medicare payments to hospitals with higher-than-expected 30-day readmission rates. Hospitals could avoid significant revenue losses by increasing their cost per heart failure admission only a little (and possibly generating additional profits from follow-up visits). In contrast, from a payer perspective, reducing readmissions has always been a clear win. Reducing readmissions improves population health and can save significant amounts of money. Medicare savings of $8.2 billion by 2020 are anticipated as a result of reductions in readmissions (Laderman, Loehrer, and McCarthy 2013).

As we will see in this chapter, the ACA has changed incentives for insurers and providers. Although focused on expanding health insurance coverage, the ACA has helped spark innovation in the federal, state, local, and private sectors. We will also examine the major uncertainties that exist in the varied political, regulatory, and market environments that define American healthcare about how to realize the Triple Aim. The barriers are not only political.

6.2 Reducing Costs

Cost per person depends on services per person and the price of each of those services, so there are two ways of reducing costs. One is to reduce service use. The other way is to reduce the price per service. Both ways require changes in behavior, and these changes in behavior require changes in incentives. As we will see in this chapter, new insurance models are being tested publicly and privately.

The Medicare Physician Group Practice Demonstration

In this demonstration, which compared outcomes for millions of Medicare beneficiaries, physician groups shared in any savings that they realized if they met quality targets (Colla et al. 2012). This demonstration was, in short, a test of the effects of an **accountable care organization** (ACO), which is one of the initiatives funded by the ACA. An ACO gives providers incentives to improve quality and reduce cost per patient, making the arrangement more like an HMO than a fee-for-service (FFS) organization.

> **Accountable care organization**
> A provider organization that contracts to be paid based on the cost and quality metrics of a patient population

About 15 percent of the demonstration's patients were eligible for both Medicare and Medicaid. Because these patients are poor and elderly or disabled, their spending was much higher than average.

Per capita savings in the demonstration group averaged just $114, but this figure may understate the potential of ACOs. First, savings among patients who were eligible for both Medicare and Medicaid averaged $532, hinting that improving the care of these patients might have a substantial payoff. Second, savings varied considerably among the group practices. Two large, well-established clinics began with lower-than-average costs and also realized greater-than-average savings. Both clinics had offered HMOs for many years, suggesting that experience in controlling costs might be important.

Savings were not linked with lower quality of care. Quality was generally better in the demonstration group, which had higher quality scores and lower readmission and emergency department use rates.

The traditional strategy for changing incentives has long focused on HMOs. In these integrated delivery models, the health plan is paid a fixed amount per member per month (perhaps with **risk adjustment**) and physicians are usually salaried. As a result, neither the organization nor the physician gains from higher use of services. In addition, HMOs increasingly exclude high-cost providers from their networks, which can result in significant savings. For example, the Massachusetts health insurer Harvard Pilgrim launched a new health plan that costs about 10 percent less than its standard plan, largely because its smaller network excludes some providers with high prices (Weisman 2012).

HMOs have elicited three main concerns. One is that HMOs will stint on needed care. A second is that HMOs will have lower costs because they can enroll low-risk customers, not because they deliver care more efficiently. A third is that Americans do not want to accept any limits on their choices and will simply reject HMOs.

HMO advocates point out that the available evidence points to **overuse of care** in FFS settings more than to underuse in HMO settings. Robust (but limited) evidence indicates that Americans in FFS settings get care that provides little value to them (Korenstein et al. 2012). For example, in a large sample of Medicare patients, 24 percent of those with normal colonoscopy results had early repeat exams with no evidence that the colonoscopy was anything but routine (Goodwin et al. 2011). Why the early colonoscopies were done is not known, but the authors of the study suspected that high colonoscopy profit margins play a role. Although FFS physicians are constrained by professional ethics, they have significant financial incentives to provide lots of care.

HMO physicians face different incentives. Most are salaried and have weak incentives to skimp on care. These weak incentives may be offset by professional ethics. The HMO itself has incentives to limit care, although this fact may be balanced by the need to keep and attract customers.

HMO patients clearly use less care than comparable FFS patients. Landon and colleagues (2012) found that utilization rates were generally lower in Medicare Advantage HMOs than in traditional Medicare. Although outpatient visit rates were virtually equal, emergency department use was a third lower in HMOs, ambulatory surgeries were 7 percent lower, hospital days were 8 percent lower, and knee replacements were also 8 percent lower. Another study (Ayanian et al. 2013) found that Medicare HMOs generally did a better job of providing recommended preventive services, such as appropriate cholesterol testing or flu vaccinations. Given ongoing concerns about overuse of emergency departments and underuse of preventive services, these differences could be viewed as evidence of better care in HMOs.

Favorable risk selection is a major concern related to HMOs. For a number of reasons, HMOs tend to attract patients who are much better risks than FFS plans do. (One reason is that healthy patients are less likely to have to end a relationship with a physician when they join an HMO.) An example of favorable risk selection is that Medicare Advantage plans have generally been able to enroll healthier beneficiaries, meaning that their costs would be lower whether or not they delivered care more efficiently. To address this imbalance, Medicare improved its risk adjustment formula and reduced options to switch plans. Newhouse and colleagues (2012) concluded that by 2008 these changes had markedly reduced differences in predicted spending and mortality. Because the ACA's insurance exchanges use similar approaches, problems with risk selection should be smaller.

The easiest of these concerns to address is acceptability. Enrollment in Medicare Advantage HMOs, which is completely voluntary, rose from 5.6 million in 2007 to 9.3 million in 2013 (Gold et al. 2013). At least some Americans are willing to choose HMOs. The "rejection" of HMOs around the turn of the twenty-first century largely came from employees who had no choice other than an HMO. As of 2013, more than 70 million Americans were enrolled in HMOs (Kaiser Family Foundation 2013), with significant growth taking place among Medicaid and Medicare enrollees. Even though the remainder of this chapter emphasizes new approaches to realizing the Triple Aim, HMOs remain a relevant strategy.

Transforming Primary Care: Geisinger's Medical Home

Geisinger Health System is an integrated, physician-led system that serves more than 2.6 million residents of Pennsylvania. In 2006 Geisinger launched a new program called ProvenCare. It stresses evidence-based medicine, bundled prices for some procedures (such as open-heart surgery), and enhanced patient engagement. ProvenHealth Navigator, Geisinger's version of a **medical home**, was launched at the same time. ProvenCare and ProvenHealth Navigator are integral parts of Geisinger's Medicare Advantage HMO (Steele 2010).

Geisinger's Medicare Advantage HMO is different from many Medicare Advantage HMOs because it is integrated with the health system and because Geisinger has years of experience in running an HMO. Begun in 1972 as a pilot program for Geisinger Medical Center employees and residents of five nearby counties, Geisinger Health Plan received state approval to operate an HMO in 1985 and approval to offer Medicare Advantage plans in 1994 (Geisinger Gold 2014).

(continued)

Medical home
A primary care model, often called a *patient-centered medical home*, that emphasizes being patient centered, comprehensive, team based, coordinated, accessible, and committed to quality and safety (A medical home devotes resources to coordinating care, improving communication, and making care available after office hours.)

(continued)

A team of researchers used the gradual rollout of ProvenHealth Navigator to examine whether it reduced costs (Maeng, Graham, et al. 2012). It did. Costs were 4.3 percent lower for patients in Proven-Health Navigator clinics. Even better, for patients receiving care from ProvenHealth Navigator clinics for more than two years, costs were 6.7 percent lower. Given that patients in ProvenHealth Navigator clinics also reported higher patient satisfaction and better clinical outcomes (Maeng, Graf, et al. 2012), these data suggest that Geisinger is close to realizing the Triple Aim.

Will medical homes work better or worse in other settings? Can medical homes be effective as independent clinics, or do they need to be part of an HMO or ACO? Stay tuned.

Bundled payment
A single payment, also called a *bundled episode payment*, that covers all services delivered during a given episode of care (Examples of an episode of care include hip replacement, a year of diabetes care, or pregnancy.)

Narrow network
A limited group of providers who have contracted with an insurance company (Patients will usually pay more if they get care from a provider not in the network. The network is usually restricted to providers with good quality who will accept low payments.)

Reference pricing
A system in which an insurer's allowed fee has an upper limit (A customer who chooses a provider with a price above the limit will pay the difference between the limit and the price.)

6.3 Innovations to Reduce the Cost of Care

How the ACA will affect the cost of care is not easy to understand. The ACA supports a broad array of initiatives, and it is not clear how well they will work. Will **bundled payments**, ACOs, medical homes, expanded insurance coverage, incentives to reduce readmissions, or reduced Medicare payments have an impact on costs? Will the ACA's changes in insurance markets have indirect effects on costs? Will state expansions of Medicaid managed care reduce costs? Will private-sector efforts to rein in costs, which include bundled payments, high-deductible plans, ACOs, **narrow networks**, medical homes, and **reference pricing**, be effective? Will healthcare organizations that offer better quality and lower costs continue to capture market share? The questions are many, and the evidence is varied and preliminary.

The sheer number and variety of efforts to bend the cost curve are hard to grasp. In addition, because of the diversity and novelty of these efforts, interpreting successes and failures is difficult. Might a minor design change turn a seeming failure into a success? Can a successful pilot be repeated elsewhere, or were the unique attributes of the patients and the providers involved responsible for the results? To offer a sense of the many cost control efforts and settings that are in play, this section looks at public and private efforts in three states: New Jersey, Missouri, and California.

6.3.1 Innovations to Reduce the Cost of Care: New Jersey

New Jersey is a high-cost state, so the fact that multiple efforts are underway is not surprising. Average spending per capita is $7,583, which is 11 percent above the national average, and the uninsured comprise 16 percent of the population, very close to the national average (Kaiser Family Foundation 2013). Twenty-two percent of the population is enrolled in an HMO, which is near the national average. As of 2013, control of the state government was split. The governor was a Republican, but both houses of the legislature had comfortable Democratic majorities (StateScape 2014).

In 2009, a handful of New Jersey hospitals joined a New Jersey Hospital Association **gainsharing** pilot program, made possible by the Medicare Modernization Act of 2003. Gainsharing means that physicians can earn bonuses if they work with a hospital to reduce the cost of caring for Medicare patients. (Examples include bonuses for physicians who agree to use the same hip prosthesis, who agree to a common time for rounds, or who adopt a standard protocol.) An earlier attempt ended before it really got started, but the 2009 program was widely believed to be successful. Participating hospitals reduced their costs of treating Medicare patients, primarily by reducing length of stay. The best evidence of the gainsharing pilot's perceived success is that it grew to 33 hospitals statewide in 2013 (Davis 2013).

> **Gainsharing**
> A strategy for rewarding those who contribute to an organization's success

Termed a form of bundled payment by Medicare, this expanded demonstration continues to emphasize gainsharing. The hospital gets a discounted payment for its services and benefits financially if it can deliver these services for less than the discounted payment. Gainsharing continues to be allowed, but Medicare will pay physicians separately.

Twenty-four New Jersey healthcare organizations will be taking part in three other bundled payment demonstrations. Twelve hospitals are testing a bundle that combines physicians' services, acute inpatient services, and all related post-acute services. (Post-acute services include care in skilled nursing facilities, inpatient rehabilitation facilities, long-term care hospitals, and home health agencies. They also include readmissions and some outpatient services.) Ten organizations (a mix of home health and skilled nursing companies) are testing a bundle that covers post-acute services, and two hospitals are testing a single prospective payment for all services during a hospitalization episode (Centers for Medicare & Medicaid Services 2014a). Only three of these New Jersey organizations are proceeding without support from a company such as Remedy Partners, which is essentially a bundled payment consulting firm (Centers for Medicare & Medicaid Services 2014b).

In addition, multiple changes are taking place in New Jersey Medicaid. New Jersey is participating in Medicaid expansion under the ACA, meaning that an additional 265,000 people will have coverage. All of those who enroll will be in managed care plans, including those eligible for Medicare and Medicaid, those receiving behavioral health services, those with developmental disabilities, and those eligible for long-term care services (National Senior Citizens Law Center 2013). In addition, New Jersey Medicaid will begin testing ACOs, will limit benefits for those newly eligible, and will change how it pays many providers. One of those changes is a requirement that all Medicaid managed care plans include patient-centered medical homes in their networks. (This chapter uses the more generic term *medical home*.)

A number of New Jersey Federally Qualified Health Centers are participating in the Advanced Primary Care Practice demonstration. This demonstration is designed to test if the medical home model can help realize the Triple Aim in these centers. In addition, the Comprehensive Primary Care Initiative, a medical home demonstration, covers the entire state of New Jersey. The demonstration allocates risk-adjusted care coordination funds to physician practices (NJBIZ 2013). An otherwise typical project of the Centers for Medicare & Medicaid Services, the Comprehensive Primary Care Initiative differs in that five major private insurers are participating. Because more insurers are participating, more practices can participate at lower cost. Improved care, better clinical outcomes, and lower costs have been shown in a number of trials (though not all), so these trials would seem to indicate projects with potential (Arend et al. 2012).

In New Jersey, as in most states, multiple ACOs have been launched in recent years. Many existing ACOs focus on the Medicare population, but private insurers are increasingly creating these arrangements (McCann 2013). The Centers for Medicare & Medicaid Services has already announced that beneficiaries in its Pioneer ACO program had better care, lower costs, and higher satisfaction than beneficiaries in its FFS programs (Centers for Medicare & Medicaid Services 2013).

Insurers are also moving aggressively toward narrow networks that exclude providers with high prices. For example, Aetna offered only narrow-network products on the exchanges in New Jersey (McQueen 2013). The assumption is that customers who buy insurance on an exchange will be price sensitive, so lower prices will be essential.

In addition, eight hospitals and health centers are taking part in the Strong Start for Mothers and Newborns initiative. Funded by the ACA, this initiative seeks to reduce the number of elective preterm deliveries as one of its goals.

In short, many innovations are being tried in New Jersey. These innovations are supported by the federal government, the state government, private insurers, provider organizations, and healthcare organizations.

6.3.2 Innovations to Reduce the Cost of Care: Missouri

Missouri is not a high-cost state, but multiple efforts are underway nonetheless. Average spending per capita is $6,967, which is 2 percent above the national average, and the uninsured comprise 14 percent of the population, slightly less than the national average (Kaiser Family Foundation 2013). Thirteen percent of the population is enrolled in an HMO, which is well below the national average.

As of 2013, control of the state government was split. The governor was a Democrat, but both houses of the legislature had large Republican majorities (StateScape 2014). The governor urged that Missouri take part in Medicaid expansion, but the legislature rejected the expansion, declined to set up a state health insurance exchange, restricted the activity of helping with ACA enrollment, and decided not to enforce the new ACA insurance regulations (Somashekhar 2013).

Given the political resistance to the ACA in Missouri, one might not anticipate that the state is home to a number of ACOs, but it is. Mercy Hospital Springfield and Mercy Clinic Springfield (Mercy Clinic was a participant in the Medicare Physician Group Practice Demonstration) have been recognized by the Centers for Medicare & Medicaid Services as an ACO. BJC HealthCare of Saint Louis, Mosaic Life Care of Saint Joseph, and the Kansas City Metropolitan Physicians Association have also been recognized (Centers for Medicare & Medicaid Services 2014b). In addition, several insurers have launched narrow-network plans, which resemble an ACO in several important ways. The insurer chooses a small number of hospitals and physicians who have demonstrated high quality (usually based on adherence to standards of care) with low costs and then markets the plan as an inexpensive alternative. For example, a series of plans from Coventry essentially limits patients to hospitals and physicians who are part of the Mercy Health System in the Saint Louis area (Doyle 2013). Insurers and healthcare organizations increasingly see ACOs and narrow networks as potentially advantageous business models (Pfannenstiel 2013a).

Narrow networks are likely to be especially attractive in Missouri because prices that insurers and patients pay vary so widely. For example, in 2011 in Kansas City the average private price for an inpatient stay was about double the Medicare price, but some hospitals were paid 50 percent more (White, Bond, and Reschovsky 2013). Hospital outpatient prices were even higher. In Kansas City and Saint Louis the average hospital outpatient price was nearly triple the Medicare price, and some hospitals were able to negotiate much higher prices. As a result, a number of insurers are experimenting with offering narrow networks on exchanges and to employers.

In 2007 the Missouri legislature passed the Missouri Health Improvement Act, which required that Missouri Medicaid provide all beneficiaries with a healthcare home (which was not defined by the law) (National Academy for State Health Policy 2014). In 2011 the Centers for Medicare & Medicaid Services approved two separate medical home programs for Missouri. One was for patients served by community mental health centers, and the other focused on patients served by Federally Qualified Health Centers, Rural Health Clinics, and hospital-based primary care clinics. As a result, more than 50 organizations (which sponsor more than 100 clinics) across the state are taking part in Medicaid-supported medical home demonstrations (Centers for Medicare & Medicaid Services 2014b).

In addition, medical home projects have been launched for patients with other insurance plans. For example, in 2009 Blue Cross and Blue Shield of Kansas City began a test of paying practices to become medical homes. Finding that hospital admissions and readmissions dropped for patients in medical homes, the insurer sharply expanded the program (Pfannenstiel 2013b). From this insurer's perspective, paying a primary care practice to coordinate and manage care is a good investment. The scientific evidence regarding medical homes shows a mix of favorable, unfavorable, and inconclusive results (Peikes et al. 2012), so the value of medical homes remains uncertain.

Eight Missouri hospitals are taking part in Medicare's bundled payment demonstration. Most are taking part in the trial that pays the hospital for all inpatient and post-acute care, but three are participating in the version in which the hospital is paid prospectively for all of the services provided (including physicians' services) during a hospital episode (Centers for Medicare & Medicaid Services 2014b). A small-scale precursor to the demonstration found that participating hospitals generally reduced costs and improved quality, primarily by standardizing how they provided some cardiac and orthopedic services (Herman 2012). Because of these results, private employers and insurers are also experimenting with bundled payments. In Missouri, Anthem Blue Cross and Blue Shield is conducting a trial of bundled payments for orthopedic services, and Wal-Mart Stores offers its employees and their families free heart and spine surgeries, while paying Mercy Hospital Springfield using a bundled payment system (Herman 2013).

Two other ACA programs are underway in Missouri. The Kansas City Quality Improvement Consortium, which operates in five Kansas and Missouri counties in the metropolitan area, is taking part in the Community-Based Care Transitions Program. This program seeks to improve transitions between settings, to improve quality of care, to reduce readmissions for high-risk beneficiaries, and to reduce Medicare spending. Two other organizations are participating in the Strong Start for Mothers and Newborns initiative, which was described in Section 6.3.1.

Even though significant political opposition to the ACA is present in Missouri, multiple innovations that are designed to bend the cost curve are being tested there. These changes are supported by the federal government, the state government, private insurers, and healthcare organizations. Although ACA innovations command the most attention, private insurers are actively exploring bundled payments, medical homes, ACOs, narrow networks, clinical feedback to providers, enhanced price transparency for consumers, and value-based insurance (Johnson 2013). Private insurers started some of these innovations before the passage of the ACA, but the pace of change certainly seems to have speeded up.

6.3.3 Innovations to Reduce the Cost of Care: California

California is a low-cost state, but multiple efforts are underway nonetheless. Average spending per capita is $6,238, which is 9 percent below the national average, and the uninsured comprise 26 percent of the population, well above the national average (Kaiser Family Foundation 2013). Forty-two percent of the population is enrolled in an HMO, which is well above the national average. As of 2013 control of the state government was solidly Democratic. The governor was a Democrat, and both houses of the legislature had comfortable Democratic majorities (StateScape 2014).

In California the ACA is likely to mean that more than 3 million residents will gain health insurance (Long and Gruber 2011). The state has agreed to expand Medicaid, which is expected to increase eligibility by 1.4 million. In addition, about 2.5 million Californians are already eligible for Medicaid but not enrolled. To increase coverage, California has already taken steps to simplify Medicaid eligibility determinations and enrollment. These steps include using a standardized application, using electronic federal and state data sources, and allowing applications in person, by mail, online, or by phone. Beginning in January 2014, Covered California (the California health benefit exchange) further simplified and expanded enrollment (Lucia et al. 2013). Bending the cost curve is a high priority in California, and expanding coverage is seen as an essential part of that effort. California's Medicaid program is also in the process of shifting most enrollees (including children, rural residents, and those also eligible for Medicare) to managed care.

Both the federal government and commercial insurers are funding medical home projects in California. Seventy Federally Qualified Health Centers are participating in the Advanced Primary Care Practice demonstration in California. In addition, Blue Shield of California has developed a narrow network that includes a medical home for patients with chronic conditions (such as cancer, heart failure, or diabetes). This combination is one tier of a product called Blue Groove being offered to large employers in Sacramento and Modesto (Burns 2012). Healthcare organizations in California are setting up medical homes as well. Just in the Bay Area, John Muir Health, Stanford HealthCare Alliance, and Sutter Health launched programs in 2012 (Kleffman 2012).

California has eleven ACOs in place. Six of these were part of the Medicare Pioneer ACO demonstration (although two withdrew in July 2013) (Gamble and Punke 2013). Most of the organizations have both Medicare and commercial ACO contracts. Most of the organizations sponsoring ACOs have participated in California's many HMOs, so profitably providing care to ACO members should not seem new.

Twenty-eight California hospitals are taking part in Medicare's bundled payment demonstration. Eight hospitals (covering 118 types of episodes) are taking part in the trial that pays the hospital for all inpatient and post-acute care. A provider of post-acute services is participating in the version of the trial that just covers post-acute services. Eighteen hospitals (covering 136 episodes of care) are testing prospective payment for all of the services provided (including physicians' services) during a hospital episode (Centers for Medicare & Medicaid Services 2014b). Participation in the prospective payment trial is different than in other states. California hospitals are testing many more episodes of care than New Jersey or Missouri hospitals, only one hospital is relying on an external consultant, and Tenet Healthcare Corporation (a large for-profit system) is sponsoring six hospitals.

A number of private bundled payment trials are also underway. Hoag Orthopedic Institute of Irvine has contracts with Kroger that cover orthopedic and spine surgery and contracts with Aetna, Cigna, and Blue Shield of California that cover orthopedics (Herman 2013). Alta Bates Summit Medical Center (a Sutter Health affiliate) has contracts with Aetna and Blue Shield for total hip and knee replacements (Stansbury and Lally 2013). A challenge is that bundled payment is an alternative to capitation, and many California providers are already capitated.

California is engaged in two other major initiatives. Nearly 400 California hospitals are taking part in the Partnership for Patients program. Its goal is to reduce hospital-acquired conditions and readmissions. In addition, the American Association of Birth Centers is testing birth centers in four locations. This trial is a part of the Strong Start for Mothers and Newborns initiative discussed previously.

In California just about everything is being tried to bend the cost curve. Not surprisingly, given insurers' and providers' extensive experience with managed care, more is being done in California than elsewhere.

Steering Patients to Less Expensive Providers

Medicare and Medicaid payments are set administratively and vary only modestly within markets. With commercial insurance, in contrast, prices may be very different for seemingly comparable services. Health systems that have large market shares or excellent reputations may be able to negotiate much higher prices than competitors. In Los Angeles, for example, commercial insurers paid some hospitals less than Medicare did, while other hospitals received more than 400 percent of the Medicare payment (Ginsburg 2010). Commercial insurers have difficulty selling plans that exclude high-priced hospitals, and these "must-have" hospitals often insist on contracts that include all of their

(continued)

(continued)

services in the insurer's network. This requirement limits insurers' cost reduction strategies.

Plan sponsors, in contrast, need have no such ambivalence, and some have begun to try to steer patients to less expensive providers. One strategy, known as *reference pricing*, caps the amount the employer will pay for a service and requires patients to pay the difference between the reference price and the allowed charge (the price negotiated with a provider). For example, suppose an employer sets the reference price for hip replacement at $30,000. An employee who goes to a hospital with an allowed charge of $32,000 will pay $2,000 out of pocket, but an employee who goes to a hospital with an allowed charge of $42,000 will pay $12,000 out of pocket. The goal is to encourage employees to use the lower-priced provider and, just possibly, to encourage the higher-priced provider to negotiate a better deal with the plan.

In January 2011 the California Public Employees' Retirement System implemented reference pricing for hip and knee replacement surgery (Robinson and Brown 2013). Before reference pricing, 52 percent of the system's procedures were in higher-priced hospitals. Within a year this share fell to 37 percent. In addition, the average price decreased by 26 percent, primarily because higher-priced facilities negotiated lower prices. This pilot study has occasioned interest within the healthcare industry.

Reference pricing could be applied more broadly. For example, the average price of a colonoscopy in the United States is $1,185, but according to the International Federation of Health Plans (2013) a quarter of providers charge $536 or less. What would happen in this market with a reference price of $500?

Some have suggested taking this idea a step further. Although a good way to detect colon cancer, colonoscopies are expensive and not very pleasant. An annual fecal immunochemical test (with a colonoscopy if abnormal results are found) can be as effective as a colonoscopy for population colon cancer screening but costs less than $25 (Flitcroft et al. 2012). What would happen in the market for colonoscopies with a reference price of $25?

6.4 Conclusion

The ACA appears to have changed the political and economic landscape. For the most part, it has done so by speeding up trials of ideas that existed before its passage. Bundled payments, medical homes, ACOs, and HMOs are not new ideas, but by supporting pilot studies of these ideas, the ACA has encouraged an explosion of these prototypes.

The innovations that seem new—narrow networks and reference pricing—have largely come out of the private sector. Both reflect old ideas, though, because insurers and plan sponsors have noted that they pay different amounts for products that seem similar. What is new is that insurers are increasingly willing to take steps to avoid high-cost providers, and some providers are willing and able to use this opportunity to capture market share. Nonetheless, the ACA appears to have had an effect on the private sector as well. By creating large markets of cost-conscious consumers, the ACA seems to have altered the strategies of insurers and some providers.

The effects of expanding insurance coverage on costs will take years to understand, but another feature of the ACA already seems to have shown positive results. The ACA incorporated incentives for hospitals to reduce readmissions (which went into effect on October 1, 2012), and readmissions for 2012 decreased (Gerhardt et al. 2013). Cost per beneficiary rose by just 0.3 percent in the first year of Medicare's Pioneer ACO, and costs for similar beneficiaries in traditional Medicare grew by only 0.8 percent (Centers for Medicare & Medicaid Services 2013). For all of these beneficiaries, reductions in hospital admissions and readmissions helped keep costs rising more slowly than general inflation.

Even more striking, Cigna, Aetna, and other insurers have publicly announced that they plan to start hundreds more ACOs during the next several years (Hastings 2013). And this statement says nothing about the hundreds of other innovations likely to be launched.

These innovations are a long way from becoming established tools for federal, state, and private policymakers. Some will work. Some will not. Early results suggest that ACOs are realizing some savings and that reductions in spending for targeted groups also reduce costs for other patients served by the same providers (McWilliams, Landon, and Chernew 2013). All of these indications seem likely to mean that healthcare managers will live in interesting times.

Exercises

6.1 An insurance market consists of high-risk patients, who average $40,000 in spending per year, and low-risk patients, who average $1,000 per year. Overall, low-risk patients represent 90 percent of the population. What would average spending be for a population like this?

6.2 Refer to Exercise 6.1. What would average spending be if low-risk patients were 92 percent of the population?

6.3 Refer to Exercise 6.1. If an insurer sold 100,000 policies at $6,000, what would revenue be? What would medical costs be if the insurer paid for everything and low-risk patients were 90 percent of the population? How would that change if low-risk patients were 92 percent of the population?

6.4 Why did hospitals have limited incentives to reduce readmissions prior to the ACA?

6.5 Refer to the box titled "Steering Patients to Less Expensive Providers" in this chapter. What would happen in the market for colonoscopies with a reference price of $500? What would happen in the market for colonoscopies with a reference price of $25?

6.6 Go to the CMS Innovation Center website (http://innovation.cms.gov) and see what ideas are being tested in a state of your choice.

6.7 Why would a system like John Muir Health launch a medical home that is intended to reduce its revenues?

6.8 How are a narrow network and an ACO different?

6.9 What recent evidence about the performance of ACOs can you find? Are they growing? Are they saving money? Do enrollees seem to like the care they get? Is the quality of care good?

6.10 What recent evidence about the performance of medical homes can you find? Are they growing? Are they saving money? Do enrollees seem to like the care they get? Is the quality of care good?

6.11 What recent evidence about bundled payment programs can you find? Are they growing? Are they saving money? Do enrollees seem to like the care they get? Is the quality of care good?

6.12 What recent evidence about Medicare Advantage HMOs can you find? Are they growing? Are they saving money? Do enrollees seem to like the care they get? Is the quality of care good?

6.13 How much did cost per Medicare beneficiary go up last year? (The Kaiser Family Foundation publishes these data on its website [http://kff.org/state-category/medicare/]).

6.14 Why would a health system want to participate in a trial of bundled payments?

6.15 What risk does a health system bear when it agrees to a bundled payment?

6.16 What risk does a health system bear when it agrees to accept capitation?

References

Arend, J., J. Tsang-Quinn, C. Levine, and D. Thomas. 2012. "The Patient-Centered Medical Home: History, Components, and Review of the Evidence." *Mount Sinai Journal of Medicine* 79 (4): 433–50.

Ayanian, J. Z., B. E. Landon, A. M. Zaslavsky, R. C. Saunders, L. G. Pawlson, and J. P. Newhouse. 2013. "Medicare Beneficiaries More Likely to Receive Appropriate Ambulatory Services in HMOs Than in Traditional Medicare." *Health Affairs* 32 (7): 1228–35.

Berwick, D. M., T. W. Nolan, and J. Whittington. 2008. "The Triple Aim: Care, Health, and Cost." *Health Affairs* 27 (3): 759–69.

Burns, J. 2012. "Narrow Networks Found to Yield Substantial Savings." *Managed Care*. Published February. www.managedcaremag.com/archives/1202/1202.narrow_networks.html.

Centers for Medicare & Medicaid Services. 2014a. "Bundled Payments for Care Improvement (BPCI) Initiative: General Information." Accessed April 23. http://innovation.cms.gov/initiatives/bundled-payments/.

———. 2014b. "Where Innovation Is Happening." Accessed April 7. http://innovation.cms.gov/initiatives/map/index.html#state=MO&model=federally-qualified-health-center-fqhc-advanced-primary-care-practice-demonstration.

———. 2013. "Pioneer Accountable Care Organizations Succeed in Improving Care, Lowering Costs." Accessed July 2, 2014. www.cms.gov/Newsroom/Media ReleaseDatabase/Press-Releases/2013-Press-Releases-Items/2013-07-16.html.

Colla, C. H., D. E. Wennberg, E. Meara, J. S. Skinner, D. Gottlieb, V. A. Lewis, C. M. Snyder, and E. S. Fisher. 2012. "Spending Differences Associated with the Medicare Physician Group Practice Demonstration." *Journal of the American Medical Association* 308 (10): 1015–23.

Davis, M. 2013. "New Program Has Mercer County Hospitals Sharing Fees with Doctors to Contain Costs." *NJ.com*. Published February 7. www.nj.com/mercer/index.ssf/2013/02/new_program_has_mercer_county.html.

Doyle, J. 2013. "Health Insurers Face an Uncertain Future." *St. Louis Post-Dispatch*. Published November 17. www.stltoday.com/business/local/health-insurers-face-an-uncertain-future/article_3850851f-bc7e-5689-b91b-b106011e3de1.html.

Flitcroft, K. L., L. M. Irwig, S. M. Carter, G. P. Salkeld, and J. A. Gillespie. 2012. "Colorectal Cancer Screening: Why Immunochemical Fecal Occult Blood Tests May Be the Best Option." *BMC Gastroenterology* 12: 183.

Gamble, M., and H. Punke. 2013. "100 Accountable Care Organizations to Know." *Becker's Hospital Review*. Published August 14. www.beckershospitalreview.com/lists/100-accountable-care-organizations-to-know.html.

Geisinger Gold. 2014. "Geisinger Gold History." www.thehealthplan.com/ Meridian/Content_With_Template/Gold/Why_Gesinger_Gold/ Geisinger_Gold_History/.

Gerhardt, G., A. Yemane, P. Hickman, A. Oelschlaeger, E. Rollins, and N. Brennan. 2013. "Medicare Readmission Rates Showed Meaningful Decline in 2012." *Medicare & Medicaid Research Review* 3 (2): E1–E12.

Ginsburg, P. B. 2010. *Wide Variation in Hospital and Physician Payment Rates Evidence of Provider Market Power.* Center for Studying Health System Change Research Brief No. 16. Published November. www.hschange.com/ CONTENT/1162/.

Gold, M., G. Jacobson, A. Damico, and T. Neuman. 2013. *Medicare Advantage 2013 Spotlight: Enrollment Market Update.* Kaiser Family Foundation Issue Brief. Published June. http://kaiserfamilyfoundation.files.wordpress. com/2013/06/8448.pdf.

Goodwin, J. S., A. Singh, N. Reddy, T. S. Riall, and Y. F. Kuo. 2011. "Overuse of Screening Colonoscopy in the Medicare Population." *Archives of Internal Medicine* 171 (15): 1335–43.

Hastings, D. 2013. "Pioneer ACOs Year One: On the Path to a Learning Health Care System." *Health Affairs Blog,* July 17. http://healthaffairs.org/ blog/2013/07/17/pioneer-acos-year-one-on-the-path-to-a-learning-health-care-system/.

Herman, B. 2013. "Which Providers and Employers Have Commercial Bundled Payments?" *Becker's Hospital Review.* Published March 8. www.beckershospital review.com/racs-/-icd-9-/-icd-10/which-providers-and-employers-have-commercial-bundled-payments.html.

———. 2012. "2 Major Lessons from CMS' Bundled Payment ACE Demonstration." *Becker's Hospital Review.* Published April 3. www.beckershospitalreview. com/hospital-physician-relationships/2-major-lessons-from-cms-bundled-payment-ace-demonstration.html.

International Federation of Health Plans. 2013. *2012 Comparative Price Report.* Accessed July 2, 2014. www.ifhp.com.

Johnson, K. 2013. Personal communication with author, September 18.

Kaiser Family Foundation. 2013. "State Health Facts." Accessed July 2, 2014. http://kff.org/statedata/.

Kleffman, S. 2012. "High-Cost Patients Across the Bay Area Get Closer Care to Keep Them Out of Hospitals." *Contra Costa Times.* Published March 5. www. contracostatimes.com/ci_20104187.

Korenstein, D., R. Falk, E. A. Howell, T. Bishop, and S. Keyhani. 2012. "Overuse of Health Care Services in the United States: An Understudied Problem." *Archives of Internal Medicine* 172 (2): 171–78.

Laderman, M., S. Loehrer, and D. McCarthy. 2013. "The Effect of Medicare Readmissions Penalties on Hospitals' Efforts to Reduce Readmissions: Perspectives from the Field." *The Commonwealth Fund Blog*, February 26. www.common wealthfund.org/Blog/2013/Feb/The-Effect-of-Medicare-Readmissions-Penalties-on-Hospitals.aspx#citation.

Landon, B. E., A. M. Zaslavsky, R. C. Saunders, L. G. Pawlson, J. P. Newhouse, and J. Z. Ayanian. 2012. "Analysis of Medicare Advantage HMOs Compared with Traditional Medicare Shows Lower Use of Many Services During 2003–09." *Health Affairs* 31 (12): 2609–17.

Long, P., and J. Gruber. 2011. "Projecting the Impact of the Affordable Care Act on California." *Health Affairs* 30 (1): 63–70.

Lucia, L., K. Jacobs, G. Watson, M. Dietz, and D. H. Roby. 2013. *Medi-Cal Expansion Under the Affordable Care Act: Significant Increase in Coverage with Minimal Cost to the State*. Los Angeles, CA: UC Berkeley Center for Labor Research and Education.

Maeng, D. D., T. R. Graf, D. E. Davis, J. Tomcavage, and F. J. Bloom Jr. 2012. "Can a Patient-Centered Medical Home Lead to Better Patient Outcomes? The Quality Implications of Geisinger's ProvenHealth Navigator." *American Journal of Medical Quality* 27 (3): 210–16.

Maeng, D. D., J. Graham, T. R. Graf, J. N. Liberman, N. B. Dermes, J. Tomcavage, D. E. Davis, F. J. Bloom, and G. D. Steele Jr. 2012. "Reducing Long-Term Cost by Transforming Primary Care: Evidence from Geisinger's Medical Home Model." *American Journal of Managed Care* 18 (3): 149–55.

McCann, E. 2013. "New Jersey Health System Builds Big ACO." *Healthcare Finance News*. Published August 9. www.healthcarefinancenews.com/news/new-jersey-health-system-builds-big-aco.

McQueen, M. P. 2013. "Less Choice, Lower Premiums: Many Exchange Plans Will Offer Narrow Networks." *ModernHealthcare.com*. Published August 17. www.modernhealthcare.com/article/20130817/MAGAZINE/308179921.

McWilliams, J., B. E. Landon, and M. E. Chernew. 2013. "Changes in Health Care Spending and Quality for Medicare Beneficiaries Associated with a Commercial ACO Contract." *Journal of the American Medical Association* 310 (8): 829–36.

National Academy for State Health Policy. 2014. "Missouri." Accessed April 24. http://nashp.org/med-home-states/missouri.

National Senior Citizens Law Center. 2013. *Medicaid Managed Long-Term Services and Supports: A Review and Analysis of Recent CMS Waiver Approvals in New Jersey and New York*. Published March. www.nsclc.org/wp-content/uploads/2013/03/MLTSS-NY-NJ-Final-030113.pdf.

Newhouse, J. P., M. Price, J. Huang, J. M. McWilliams, and J. Hsu. 2012. "Steps to Reduce Favorable Risk Selection in Medicare Advantage Largely Succeeded, Boding Well for Health Insurance Exchanges." *Health Affairs* 31 (12): 2618–28.

NJBIZ. 2013. "N.J. Primary Care Practices Strive to Improve Quality, Lower Cost of Care." *NJBIZ*. Published January 14. www.njbiz.com/article/20130114/NJBIZ01/130119965/NJ-primary-care-practices-strive-to-improve-quality-lower-cost-of-care.

Peikes, D., A. Zutshi, J. L. Genevro, M. L. Parchman, and D. S. Meyers. 2012. "Early Evaluations of the Medical Home: Building on a Promising Start." *American Journal of Managed Care* 18 (2): 105–16.

Pfannenstiel, B. 2013a. "Accountable Care Organizations: Can This Payment Model Help Save Kansas City's Independent Physician Practices?" *Kansas City Business Journal*. Published June 12. www.bizjournals.com/kansascity/news/2013/06/12/accountable-care-organizations-can.html.

———. 2013b. "Patient-Centered Medical Homes: Can Changing How Doctors Get Paid Mean Better Care?" *Kansas City Business Journal*. Published May 29. www.bizjournals.com/kansascity/news/2013/05/29/patient-centered-medical-homes-can.html?page=all.

Robinson, J. C., and T. T. Brown. 2013. "Increases in Consumer Cost Sharing Redirect Patient Volumes and Reduce Hospital Prices for Orthopedic Surgery." *Health Affairs* 32 (8): 1392–97.

Ryan, J., R. Andrews, M. B. Barry, S. Kang, A. Iskander, P. Mehla, and R. Ganeshan. 2013. "Preventability of 30-Day Readmissions for Heart Failure Patients Before and After a Quality Improvement Initiative." *American Journal of Medical Quality*. Published online August 16. doi:10.1177/1062860613496135.

Somashekhar, S. 2013. "States Find New Ways to Resist Health Law." *Washington Post*. Published August 28. www.washingtonpost.com/national/health-science/states-find-new-ways-to-resist-health-law/2013/08/28/c63f8498-0a93-11e3-8974-f97ab3b3c677_story.html.

Stansbury, J., and S. Lally. 2013. "AHRQ Bundled Episode Payment and Gainsharing Demonstration: Overview." Integrated Healthcare Association. Published June. www.iha.org/pdfs_documents/AHRQ_BPDemonstration_Overview_June2013.pdf.

StateScape. 2014. "Legislative Control 2014." Accessed July 2. www.statescape.com/resources/partysplits/partysplits.aspx.

Steele, G. 2010. "Geisinger Chief Glenn Steele: Seizing Health Reform's Potential to Build a Superior System. Interview by Susan Dentzer." *Health Affairs* 29 (6): 1200–1207.

Takeda, A., S. J. Taylor, R. S. Taylor, F. Khan, H. Krum, and M. Underwood. 2012. "Clinical Service Organisation for Heart Failure." *Cochrane Database of Systematic Reviews* 9: CD002752. doi:10.1002/14651858.CD002752.pub3.

Weisman, R. 2012. "Harvard Pilgrim Set to Launch a Lower Cost Network." *Boston Globe*. Published March 18. www.bostonglobe.com/business/2012/03/17/insurer-set-launch-lower-cost-network/DebRXmeoDz0HyCVIzjkB6I/story.html.

White, C., A. M. Bond, and J. D. Reschovsky. 2013. *High and Varying Prices for Privately Insured Patients Underscore Hospital Market Power*. Center for Studying Health System Change Research Brief No. 27. Published September. www.hschange.org/CONTENT/1375/.

THE DEMAND FOR HEALTHCARE PRODUCTS

Learning Objectives

After reading this chapter, students will be able to

- calculate sales and revenue using simple models,
- discuss the importance of demand in management decision making,
- articulate why consumer demand is an important topic in healthcare,
- apply demand theory to anticipate the effects of a policy change,
- use standard terminology to describe the demand for healthcare products, and
- discuss the factors that influence demand.

Key Concepts

- The *quantity demanded* is the amount of a good or service purchased at a specific price when all other factors are held constant.
- When a product's price rises, the quantity demanded usually falls.
- *Demand* (a demand curve) describes the amounts of a good or service that will be purchased at different prices when all other factors are held constant.
- An *increase or decrease in demand* reflects a shift in the entire list of amounts purchased at different prices. An increase or a decrease in demand results when another factor that influences consumer decisions changes.
- Other factors that influence demand for healthcare products include consumer income, insurance coverage, perceptions of health status, perceptions of the productivity of goods and services, prices of other goods and services, and tastes.
- The amount of money a consumer pays for a good or service is called the *out-of-pocket price* of that good or service.
- Because of insurance, the total price and the out-of-pocket price can differ quite a bit.

- A *complement* is a good or service that is used in conjunction with another good or service. Demand for a good falls if the price of a complement increases.
- A *substitute* is a good or service used instead of another good or service. Demand for a good rises if a substitute increases in price.

7.1 Introduction

Demand
The amounts of a good or service that will be purchased at different prices when all other factors are held constant

Demand is one of the central ideas of economics. It underpins many of the contributions of economics to public and private decision making. Analyses of demand tell us that human wants are seldom absolute. More often they are conditioned by questions: "Is it really worth it?" "Is its value greater than its cost?" These questions are central to understanding healthcare economics.

Demand forecasts are essential to management. Most managerial decisions are based on revenue projections. Revenue projections in turn depend on estimates of sales volume, given prices that managers set. A volume estimate is an application of demand theory. An understanding of the relationship between price and quantity must be part of every manager's tool kit. On an even more fundamental level, demand forecasts help managers decide whether to produce a certain product at all and how much to charge. Suppose you conclude that the direct costs of providing therapeutic massage are $48 and that you will need to charge at least $75 to cover other costs and offer an attractive profit margin. Will you have enough customers to make this service a sensible addition to your product line? Demand analyses are designed to answer such questions.

7.1.1 Rationing

On an abstract level, we need to ration goods and services (including medical goods and services) somehow. Human wants are infinite, or nearly so. Our capacity to satisfy those wants is finite. We must develop a system for determining which wants will be satisfied and which will not. **Market systems** use prices to ration goods and services. A price system costs relatively little to operate, is usually self-correcting (e.g., prices fall when the quantity supplied exceeds the **quantity demanded**, which tends to restore balance), and allows individuals with different wants to make different choices. These advantages are important. The problem is that markets work by limiting the choices of some consumers. As a result, even if the market *process* is fair, the market *outcome* may seem unfair. Wealthy societies typically view exclusion of some consumers from valuable medical services, perhaps because of low income or perhaps because of previous catastrophic medical expenses, as unacceptable.

Market system
A system that uses prices to ration goods and services

Quantity demanded
The amount of a good or service that will be purchased at a specific price when all other factors are held constant

The implications of demand are not limited to market-oriented systems. Demand theory predicts that if care is not rationed by price, it will be rationed by other means, such as waiting times, which are often inconvenient for consumers. In addition, careful analyses of consumer use of services have convinced most analysts that medical goods and services should not be free. If care were truly costless for consumers, they would use it until it offered them no additional value. Today this understanding is reflected in the public and private insurance plans of most nations.

Value-Based Insurance

Consumers buy more when prices drop. Insurance plans have long used this principle to keep spending down. Unfortunately, consumers are as likely to reduce use of highly effective products as they are to reduce use of fairly ineffective products. This result is even more apt to be true if the benefits of a service are subtle or accrue over time. For example, taking a drug called a *statin* can lower your cholesterol and may reduce plaque in arteries, which can lower the risk of heart attack. However, you do not feel any better if you take a statin, and you do not feel any worse if you stop. Adherence, which involves getting people to fill their prescriptions for statins and take their medicine, is not easy. From an insurance perspective, however, improving adherence can reduce the odds of a very expensive heart attack.

Value-based insurance sharply reduces the prices that consumers pay for effective treatments, hoping to improve adherence. At Pitney Bowes, statin adherence for a group of high-risk employees had steadily declined to about 71 percent. To try to increase adherence, Pitney Bowes reduced copayments from more than $24 per month to less than $1 (Choudhry et al. 2010). It worked.

This study and others suggest that insurers can use copayments to steer consumers to high-value services. It seems fairly clear that doing so can improve health outcomes. It is less clear whether value-based insurance can reduce spending.

Care cannot really be free. Someone must pay, somehow. Modern healthcare requires the services of highly skilled professionals, complex and elaborate equipment, and specialized supplies. Even the resources for which there is no charge represent a cost to someone.

7.1.2 Indirect Payments and Insurance

Because the burden of healthcare costs falls primarily on an unfortunate few, health insurance is common. Insurance creates another use for demand analyses. To design sensible insurance plans, we need to understand the public's valuation of services. Insurance plans seek to identify benefits the public is willing

Out-of-pocket price
The amount of money a consumer pays for a good or service

to pay for. The public may pay directly (through the **out-of-pocket price**) or indirectly. Indirect payments can take the form of health insurance premiums, taxes, wage reductions, or higher prices for other products. Understanding the public's valuation is especially important in the healthcare sector because indirect payments are so common. When consumers pay directly, valuation is not very important (except for making revenue forecasts). Right or wrong, a consumer who refuses to buy a $7.50 bottle of aspirin from an airport vendor because it is "too expensive" is making a clear statement about value. In contrast, a Medicare patient who thinks coronary artery bypass graft surgery is a good buy at a cost of $1,000 is not providing us with useful information. The surgery costs more than $30,000, but the patient and taxpayers pay most of the bill indirectly. Because consumers purchase so much medical care indirectly, with the assistance of public or private insurance, assessing whether the values of goods and services are as large as their costs is often difficult.

7.2 Why Demand for Healthcare Is Complex

The demand for medical care is more complex than the demand for many other goods for four reasons.

1. The price of care often depends on insurance coverage. Insurance has powerful effects on demand and makes analysis more complex.
2. Healthcare decisions are typically quite perplexing. Consumers would prefer to be healthy and use no medical services. Medical services have value largely because of their impact on health. The links between medical care and health outcomes are often difficult to ascertain at the population level (where the average impact of care is what matters) and stunningly complex at the individual level (where what happens to oneself is what matters). Forced to make hard choices, consumers may make bad choices.
3. This complexity contributes to consumers' poor information about costs and benefits of care. Such "rational ignorance" is natural. Because most consumers will not have to make most healthcare choices, it makes no sense for them to be prepared to do so.
4. The net effect of complexity and consumer ignorance is that producers have significant influence on demand. Consumers naturally turn to healthcare professionals for advice. Unfortunately, because they are human, professionals' choices are likely to reflect their values and incentives as well as those of their patients.

Demand is complicated by itself. To keep things simple, we will first examine the demand for medical goods and services in cases where insurance and the guidance of healthcare professionals play no role. The demand for over-the-counter pharmaceuticals, such as aspirin, is an example. We will then add insurance to the mix but keep professional advice out. The demand for dental prophylaxis will be the example in this case. Finally, we will add the role of professional advice.

7.3 Demand Without Insurance and Healthcare Professionals

In principle, a consumer's decision to buy a particular good or service reflects a maddening array of considerations. For example, a consumer with a headache who is considering buying a bottle of aspirin must compare its benefits, as he or she perceives them, to those of the other available choices. Those choices might include taking a nap, going for a walk, taking another nonprescription analgesic, and consulting a physician.

Economic models of demand radically simplify descriptions of consumer choices by stressing three key relationships that affect the amounts purchased:

1. The impact of changes in the price of a product
2. The impact of changes in the prices of related products
3. The impact of changes in consumer incomes

Demand curve
A graphic depiction of how much consumers are willing to buy at different prices

This simplification is valuable to firms and policymakers, who cannot change much besides prices and incomes. This focus can be misleading, however, if it obscures the potential impact of public information campaigns (including advertising).

7.3.1 Changes in Price

The fundamental prediction of demand theory is that the quantity demanded will decrease when the price of a good or service rises. The quantity demanded may decrease because some consumers buy smaller amounts of a product (as might be the case with analgesics) or because a smaller proportion of the population chooses to buy a product (as might be the case with dental prophylaxis). Exhibit 7.1 illustrates this sort of relationship. On **demand curve** D_1 a price reduction from P_1 to P_2 increases the quantity demanded from Q_1 to Q_2.

Exhibit 7.1 also illustrates a **demand shift** (or shift in demand). At each price, demand curve D_2 indicates a lower quantity demanded than demand curve D_1. (Alternatively, at each volume, willingness to pay will be smaller with D_2.) This shift might be due to a drop in income, a drop in the price of a **substitute**, an increase in the price of a **complement**, a change in demographics or consumer information, or other factors.

Demand shift
A shift that occurs when a factor other than the price of the product itself (e.g., consumer incomes) changes

Substitute
A product used instead of another product

Complement
A product used in conjunction with another product

EXHIBIT 7.1
Linear Demand

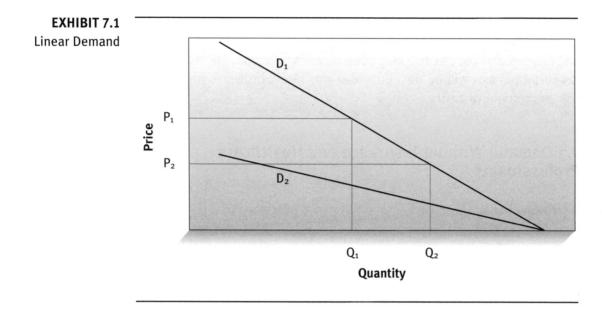

Demand curves can also be interpreted to mean that prices will have to be cut to increase the sales volume. Consumers who are not willing to pay what the product now costs may enter the market at a lower price, or current consumers may use more of the product at a lower price. Demand curves are important economic tools. Analysts use statistical techniques to estimate how much the quantity demanded will change if the price of the product, income, or other factors change.

Like Exhibit 7.1, Exhibit 7.2 illustrates a shift in demand. In Exhibit 7.2, however, the demand curves are not straight lines.

EXHIBIT 7.2
Nonlinear
Demand

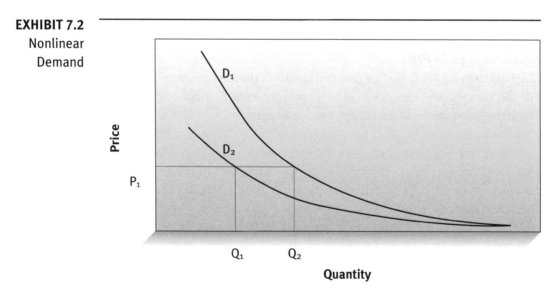

Substitution explains why demand curves generally slope down, that is, why consumption of a product usually falls if its price rises. Substitutes exist for most goods and services. When the price of a product is higher than that of its substitute, more people choose the substitute. Substitutes for aspirin include taking a nap, going for a walk, taking another nonprescription analgesic, and consulting a physician. If close substitutes are available, changes in a product's price could lead to large changes in consumption. If none of the alternatives are close substitutes, changes in a product's price will lead to smaller changes in consumption. Taking another nonprescription analgesic is a close substitute for taking aspirin, so we would anticipate that consumers would be sensitive to changes in the price of aspirin.

Substitution is not the only result of a change in price. When the price of a good or service falls, the consumer has more money to spend on all goods and services. Most of the time this income effect reinforces the substitution effect, so we can predict with confidence that a price reduction will cause consumers to buy more of that good. In a few cases, things get murkier. A rise in the wage rate, for example, increases the income you would forgo by reducing your work week. At first blush, you might expect that a higher wage rate would reduce your demand for time off. At the same time, though, a higher wage rate increases your income, which may mean more money for travel and leisure activities, increasing the amount of time you want off. In these cases empirical work is necessary to predict the impact of a change in prices.

Two points about price sensitivity need to be made here. First, a general perception that use of most goods and services will fall if prices rise is a useful notion to keep tucked away. Second, managers need more precise guidance. How much will sales increase if I reduce prices by 10 percent? Will my total revenue rise or fall as a result? To answer these questions takes empirical analysis. Fleshing out general notions about price sensitivity with estimates is one of the tasks of economic analysis. We also need an agreed-upon terminology to talk about how much the quantity demanded will change in response to a change in income, the price of the product, or the prices of other products. Economists describe these relationships in terms of elasticities, which we will talk more about later.

7.3.2 Factors Other Than Price

Changes in factors other than the price of a product shift the entire demand curve. Changes in beliefs about the productivity of a good or service, preferences, the prices of related goods and services, and income can shift the demand curve.

Consumers' beliefs about the health effects of products are obviously central to discussions of demand. Few people want aspirin for its own sake.

The demand for aspirin, as for most medical goods and services, depends on consumers' expectations about its effects on their health. These expectations have two dimensions. One dimension consists of consumers' beliefs about their own health. If they believe they are healthy, they are unlikely to purchase goods and services to improve their health. The other dimension consists of their perception of how much a product will improve health. If I have a headache but do not believe that aspirin will relieve it, I will not be willing to buy aspirin. Health status and beliefs about the capacity of goods and services to improve health underpin demand.

Demand is a useful construct only if consumer preferences are stable enough to allow us to predict responses to price and income changes and if price and income changes are important determinants of consumption decisions. If on Tuesday 14 percent of the population thinks aspirin is something to avoid (whether it works or not) and on Friday that percentage has risen to 24 percent, demand models will be of little use. We would need to track changes in attitude, not changes in price. Alternatively, if routine advertising campaigns could easily change consumers' opinions about aspirin, tracking data on incomes and prices would be of little use. Preferences are usually stable enough for demand studies to be useful, so managers can rely on them in making pricing and marketing decisions.

Increase or decrease in demand
A shift in the entire price-quantity schedule (a new demand curve, not a movement along an existing curve)

Changes in income and wealth usually result in **increases or decreases in demand**. In principle, an increase in income or wealth could shift the demand curve either out (more consumption at every price) or in (less consumption at every price). Overall spending on healthcare clearly increases with income (Farag et al. 2012), but spending on some products falls with income. For example, nursing home use decreases for consumers with higher incomes (Goda, Golberstein, and Grabowski 2011). For the most part, however, consumers with larger budgets buy more healthcare products.

Changes in the prices of related goods also shift demand curves. Related goods are substitutes (products used instead of the product in question) and complements (products used in conjunction with the product in question). A substitute need not be a perfect substitute; in some cases it is simply an alternative. For example, ibuprofen is a substitute for aspirin. A reduction in the price of a substitute usually shifts the demand curve in (reduced willingness to pay at every volume). If the price of ibuprofen fell, some consumers would be tempted to switch from aspirin to ibuprofen, and the demand for aspirin would shift in. Conversely, an increase in the price of a substitute usually shifts the demand curve out (increased willingness to pay at every volume). If the price of ibuprofen rose, some consumers would be tempted to switch from ibuprofen to aspirin, and the demand for aspirin would shift out.

CASE 7.1   MinuteClinic

Mentioning a nationwide shortage of primary care providers, millions of newly insured patients through the Affordable Care Act, and an aging population, Dr. Andrew Sussman, president of CVS's MinuteClinic division, said in November 2013, "MinuteClinic can help to meet that demand, collaborating with local provider groups, as part of a larger health care team" (Nesi 2014).

MinuteClinic started in 2000 and as of early 2014 has more than 600 locations. Its clinics are staffed by nurse practitioners and physician assistants, rather than physicians. The clinics are open seven days a week and appointments are not needed. The nurse practitioners and physician assistants diagnose, treat, and write prescriptions for a variety of common illnesses. The clinics show customers the prices of care (typically less than the prices in a physician's office) and usually accept insurance. Most clinics are in CVS pharmacies (CVS Caremark 2013).

Of course, not everyone thinks MinuteClinic is a good idea. CVS has made three attempts to establish MinuteClinic locations in Rhode Island (where it is headquartered). Its first attempt was rebuffed in the face of opposition from the Rhode Island Medical Society. In 2005 the Society's president wrote that "by skimming away a certain volume of less complex and routine work, MinuteClinic will compromise the economic viability of some primary care practices" (Nesi 2014). The American Academy of Family Physicians continues to have reservations about MinuteClinic and similar retail clinics, noting that while they "may provide a limited scope of health care services for patients, this can ultimately lead to fragmentation of the patient's health care unless it is coordinated with the patient's primary care physician's office" (American Academy of Family Physicians 2014).

Discussion questions:
- For what products is MinuteClinic a substitute?
- For what products is it a complement?
- In what sense is MinuteClinic designed to meet the needs of patients?
- Do you share the Rhode Island Medical Society's concerns?
- Why might they be right?
- Why might they be wrong?
- A common criticism is that MinuteClinic locates its clinics in well-to-do areas. Is this a concern?

7.4 Demand with Insurance

Insurance changes demand by reducing the price of covered goods and services. For example, a consumer whose dental insurance plan covers 80 percent of the cost of a routine examination will need to pay only $10 instead of the full $50. The volume of routine examinations will usually increase as a result of an increase in insurance coverage, primarily because a higher proportion of the covered population will seek this form of preventive care. The response will not typically be large, however. Most consumers will not change their decisions to seek care because prices have changed. But managers should recognize that some consumers will respond to price changes caused by insurance. (We will develop tools for describing responses to price changes and review the evidence on this score in the next chapter.)

Exhibit 7.3 depicts standard responses to increases in insurance. An increase in insurance (a higher share of the population covered or a higher share of the bill covered) rotates the demand curve from D_1 to D_2. As a result, the quantity demanded will rise from Q_1 to Q_2 if the price remains at P_1. Or, if the quantity remains at Q_1, the price could rise from P_1 to P_2.

For provider organizations, an increase in insurance represents an opportunity to increase prices and margins. The rotation of D_2 has made it steeper, meaning that demand has become less sensitive to price. As demand becomes less sensitive to price, profit-maximizing firms will seek higher margins. (Higher margins mean that the cost of production will represent a smaller share of what consumers pay for a product.) Higher prices and increased quantity mean that the expansion of unmanaged insurance will result in substantial increases in spending.

EXHIBIT 7.3
The Impact of Insurance on Demand

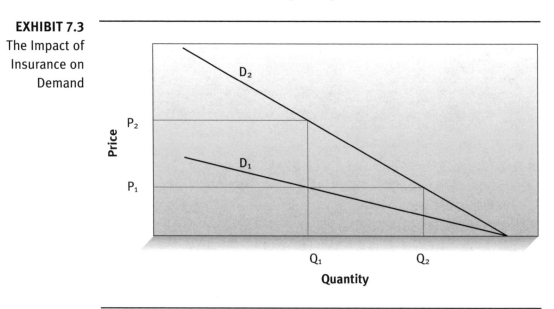

7.5 Demand with Advice from Providers

Consumers are often rationally ignorant about the healthcare system and the particular decisions they need to make. They are ignorant because medical decisions are complex, because they are unfamiliar with their options, because they lack the skills and information they need to compare their options, and because they lack time to make a considered judgment. This ignorance is rational because consumers do not know what choices they will have to make, because the cost of acquiring skills and information is high, and because the benefits of acquiring these skills and information are unknown.

Increased Cost Sharing

Demand theory implies that having patients pay a larger share of the bill (usually termed increased **cost sharing**) should reduce consumption of care. Does it? A landmark study by the RAND Corporation tells us that it does (Manning et al. 1987). The RAND Health Insurance Experiment randomly assigned consumers to 15 different health plans in six locations and then tracked their use of care (see Exhibit 7.4). Its fee-for-service sites had coinsurance rates of 0 percent, 25 percent, 50 percent, and 95 percent. The health plans fully covered expenses above *stop-loss limits* (the maximum amount a consumer would have to pay out of pocket), which varied from 5 percent to 15 percent of income. Spending was substantially lower for consumers who shared in the cost of their care. Increasing the coinsurance rate (the share of the bill that consumers pay) from 0 percent to 25 percent reduced total spending by nearly a fifth. This reduction had minimal effects on health.

Cost sharing
The general term for direct payments to providers by insurance beneficiaries (Deductibles, copayments, and coinsurance are forms of cost sharing.)

Coinsurance Rate	Spending	Any Use of Care	Hospital Admission
0%	$750	87%	10%
25%	$617	79%	8%
50%	$573	77%	7%
95%	$540	68%	8%

Source: Manning et al. (1987).

EXHIBIT 7.4
Effect of Co-insurance Rate

(continued)

(continued)

Costs were lower because consumers had fewer contacts with the healthcare system. The experiment went on for a number of years, and the suspicion that reducing use of care would increase spending later was not borne out. Based on the results of this study, virtually all insurance plans now incorporate some form of cost sharing for care initiated by patients. Recall that the box titled "Value-Based Insurance" noted that consumers cut use of both effective care and ineffective care, leading many insurers to redesign their plans.

Agent
A person who takes actions on behalf of another person (the principal)

Principal
The organization or individual represented by an agent

Agency
An arrangement in which one person (the agent) takes actions on behalf of another (the principal)

Consumers routinely deal with situations in which they are ignorant. Few consumers really know whether their car needs a new constant velocity joint, whether their roof should be replaced or repaired, or whether they should sell their stock in Cerner Corporation. Of course, consumers know they are ignorant. They often seek an **agent**, someone who is knowledgeable and can offer advice that advances the consumers' interests. Most people with medical problems choose a physician to be their agent.

Using an agent reduces, but does not eliminate, the problems associated with ignorance. Agents sometimes take advantage of **principals** (the ignorant consumers they represent). Taking advantage can range from out-and-out fraud (e.g., lying to sell a worthless insurance policy) to simple shirking (e.g., failing to check the accuracy of ads for a property). If consumers can identify poor agent performance, fairly simple remedies further reduce the problems associated with ignorance. In many cases an agent's reputation is of paramount importance, so agents have a strong incentive to please principals. In other cases simply delaying payment until a project has been successfully completed substantially reduces **agency** problems.

The most difficult problems arise when consumers have difficulty distinguishing bad outcomes from bad performance on the part of an agent. This problem is fairly common. Did your house take a long time to sell because the market weakened unexpectedly or because your agent recommended that you set the price too high? Was your baby born via cesarean section to preserve the baby's health or to preserve your physician's weekend plans? Most contracts with agents are designed to minimize these problems by aligning the interests of the principal and the agent. For example, real estate agents earn a share of a property's sale price so that both the agent and the seller profit when the property is sold quickly at a high price. In similar fashion, earnings of mutual fund managers are commonly based on the total assets they manage, so managers and investors profit when the value of the mutual fund increases.

Agency models have several implications for our understanding of demand. First, what consumers demand may depend on incentives for providers. Agency models suggest that changes in the amount paid to providers, the way providers are paid, or providers' profits may change their recommendations for consumers. For example, consumers may respond to a lower price for generic drugs only because pharmacists have financial incentives to recommend them. Second, provider incentives will affect consumption of some goods and services more than others. Provider recommendations will not affect patients' initial decisions to seek care. And where standards of care are clear and generally accepted, providers are less apt to change their recommendations when their incentives change. When a consensus about standards of care exists, providers who change their recommendations in response to financial incentives risk denial of payment, identification as a low-quality provider, or even malpractice suits. Third, patients with chronic illnesses are often quite knowledgeable about the therapies they prefer. When patients have firm preferences, agency is likely to have less effect on demand. In short, agency makes the demand for medical care more complex.

Agency is one of the most important factors that makes managed care necessary. (That insurance plans must protect consumers from virtually all of the costs of some very expensive procedures, so out-of-pocket costs need to fall to near zero, is the other main factor.) If all the parties to a healthcare transaction had all the same information, expenditures could be limited simply by changing consumer out-of-pocket payments. In many cases, though, provider incentives need to be aligned with consumer goals. (Of course, health plans also have an agency relationship with beneficiaries, and nothing guarantees that plans will be perfect agents.) Most of the features of managed care address the agency problem in one way or another. For example, bundled payments are intended to increase physicians' incentives to be efficient in improving the health of their patients. Likewise, ACOs pay quality and cost bonuses to increase incentives for providers to share information and coordinate care.

7.6 Conclusion

Demand is one of the central ideas of economics, and managers need to understand the basics of demand. In most cases, consumption of a product falls when its price increases, and studies of healthcare products confirm this generalization. An understanding of this relationship between price and quantity is part of effective management. Without it, managers cannot predict sales, revenues, or profits.

To make accurate forecasts, managers also must be aware of the effects of factors they do not control. Demand for their products will be higher when the price of complements is lower or the price of substitutes is higher. In most cases, demand will be higher in areas with higher incomes. We will explore how to make forecasts in more detail in Chapter 8.

The demand for healthcare products is complex. Insurance and professional advice have significant effects on demand. Insurance means that three prices exist: the out-of-pocket price the consumer pays, the price the insurer pays, and the price the provider receives. The quantity demanded will usually fall when out-of-pocket prices rise but may not change when the other prices do. Because professional advice is important in consumers' healthcare decisions, the incentives professionals face can influence consumption of some products. How and how much professionals are paid can affect their recommendations, and recognition of this effect has helped spur the shift to managed care. To change patterns of consumption, managers may need to change incentives for patients and providers.

Exercises

7.1 Is the idea of demand useful in healthcare, given the important role of agents?

7.2 Should medical services be free? Justify your answer.

7.3 Why might a consumer be "rationally ignorant" about the proper therapy for gallstones?

7.4 Why do demand curves slope down (i.e., sales volume usually rises at lower prices)?

7.5 Why would consumers ever choose insurance plans with large deductibles?

7.6 During the last five years, average daily occupancy at Autumn Acres nursing home has slid from 125 to 95 even though Autumn Acres has cut its daily rate from $125 to $115. Do these data suggest that occupancy would have been higher if Autumn Acres had raised its rates? What changes in nonprice demand factors might explain this change? (The supply, or the number of nursing home beds in the area, has not changed during this period.)

7.7 Your hospital is considering opening a satellite urgent care center about five miles from your main campus. You have been charged with gathering demographic information that might affect the demand for the center's services. What data are likely to be relevant?

7.8 How would each of the following changes affect the demand curve for acupuncture?

a. The price of an acupuncture session increases.

b. A reduction in back problems occurs as a result of sessions on stretching on a popular television show.

  c. Medicare reduces the copayment for acupuncture from $20 to
  $10.

  d. The surgeon general issues a warning that back surgery is
  ineffective.

  e. Medicare stops covering back surgery.

7.9 Your boss has asked you to describe how the demand for an over-
the-counter sinus medication would change in the following
situations. Assuming the price does not change, forecast whether the
sales volume will go up, remain constant, or go down.

  a. The local population increases.

  b. A wet spring leads to a bumper crop of ragweed.

  c. Factory closings lead to a drop in the area's average income.

  d. A competing product with a different formula is found to be
  unsafe.

  e. A research study showing that the medication causes severe
  dizziness is published.

  f. The price of another sinus medication drops.

7.10 A community has four residents. The table shows the number of
dental visits each resident will have. Calculate the total quantity
demanded at each price. Then graph the relationship between price
and total quantity, with total quantity on the horizontal axis.

Price	Abe's Quantity	Beth's Quantity	Cal's Quantity	Don's Quantity
$40	0	0	0	1
$30	0	1	0	1
$20	0	1	0	2
$10	1	2	1	2
$0	1	2	1	3

7.11 A clinic focuses on three services: counseling for teens and young
adults, smoking cessation, and counseling for young parents. An
analyst has developed a forecast of the number of visits each group
will make at different prices. Calculate the total quantity demanded
at each price. Then graph the relationship between price and total
quantity, putting total quantity on the horizontal axis.

Price	Teen Counseling	Smoking Cessation	Parent Counseling
$80	10	0	0
$60	15	1	0
$40	20	2	0
$20	40	4	6
$0	50	6	8

7.12 The price–quantity relationship has been estimated for a new prostate cancer blood test: $Q = 4,000 - 20 \times P$. Use a spreadsheet to calculate the quantity demanded and total spending for prices ranging from $200 to $0, using $50 increments. For each $50 drop in price, calculate the change in revenue, the change in volume, and the additional revenue per unit. (Call the additional revenue per unit *marginal revenue*.)

7.13 A physical therapy clinic faces a demand equation of $Q = 200 - 1.5 \times P$, where Q is sessions per month and P is the price per session.

   a. The clinic currently charges $80. What is its sales volume and revenue at this price?

   b. If the clinic raised its price to $90, what would happen to volume and revenue?

   c. If the clinic lowered its price to $70, what would happen to volume and revenue?

7.14 Researchers have concluded that the demand for annual preventive clinic visits by children with asthma equals $1 + 0.00004 \times Y - 0.04 \times P$. In this equation Y represents family income and P represents price.

   a. Calculate how many visits a child with a family income of $100,000 will make at prices of $200, $150, $100, $50, and $0. If you predict that visits will be less than zero, convert your answer to zero.

   b. Now repeat your calculations for a child with a family income of $35,000.

   c. How do your predictions for the two children differ?

   d. Assume that the market price of a preventive visit is $100. Does this system seem fair? What fairness criteria are you using?

   e. Would your answer change if the surgeon general recommended that every child with asthma have at least one preventive visit each year?

References

American Academy of Family Physicians. 2014. "Retail Clinics." Accessed July 2. www.aafp.org/about/policies/all/retail-clinics.html.

Choudhry, N. K., M. A. Fischer, J. Avorn, S. Schneeweiss, D. H. Solomon, C. Berman, S. Jan, J. Liu, J. Lii, M. A. Brookhart, J. J. Mahoney, and W. H. Shrank. 2010. "At Pitney Bowes, Value-Based Insurance Design Cut Copayments and Increased Drug Adherence." *Health Affairs* 29 (11): 1995–2001.

CVS Caremark. 2013. *2012 Annual Report.* Accessed July 2, 2014. http://investors. cvscaremark.com/~/media/Files/C/CVS-IR/reports/cvs-ar-2012.pdf.

Farag, M., A. K. NandaKumar, S. Wallack, D. Hodgkin, G. Gaumer, and C. Erbil. 2012. "The Income Elasticity of Health Care Spending in Developing and Developed Countries." *International Journal of Health Care Finance and Economics* 12 (2): 145–62.

Goda, G. S., E. Golberstein, and D. C. Grabowski. 2011. "Income and the Utilization of Long-Term Care Services: Evidence from the Social Security Benefit Notch." *Journal of Health Economics* 30 (4): 719–29.

Manning, W. G., A. Leibowitz, M. S. Marquis, J. P. Newhouse, N. Duan, and E. B. Keeler. 1987. "Health Insurance and the Demand for Medical Care: Evidence from a Randomized Experiment." *American Economic Review* 77 (3): 251–77.

Nesi, T. 2014. "CVS Aiming to Open MinuteClinics in RI This Year." *WPRI.com.* Published February 19. wpri.com/2014/02/19/cvs-aiming-to-open-minute clinics-in-ri-this-year/.

ELASTICITIES

After reading this chapter, students will be able to

- calculate an arc elasticity,
- use elasticities to describe economic data,
- apply elasticities to make simple forecasts, and
- use elasticity terms appropriately.

Key Concepts

- Economists use elasticities to avoid confusion about units.
- An elasticity is the percentage change in one variable that is associated with a 1 percent change in another.
- Elasticities allow quick calculations of the effects of strategic choices.
- Managers can use elasticities to forecast sales.
- To avoid ambiguities, use arc elasticities (which use the average of the starting and ending values as the denominator of percentage change calculations).
- An income elasticity of demand is the percentage change in the quantity demanded that is associated with a 1 percent change in consumer income.
- A price elasticity of demand is the percentage change in the quantity demanded that is associated with a 1 percent change in the price of a product.
- A cross-price elasticity is the percentage change in the quantity demanded that is associated with a 1 percent change in the price of a substitute or complement.

8.1 Introduction

Elasticity
The percentage change in a dependent variable associated with a 1 percent change in an independent variable

Elasticities are valuable tools for managers. Armed only with basic marketing data and reasonable estimates about elasticities, managers can make sales, revenue, and marginal revenue forecasts. In addition, elasticities are ideal for analyzing "what if" questions. What will happen to revenues if we raise prices by 2 percent? What will happen to our sales if the price of a substitute drops by 3 percent?

Elasticities reduce confusion in descriptions. For example, suppose the price of a 500-tablet bottle of generic ibuprofen rose from $7.50 to $8.00. Someone who was seeking to downplay the size of this increase (or someone whose focus was on the cost per tablet) would say that the price rose from 1.5 cents to 1.6 cents per tablet. Describing this change in percentage terms would eliminate any confusion about price per bottle or price per tablet, but a potential source of confusion remains. The change could be described as an increase of 6.67 percent (by dividing the increase, 50 cents, into $7.50) or 6.25 percent (by dividing the increase into $8.00).

To avoid confusion in calculating percentages, economists recommend two courses of action. One is to be very explicit about the values used to calculate percentage changes. For example, one might say that the price increase to $8.00 represents a 6.67 percent increase from the starting value of $7.50. In our view, the best course of action is to use the average of the starting and ending values to calculate percentage changes because that approach avoids some complications that may confuse the unwary. This method finds the **arc elasticity**. In this case, using the average price of $7.75 to calculate the percentages means that only one answer is possible: Prices increased 6.45 percent.

Arc elasticity
A ratio of percentage changes that is calculated using the average of two points (For example, a percentage change in price between $8 and $2 would be calculated by subtracting $2 from $8 and then dividing the result by $5, the average of the two values.)

8.2 Elasticities

An *elasticity* is the percentage change in one variable associated with a 1 percent change in another. For example, Newhouse and Phelps (1976) used statistical techniques to estimate that the income elasticity for physician visits was 0.04. The base for this estimate is average income, so an income 1 percent above the average is associated with an average level of physician visits that is 0.04 percent above average. As we shall see, these apparently esoteric estimates can be valuable to managers.

First we need to learn a little more about elasticities. Economists routinely calculate three demand elasticities:

1. income elasticity: the percentage change in the quantity demanded that is associated with a 1 percent change in consumer income

2. price elasticity: the percentage change in the quantity demanded that is associated with a 1 percent change in a product's price

3. **cross-price elasticity**: the percentage change in the quantity demanded that is associated with a 1 percent change in the price of a substitute or complement

All of these elasticities can be represented as ratios of percentage changes. For example, the **income elasticity of demand** for visits would equal the ratio of the percentage change in visits (dQ/Q) associated with a given percentage change in income (dY/Y). (The mathematical terms dQ and dY identify small changes in consumption and income.) So, the formula for an income elasticity would be $E_Y = (dQ/Q)/(dY/Y)$. The formula for a price elasticity would be $E_P = (dQ/Q)/(dP/P)$, and the formula for cross-price elasticity would be $E_R = (dQ/Q)/(dR/R)$. (A cross-price elasticity measures the response of demand to changes in the price of a substitute or complement, so R is the price of a related product.)

Now recall that the Newhouse and Phelps (1976) estimate of the income elasticity for physician visits is 0.04. This implies that $0.04 = (dQ/Q)/(dY/Y)$. Suppose we wanted to know how much higher than average the visits per person would be in an area where the average income is 2 percent higher than the national average. Because we are considering a case in which $dY/Y = 0.02$, we multiply both sides of the equation by 0.02 and find that visits should be 0.0008 (0.08 percent) higher in an area with income 2 percent above the national average. From the perspective of a working manager, what matters is the conclusion that visits will be only slightly higher in the wealthier area.

Cross-price elasticity
The percentage change in the quantity demanded associated with a 1 percent change in the price of a related product

Income elasticity of demand
The percentage change in the quantity demanded associated with a 1 percent increase in income

8.3 Income Elasticities

Consumption of most healthcare products increases with income, but only slightly. As Exhibit 8.1 shows, consumption of healthcare products appears to increase more slowly than income. As a result, healthcare spending will represent a smaller proportion of income among high-income consumers than among low-income consumers.

Source	Date	Variable	Point Estimate
Farag et al.	2012	Spending per person	0.83 to 0.90
Newhouse and Phelps	1976	Hospital admissions	0.02 to 0.04
Newhouse and Phelps	1976	Physician visits	0.01 to 0.04

EXHIBIT 8.1
Selected Estimates of the Income Elasticity of Demand

8.4 Price Elasticities of Demand

Price elasticity of demand
The percentage change in sales volume associated with a 1 percent change in a product's price

The **price elasticity of demand** is even more useful because prices depend on choices managers make. Estimates of the price elasticity of demand will guide pricing and contracting decisions, as Chapter 9 explores in more detail. Managers need to be careful in using the price elasticity of demand for three reasons. First, because the price elasticity of demand is almost always negative, we need a special vocabulary to describe the responsiveness of demand to price. For example, –3.00 is a smaller number than –1.00, but –3.00 implies that demand is more responsive to changes in prices (a 1 percent rise in prices results in a 3 percent drop in sales rather than a 1 percent drop in sales). Second, changes in prices affect revenues directly and indirectly, via changes in quantity. Managers need to keep this fact in mind when using the price elasticity of demand. Third, managers need to think about two very different price elasticities of demand: the overall price elasticity of demand and the price elasticity of demand for his or her firm's products.

Inelastic
A term used to describe demand when the quantity demanded falls by less than 1 percent when the price rises by 1 percent (This term is usually applied only to price elasticities of demand.)

Economists usually speak of price elasticities of demand (but not other elasticities) as being *inelastic* or *elastic*. When a 1 percent increase in price results in a reduction of less than 1 percent in the quantity demanded, the price elasticity of demand will be between 0.00 and –1.00, and demand is said to be **inelastic**. When a 1 percent increase in price results in a reduction of more than 1 percent in the quantity demanded, the price elasticity of demand will be smaller than –1.00, and demand is said to be **elastic**.

Elastic
A term used to describe demand when the quantity demanded falls by more than 1 percent when the price rises by 1 percent (This term is usually applied only to price elasticities of demand.)

Inelastic demand does not mean that consumption will be unaffected by price changes. Suppose that, in forecasting the demand response to a 3 percent price cut, we use an elasticity of –0.20. Predicting that sales will drop by 0.6 percent, this elasticity implies that demand is inelastic but not unresponsive. Recall that a price elasticity of demand equals the ratio of the percentage change in quantity that is associated with a percentage change in price, or $(dQ/Q)/(dP/P)$. Using this formula and our elasticity estimate gives us $-0.20 = (dQ/Q)/(-0.03)$. After solving for the percentage change in quantity, we forecast that a 3 percent price cut will increase consumption by 0.006 (or 0.6 percent), which is equal to -0.20×-0.03. Exhibit 8.2 shows that the demand for medical care is usually inelastic.

EXHIBIT 8.2
Selected Estimates of the Price Elasticity of Demand

Source	Date	Variable	Point Estimate
Manning et al.	1987	Total spending	−0.17 to −0.22
Newhouse and Phelps	1976	Hospital admissions	−0.02 to −0.04
Newhouse and Phelps	1976	Physician visits	−0.08
Danyliv et al.	2014	Physician visits	−0.17 to −0.39

CASE 8.1	**Mental Health Parity**

Presenting to the board, Chris spoke with passion. "Our insurance plan should provide the same coverage for mental health services as for other medical services. It's the right thing to do, and it's good business. If our employees or their dependents have untreated mental health problems, the employees become less productive and waste money getting treated for other stuff."

"Thank you, Chris," said Kerry, the company's CEO. "This is an important question for us, and the Benefits Committee will carefully consider it." After Chris left the room, Kerry turned to Jordan, the director of human resources, and said, "Jordan, what's your take on this?"

"There are actually two questions here," said Jordan. "First, how elastic is the demand for ambulatory mental health services? How much will use of mental health services increase if coverage improves? Second, how effective is mental health care? This second question is the more important one because good mental health care can have such powerful effects.

"Now, a number of studies have concluded that use of mental health services is more price sensitive than use of other ambulatory care. Analyses of ambulatory mental health services have found elasticities ranging from −0.44 to −1.00. These results could be statistical flukes. Consumers who expect to use mental health services may choose insurance plans that offer generous coverage for those services. However, the RAND Corporation researchers Keeler, Manning, and Wells in 1988 used data from the RAND Health Insurance Experiment, which randomly assigned respondents to insurance plans, to resolve this issue.

"The RAND analysis generally confirmed that the demand for mental health services is more price sensitive than the demand for general ambulatory medical services. Demand for each is inelastic, but the elasticity for mental health services is −0.8 and the elasticity for other outpatient services is −0.3. Most consumers will not use any mental health services, but plans that offer generous mental health benefits will cost more. We can't ignore this."

"I'm confused," said Addison, an internist on the board. "In 2012 McConnell and colleagues published a study showing that Oregon's law requiring mental health parity in commercial insurance plans had

(continued)

CASE 8.1
(continued)

little effect on spending. How could that be? Real life appears to be contradicting the RAND study."

"I'm sure the plans for federal employees used managed care techniques to control spending," Jordan jumped in. "And mental health spending isn't the issue. The issues are what happens to other healthcare spending and what happens to our workers. I'm pretty sure there's good evidence showing that effective mental health treatment can reduce other costs and improve productivity."

Discussion questions:
- Why does it matter whether demand for mental health services is more elastic than demand for other services?
- The price elasticity of demand for ambulatory mental health services appears to be about −0.8, and the price elasticity for general ambulatory medical services appears to be about −0.3. How much would spending increase for each type of care if copayments were cut from $40 to $25?
- What managed care techniques do insurers use to control spending?
- Is there evidence that better treatment of mental health problems reduces other spending?
- Is there evidence that better treatment of mental health problems improves productivity?
- What is your recommendation to the Benefits Committee?

8.5 Using Elasticities

Elasticities are useful forecasting tools. With an estimate of the price elasticity of demand, a manager can quickly estimate the impact of a price cut on sales and revenues. As noted previously, though, managers need to use the correct elasticity. Most estimates of the overall price elasticity of demand fall between −0.10 and −0.40. For the market as a whole, the demand for healthcare products is typically inelastic. For individual firms, in contrast, demand is usually elastic. The reason is simple. Most healthcare products have few close substitutes, but the products of one healthcare organization represent close substitutes for the products of another.

The price elasticity of demand that individual firms face typically depends on the overall price elasticity and the firm's market share. If the price elasticity of demand for hospital admissions is −0.17 and a hospital has a 12 percent share of the market, the hospital needs to anticipate that it faces a price elasticity of –0.17/0.12, or –1.42. This rule of thumb need not hold exactly, but good evidence indicates that individual firms confront elastic demand. For example, Lee and Hadley (1981) estimated that the price elasticity of demand for the services of individual physicians ranged from –2.80 to –5.07. Indeed, as we will show in Chapter 9, profit-maximizing firms should set prices high enough that demand for their products is elastic.

Armed with a reasonable estimate of the price elasticity of demand, we will now predict the impact of a 5 percent price cut on volume. If the price elasticity faced by a physician practice were –2.80, a 5 percent price cut should increase the number of visits by 14 percent, which is the product of –0.05 and –2.80. (A prudent manager will recognize that his or her best guess about the price elasticity will not be exactly right and repeat the calculations with other values. For example, if the price elasticity is really –1.40, volume will increase by 7 percent. If the price elasticity is really –4.20, volume will increase by 21 percent.)

How much will revenues change if we cut prices by 5 percent and the price elasticity is –2.80? Obviously revenues will rise less than volume does because we have reduced prices. A rough, easily calculated estimate of the change in revenues is the percentage change in prices plus the percentage change in volume. Prices will fall by 5 percent and quantity will rise by 7 to 21 percent, so revenues should rise by approximately 2 to 16 percent. Our baseline estimate is that revenues will rise by 9 percent. If costs rise by less than this percentage, profits will rise.

CASE 8.2   Reducing Waiting Time

One of the few determinants of demand that healthcare managers can control is waiting time. Ample evidence indicates that long waits discourage patients and drive up costs. Acton (1975) estimated that the elasticity of demand with respect to waiting time was –0.96 in clinics (where waits tended to be long) and –0.25 in physicians' offices (where waits tended to be shorter). This finding suggests that reducing waits by 10 percent could increase volume by 3 to 10 percent. In an environment in which many providers would like to add patients, reducing waits represents a strategy worth considering.

Christie Clinic in Champaign, Illinois, uses a simple management technique called a *huddle* to increase efficiency. Each day the staff,

(continued)

CASE 8.2
(continued)

including physicians, meets briefly to identify problems and review potential solutions. In less than a year after starting the huddles, waits for appointments decreased by 28 percent, volume rose by 10 percent with no increase in head count (meaning that costs went down), and patient satisfaction rose by 9 percent (Toussaint and Berry 2013).

More volume may not be the only benefit of reducing waiting time. Long waits for patients often mean long waits and wasted time for staff as well. Another hospital experienced unacceptable wait times for intravenous pumps in the emergency department. Initially diagnosed as an inadequate number of pumps, the problem turned out to be a poorly defined process for making pumps available. In fact, the hospital had more pumps than it needed. It was able to reduce waits for pumps while decreasing its inventory by 20 percent, saving $300,000 in the process. The new process also sharply reduced the amount of time nurses spent looking for pumps, increasing their time with patients (Toussaint and Berry 2013).

Both of these examples took place in organizations that were using Lean approaches to performance improvement. Lean emphasizes eliminating steps in production that do not add value for customers and can lead to major gains. The major alternative to Lean is Six Sigma, which can also result in significant improvements. Six Sigma is a structured approach that stresses defining the organization's problem from the perspective of internal and external customers, measuring key aspects of performance, analyzing the data, and implementing an improvement plan (McLaughlin and Olson 2012). Organizations that are not using Lean or Six Sigma to become more efficient will find it increasingly hard to compete with organizations that are.

Discussion questions:
- Acton's estimates suggest that demand is more sensitive to waiting time than to out-of-pocket price. Why might that be the case?
- For the sake of argument, assume that the entire 10 percent increase in volume at Christie Clinic is due to the 28 percent reduction in waits for appointments. What elasticity of demand with respect to appointment waits do the data for the Christie Clinic imply?
- Why would waits for patients result in waits for staff?

8.6 Conclusion

An elasticity is the percentage change in one variable that is associated with a 1 percent change in another variable. Elasticities are simple, valuable tools that managers can use to forecast sales and revenues. Elasticities allow managers to apply the results of sophisticated economic studies to their organizations.

Three elasticities are common: income elasticities, price elasticities, and cross-price elasticities. Income elasticities measure how much demand varies with income, price elasticities measure how much demand varies with the price of the product itself, and cross-price elasticities measure how much demand varies with the prices of complements and substitutes. Of these, price elasticity is the most important because it guides pricing and contracting decisions.

Virtually all price elasticities of demand for healthcare products are negative, reflecting that higher prices generally reduce the quantity demanded. The overall demand for most healthcare products is inelastic, meaning that a 1 percent increase in a product's price results in a reduction of less than 1 percent in the quantity sold. In most cases, though, the demand for an individual organization's products will be elastic, meaning that a 1 percent increase in a product's price results in a reduction of more than 1 percent in the quantity sold. This difference is based on ease of substitution. Few good substitutes are available for broadly defined healthcare products, so demand is inelastic. In contrast, the products of other healthcare providers are usually good substitutes for the products of a particular provider, so demand is elastic. When making decisions, managers must consider that their organization's products face elastic demands.

Exercises

8.1 Why are elasticities useful for managers?

8.2 Why are price elasticities called "elastic" or "inelastic" when other elasticities are not?

8.3 Why is the demand for healthcare products usually inelastic?

8.4 Why is the demand for an individual firm's healthcare products usually elastic?

8.5 Average visits per week equal 640 when the copayment is $40 and 360 when the copayment is $60.

    a. Calculate the percentage change in visits, percentage change in price, and price elasticity of demand using 640 and $40 as the denominators for percentage change calculations.

b. Calculate the percentage change in visits, percentage change in price, and price elasticity of demand using 360 and $60 as the denominators for percentage change calculations.

c. Calculate the percentage change in visits, percentage change in price, and price elasticity of demand using 500 and $50 as the denominator for percentage change calculations. (This calculation finds the arc elasticity.)

d. How do your answers differ?

8.6 Sales are 3,100 at a price of $200 and 2,400 at a price of $300. Calculate the price elasticities of demand using $200 as the base value; then use $300 as the base value. Calculate the arc price elasticity and compare the three calculations. How do your answers differ?

8.7 Per capita income in County A is $45,000. Per capita income in County B is $38,000. Physician visits average 3.4 per year in County A and 3.2 per year in County B. What is the arc income elasticity of demand for visits?

8.8 Median household income in County C is $54,021. Median household income in County D is $28,739. In County C, 17.4 percent of residents smoke. In County D, 28.4 percent of residents smoke. What is the arc income elasticity of demand for tobacco use?

8.9 The price elasticity of demand is –1.2. Is demand elastic or inelastic?

8.10 The price elasticity of demand is –0.12. Is demand elastic or inelastic?

8.11 If the income elasticity of demand is 0.2, how would the volume of services change if income rose by 10 percent?

8.12 You are a manager in a regional health system. Using an estimate of the price elasticity of demand of –0.25, calculate how much ambulatory visits will change if you raise prices by 5 percent.

8.13 If the cross-price elasticity of clinic visits with respect to pharmaceutical prices is –0.18, how much will ambulatory visits change if pharmacy prices rise by 5 percent? Are pharmaceuticals substitutes for or complements to clinic visits?

8.14 If the cross-price elasticity of clinic visits with respect to emergency department prices is 0.21, how much will ambulatory visits change if emergency department prices rise by 5 percent? Are emergency department visits substitutes for or complements to clinic visits?

8.15 If the income elasticity of demand is 0.03, how much will ambulatory visits change if incomes rise by 4 percent?

8.16 A study estimates that the price elasticity of demand for drug E is –3.41, but the price elasticity of demand for its class of drugs as a whole is –0.22.

    a. Why is demand for drug E more elastic than for the whole class of drugs?

    b. What would happen to revenues if the makers of drug E raised prices by 10 percent?

    c. What would happen to industry revenues if all manufacturers raised prices by 10 percent?

    d. Why are the answers so different? Does this difference make sense?

8.17 The price elasticity of demand for the services of Kim Jones, MD, is –4.0. The price elasticity of demand for physicians' services overall is –0.1.

    a. Why is demand so much more elastic for the services of Dr. Jones than for the services of physicians in general?

    b. If Dr. Jones reduced prices by 10 percent, how much would volume and revenue change?

    c. Suppose that all the physicians in the area reduced prices by 10 percent. How much would the total number of visits and revenue change?

    d. Why are your answers to questions b and c so different?

References

Acton, J. P. 1975. "Nonmonetary Factors in the Demand for Medical Services: Some Empirical Evidence." *Journal of Political Economy* 83 (3): 595–614.

Danyliv, A., W. Groot, I. Gryga, and M. Pavlova. 2014. "Willingness and Ability to Pay for Physician Services in Six Central and Eastern European Countries." *Health Policy.* Published March 14. www.sciencedirect.com/science/article/pii/S0168851014.

Farag, M., A. K. NandaKumar, S. Wallack, D. Hodgkin, G. Gaumer, and C. Erbil. 2012. "The Income Elasticity of Health Care Spending in Developing and Developed Countries." *International Journal of Health Care Finance and Economics* 12 (2): 145–62.

Keeler, E., W. G. Manning, and K. B. Wells. 1988. "The Demand for Episodes of Mental Health Services." *Journal of Health Economics* 7 (4): 369–92.

Lee, R. H., and J. Hadley. 1981. "Physicians' Fees and Public Medical Care Programs." *Health Services Research* 16 (2): 185–203.

Manning, W. G., A. Leibowitz, M. S. Marquis, J. P. Newhouse, N. Duan, and E. B. Keeler. 1987. "Health Insurance and the Demand for Medical Care: Evidence from a Randomized Experiment." *American Economic Review* 77 (3): 251–77.

McConnell, K. J., S. H. Gast, M. S. Ridgely, N. Wallace, N. Jacuzzi, T. Rieckmann, B. H. McFarland, and D. McCarty. 2012. "Behavioral Health Insurance Parity: Does Oregon's Experience Presage the National Experience with the Mental Health Parity and Addiction Equity Act?" *American Journal of Psychiatry* 169 (1): 31–38.

McLaughlin, D. B., and J. R. Olson. 2012. *Healthcare Operations Management*, second edition. Chicago: Health Administration Press.

Newhouse, J. P., and C. E. Phelps. 1976. "New Estimates of Price and Income Elasticities of Medical Care Services." In *The Role of Health Insurance in the Health Services Sector*, edited by Richard Rosett, 261–320. New York: Neal Watson.

Toussaint, J. S., and L. L. Berry. 2013. "The Promise of Lean in Health Care." *Mayo Clinic Proceedings* 88 (1): 74–82.

FORECASTING

9.1 Introduction

Making and interpreting forecasts are important jobs for managers. Sales forecasts are especially important because many decisions hinge on what the organization expects to sell. Pricing decisions, staffing decisions, product launch decisions, and other crucial decisions are based on the organization's revenue and sales forecasts.

Inaccurate or misunderstood forecasts can hurt businesses. The organization can hire too many workers or too few. It can set prices too high or too low. It can add too much equipment or too little. At best, these sorts of forecasting problems will cut into profits; at worst, they may drive an organization out of business.

The consequences of bad or misapplied forecasts are particularly serious in healthcare. For example, underestimating the level of demand in the short term may result in stock shortages at a pharmacy or too few nurses on duty at a hospital. In both cases, the healthcare organization will suffer financially and, more important, put patients at risk. It will suffer because the costs of meeting unexpected demand are high and because the long-term consequences of failing to meet patients' needs are significant. The best outcome in this case will be unhappy patients; the worst outcome will be that physicians stop referring patients to the organization.

Overestimating sales can also have serious long-term effects. A hospital may add too many beds because its census forecast was too high. This surplus will depress profits for some time because the facility will have hired staff and added equipment to meet its overestimated forecast, and the costs of hiring and paying new employees and buying new equipment will substantially exceed actual sales profits. In extreme cases, bad forecasts may drive a firm out of business. A facility that borrows heavily in anticipation of higher sales that do not materialize may be unable to repay those debts. Bankruptcy may be the only option.

Sales and revenue forecasts are applications of demand theory. The factors that change sales and revenues also change demand. The most important influences on demand are the price of the product, rivals' prices for the product, prices for complements and substitutes, and demographics. Recognizing these influences can simplify forecasting considerably because it focuses our attention on tracking what has changed.

9.2 What Is a Sales Forecast?

A sales forecast is a projection of the number of units (e.g., bed days, visits, doses) an organization expects to sell. The forecast must specify the time frame, marketing plan, and expected market conditions for which it is valid.

A forecast is a planning tool, not a rigid goal. Conditions may change. If they do, the organization's plan needs to be reassessed. Good management usually involves responding effectively to changes in the environment, not forging ahead as though nothing has shifted. In addition, fixed sales goals create incentives to behave opportunistically (that is, for employees to try to meet their goals instead of the organization's goals). For example, sales staff may harm the organization by making overblown claims of a product's effectiveness to meet their sales goals, even though their actions will harm the company in the long run. Alternatively, sales managers may bid on unprofitable managed care contracts just to meet goals.

Whenever possible, a sales forecast should estimate the number of units expected to be sold, not revenues. The number of units to be sold determines staffing, materials, working capital, and other needs. In addition, costs often vary unevenly with volume. A small reduction in sales volume may save an entire shift's worth of wages (thereby avoiding considerable cost), or an increase in sales may incur an insignificant cost increase if it requires no additional staff or equipment.

CASE 9.1   Building a New Urgent Care Center

"It's a slam dunk," said Kim, the marketing analyst. "The volumes we've forecasted ensure that the new urgent care center will be profitable within six months."

"Great," replied Angel, vice president of strategic management, "but I think it would be useful to walk through those numbers to put everyone at ease."

"OK, here's how we forecasted visits," said Kim. "There are 40,000 people living in our primary market area. National rates suggest that a population of this size will make 6,000 urgent care visits each year. Right now, our emergency department sees 2,500 urgent—but not emergent—visits each year. We believe that 1,500 of them will come to the urgent care center. Our seat-of-the-pants estimate is that Providence, the other hospital serving our primary market area, sees 2,000 urgent care patients per year in its emergency department. We expect to get half of those visits. We also expect that the added convenience of the urgent care center will bring in an additional 500 visits each year. So, 3,000 visits per year, each yielding revenue of $125, give us $375,000 in total revenue. We have fixed costs of $200,000. Our best estimate is that each visit has variable costs of $20, so we're talking profits of $115,000, for a margin on sales of 30 percent."

"That's nice and clear," said Angel, "but I'd like to take a closer look. About half of the patients Providence sees would have to drive past Providence to get to our urgent care center. Do we have any indication that those folks will do that? My second concern is that our emergency department is open 24/7. The urgent care center will be open 82 hours per week. Can we really hope to capture 60 percent of the emergency department's urgent care patients?"

(continued)

CASE 9.1
(continued)

Discussion questions:
- What happens to profits if the urgent care center has only 2,000 visits?
- To what extent does Kim's forecast rely on judgment rather than data? Would additional information help resolve Angel's concerns? What sort of data would you suggest gathering?
- Does building the urgent care center seem risky? Could you do anything to reduce the amount of risk?
- Would there be any advantages to planning for a small patient volume and letting your customers surprise you? Suppose you plan for 2,000 visits but volume turns out to be 3,000. What happens? Would underestimating the volume be better or worse than planning for 3,000 and getting only 2,000?

The dollar volume of sales can vary in response to factors that do not affect the resources needed to produce, market, or service sales. Discounts and price increases are examples of such factors. Revenues can vary even though neither volume nor costs change. Finally, managers can easily forecast revenue given a volume forecast. In general, managers should build their revenue estimates on sales volume estimates.

Good forecasts have five attributes. They should be

1. easy to understand,
2. easy to modify,
3. accurate (i.e., they contain the most probable actual values),
4. transparent about how variable they are, and
5. precise (i.e., they give the analyst as little wiggle room as possible).

These attributes often conflict. Managers may need to underplay how imprecise simple forecasts are because their audience is not prepared to consider variation. As Aven (2013) points out, many decision makers are more comfortable working with a single, very precise estimate, even though it may be inaccurate. Precision and accuracy always conflict because a more precise forecast (80 to 85 visits per day) will always be less accurate than a less precise forecast (70 to 95 visits per day). Offering decision makers several precise scenarios is usually a good compromise. For example, busy decision makers generally can use a forecast such as "Our baseline forecast is 82 visits per day for the next three months; our low forecast is 75 visits per day, and our high forecast is 89 visits per day."

9.3 Forecasting

All forecasts combine history and judgment. History is the only real source of data. For example, sales can be forecasted only on the basis of data on past sales of a product, past sales of similar products, past sales by rivals, or past sales in other markets. History is an imperfect guide to the future, but it is an essential starting point.

Judgment is also essential. It provides a basis for deciding what data to use, how to use the data, and what statistical techniques, if any, to use. In many cases (such as introductions of new products or new competitive situations), managers who have insufficient data have to base their forecasts mainly on judgment.

As mentioned in Section 9.2, a forecast must specify the time frame, marketing plan, and expected market conditions for which it is valid. Changes in any of these factors will change the forecast.

A forecast applies to a given period. Extrapolating to a longer or shorter period is risky; conditions may change. The time frame varies according to the forecast's use. For example, a staffing plan may need a forecast for only the next few weeks. Additional staff can be hired over a longer time horizon. In contrast, budget plans usually need a forecast for the coming year. Organizations usually set their budgets a year in advance on the basis of projected sales. Strategic plans usually need a forecast for the next several years. Longer forecasts are generally less detailed and less reliable, but managers know to take these factors into account when they develop and use them.

Forecasts should be as short term as possible. A forecast for next month's sales will usually be more accurate than forecasts for the distant future, which are likely to be less accurate because important facts will have changed. Your competitors today are likely to be your competitors in a month. Your competitors in two years are likely to be different from your competitors today, so a forecast based on current market conditions will be poor.

Marketing plan changes will influence the forecast. A clinic that increases its advertising expects visits to increase. A forecast that does not consider this increase will usually be inaccurate. Increasing discounts to pharmacy benefits managers should result in increased sales for a pharmaceutical firm. Again, a forecast that does not account for additional discounts will usually be deficient. Any major changes in an organization's marketing efforts should change forecasts. If they do not, the organization should reassess the usefulness of its marketing initiatives.

Changes in market conditions also influence forecasts. For example, a major plant closing would probably reduce a local plastic surgeon's volume. Plant employees who had intended to undergo plastic surgery may opt to delay this elective procedure, and prospective patients who work for similar plants may defer discretionary spending in fear that they too may lose their jobs. Alternatively, a hospital closure will probably cause a competing hospital to forecast more inpatient days. Historical data have limited value in projecting such an effect if a similar closure has not occurred in the past. Approval of a new drug by the Food and Drug Administration should cause a pharmaceutical firm to forecast a decrease in sales for its competing product. This sort of change in market conditions is familiar, and the firm's marketing staff will probably draw on experience to predict the loss.

Analysts routinely use three forecasting methods: **percentage adjustment, moving averages**, and **seasonalized regression analysis**. If the data are adequate and the market has not changed too much, seasonalized regression analysis is the preferred method. However, whether the data are adequate and whether the market has changed too much are judgment calls.

Percentage adjustment increases or decreases the last period's sales volume by a percentage the analyst deems sensible. For example, if a hospital had an average daily census of 100 the previous quarter, and an analyst expects the census to fall an average of 1 percent per quarter, a reasonable forecast would be a census of 99. Because of its simplicity, managers often use percentage adjustment; however, this simplicity is also a shortcoming. In principle, a manager can use any percentage adjustment that he or she wants to. Without some requirement that percentage adjustments be well justified, this approach may not yield accurate forecasts. For example, a manager might justify a request for a new position based on a forecast that average daily census will increase by 5 percent, even though the average daily census had been falling for the last 14 quarters. In addition, percentage adjustment does not allow for seasonal effects. (*Seasonal effects* are systematic tendencies for particular days, weeks, months, or quarters to have above- or below-average volume.)

Demand theory can be used to add rigor to percentage adjustment. For example, if the price of a product has changed, an estimate of the percentage change in sales can be calculated by multiplying the percentage change in price by the price elasticity of demand. So, if an organization has chosen to raise prices by 3 percent and faces a price elasticity of demand of –4, sales will drop by 12 percent. Similar calculations can be used if the price of a substitute, the price of a complement, or consumer income has changed.

The moving-average method uses the average of data from recent periods to forecast sales. This method works well for short-term forecasts, although it tends to hide emerging trends and seasonal effects. Exhibit 9.1 shows census data and a one-year moving average for a sample hospital.

Exhibit 9.1 also illustrates the calculation of a seasonalized regression format. Excel was used to estimate a regression model with a trend (a variable that increases in value as time passes) and three quarter indicators. The variable Q_1 has a value of one if the data are from the first quarter; otherwise, its value is zero. Q_2 equals one if the data are from the second quarter, and Q_3 equals one if the data are from the third quarter. For technical reasons,

Percentage adjustment
Percentage adjustment of the past *n* periods of historic demand (The adjustment is essentially a best guess of what is expected to happen in the next year.)

Moving average
The unweighted mean of the previous *n* data points

Seasonalized regression analysis
A least squares regression that includes variables that identify subperiods (e.g., weeks) that historically have had above- or below-trend sales

Quarter	Census	Moving Average	First	Second	Third	Trend
1	99		1	0	0	1
2	109		0	1	0	2
3	101		0	0	1	3
4	107		0	0	0	4
5	104	104.0	1	0	0	5
6	116	105.3	0	1	0	6
7	100	107.0	0	0	1	7
8	106	106.8	0	0	0	8
9	103	106.5	1	0	0	9
10	107	106.3	0	1	0	10
11	90	104.0	0	0	1	11
12	105	101.5	0	0	0	12
13	102	101.3	1	0	0	13
14	94	101.0	0	1	0	14
15	98	97.8	0	0	1	15
16	104	99.8	0	0	0	16
17	99	99.5	1	0	0	17
18	105	98.8	0	1	0	18
19	94	101.5	0	0	1	19
20	102	100.5	0	0	0	20
21	100	100.0	1	0	0	21
22		100.3				

EXHIBIT 9.1
Census Data for a Sample Hospital

Seasonalized Regression Model

	Coefficient	t-statistic	
Intercept	108.811	40.90	$R^2 = 0.55$
First quarter	−3.968	−1.53	$F_{(4,20)} = 4.98$
Second quarter	0.732	0.27	$p = 0.01$
Third quarter	−8.534	−3.16	
Trend	−0.334	−2.16	

Mean absolute deviation

The average absolute difference between a forecast and the actual value (It is absolute because it converts both 9 and −9 to 9. The Excel function *ABS()* performs this conversion.)

the average response in the fourth quarter is represented by the constant. A negative regression coefficient for trend indicates that the census is in a downward trend. The results also show that the typical third-quarter census is smaller than average because the coefficient for Q_3 is large, negative, and statistically significant.

The forecast based on seasonalized regression analysis is calculated as follows: $108.811 + (−0.334 \times 22) + 0.732$. Here, 108.811 is the estimate of the constant, −0.334 is the estimate of the trend coefficient, 22 is the quarter to which the forecast applies, and 0.732 is the estimate of the Q_2 coefficient. Therefore, the seasonalized forecast is 102.2, slightly higher than the forecast based on the moving average. Overall the seasonalized forecast is a little more accurate than the one-year moving average. The **mean absolute deviation** for the regression is 2.3 for periods 5 through 21, and the mean absolute deviation for the moving average is 4.0.

Exhibit 9.2 shows an overview of the forecasting process. The main message of this exhibit is that a forecast is one part of the overall product

EXHIBIT 9.2

An Overview of the Forecasting Process

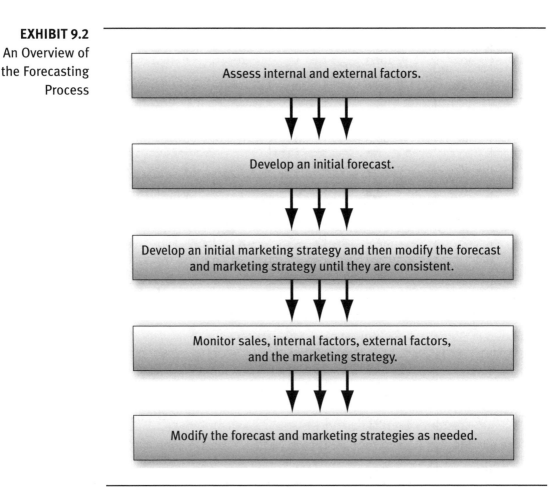

Assess internal and external factors.

Develop an initial forecast.

Develop an initial marketing strategy and then modify the forecast and marketing strategy until they are consistent.

Monitor sales, internal factors, external factors, and the marketing strategy.

Modify the forecast and marketing strategies as needed.

management process. In addition, the forecast will change as managers' assessments of relevant internal factors (e.g., cost and quality), external factors (e.g., the competitive environment and reimbursement levels), and the marketing plan change.

Simple Forecasting Techniques

A naïve forecast uses the value for the last period as the forecast for the next period—in other words, a 0 percent adjustment forecast. Exhibit 9.3 shows an example of a naïve forecast. A moving-average forecast uses the average of the last *n* values, where *n* is the number of preceding values used in the forecast. For example, the first entry in the Two-Period Moving Average column in Exhibit 9.3 equals (189 + 217) ÷ 2, or 203.

Month	Sales	Naïve Forecast	Two-Period Moving-Average Forecast
February	189		
March	217	189	
April	211	217	203
May	239	211	214
June	234	239	225
July	243	234	236.5

EXHIBIT 9.3
Naïve and Moving-Average Forecasting Techniques

To compare forecasting techniques, analysts sometimes use the mean absolute deviation, which is the average of the forecast's absolute deviations from the actual value. (When using the absolute deviation, it doesn't matter if a value is higher or lower than the actual value; all the deviations are positive numbers.) For April through July, the naïve forecast above has a mean absolute deviation of 12.0, and the two-period moving-average forecast has a mean absolute deviation of 12.1. From this perspective, the naïve forecast performs a little better.

These (and other) mechanistic forecasting methods do not allow managers to explore how changes in the environment are likely to affect sales. How would changes in insurance coverage change sales? Naïve forecasts and moving-average forecasts are little help in such situations.

9.4 What Matters?

Assessment of external factors (i.e., factors beyond the organization's control) is vital to forecasting. General economic conditions are a prime example. Expected inflation and interest rates are good indicators of the state of the economy. Local market conditions, such as business rents and local wages, also play an important role.

Government actions also can have a major impact on healthcare firms. For example, changes in Medicare rates affect most healthcare firms. Alternatively, regulations can have a significant effect on costs. Expansion of Medicaid eligibility can have major effects on some hospitals and minor effects on others. These sorts of changes will also affect most of your competitors, but forecasters would be ill advised to ignore changes in government policy.

The plans of key competitors must also be considered. Closure of a competing clinic or hospital can increase volume significantly and quickly. Introduction of a generic drug can have a dramatic effect on a pharmaceutical manufacturer. Changes in competitors' pricing policies can have a major impact on sales.

Technological change is always an important issue. If a rival gains a technological advantage, your sales can drop sharply. For example, if a rival introduces minimally invasive coronary artery bypass graft surgery, admissions to your cardiac unit will probably drop significantly until you adopt similar technology. In other cases, your own advances may affect sales of substitute products. For example, introduction of highly reliable MRI may sharply reduce the demand for conventional colonoscopy. Keep in mind, however, that if you don't introduce technologies that add value for your customers, someone else will. A decision not to introduce an attractive product because it will cannibalize sales is usually a mistake.

Finally, although markets usually change slowly, differences in general market characteristics (e.g., median income and percentage with insurance coverage) may be important in forecasting sales of a new product.

Developing a Five-Year Forecast

Beech (2001) shows how to develop a five-year forecast for a hospital's strategic financial plan. He begins the analysis by defining the hospital's service area and then estimating how the population of the service area will change during the next five years in terms of gender and

(continued)

(continued)

age. Next, Beech uses several data sources to forecast admission rates and length of stay for the services used by these population groups. (The hospital characterizes these services as medical and surgical, obstetrics and gynecology, pediatric, and psychiatric.) He then uses the hospital's own data and his estimates of overall admission rates and length of stay to calculate the hospital's market share for medical and surgical services, obstetric and gynecological services, pediatric services, and psychiatric services.

On the basis of these market share estimates, Beech develops four demand forecasts. His baseline forecast predicts that the hospital's market share and overall utilization will not change. His decreased utilization forecast predicts that overall days of care will drop by 10 percent but that the hospital will maintain its market share. His decreased market share forecast predicts that the hospital's market share will fall by 2 percent, and his increased market share forecast predicts that the hospital's market share will rise by 2 percent. (The decreased market share and increased market share forecasts predict that utilization rates will not change.) History suggests that Beech's decreased utilization forecast is most likely to occur. To the relief of the hospital's management, the area's population growth will offset most of the drop in days of care per thousand residents, so overall days of care will drop by less than 1 percent. However, this scenario implies that pediatric days will drop by more than 7 percent, so the hospital will need to look carefully at costs in this service line.

Assessment of internal factors (i.e., factors within an organization's control) is also vital to forecasting. For example, existing production may limit sales, or may have limited sales in the past. If so, changes in capacity or productivity need to be considered. Changes in the availability of resources and personnel can also have a powerful effect on sales. For many healthcare organizations, the entry or exit of a key physician can dramatically shape volume. In addition, changes in the size, support, composition, and organization of the sales staff can affect sales dramatically. For instance, a small drug firm may experience a large increase in sales if one of its products is marketed by a larger firm's sales staff.

Failures or improvements in key systems can also have dramatic effects on sales. Breakdowns in a clinic's phone or scheduling system may drive away potential customers. Fixing the phone system, in contrast, might be the most effective marketing campaign the clinic ever launched.

CASE 9.2   Forecasting the Demand for Transfusions

"Our blood inventories are shrinking," said Drew, the director of trans-fusion services, "and I'm worried that we might not be able to supply our customers if there's a surge in demand. We need to do something. And it needs to be smart, because the shelf life of blood is only six weeks. Simply collecting more may not solve our problem."

At this point, Kim, the marketing analyst, chimed in, "We need to do more than just predict our annual volume. We need a monthly forecast. That way we can target our drives so that we collect enough blood shortly before we expect to use it. Less blood will expire, and we will only need to address unexpected spikes in use."

"The good news," said Taylor, the assistant director of transfu-sion services, "is that we have monthly data for the last six years. We should be able to use them. I know that in 2004 Dr. Pereira tested a number of time-series models and suggested several that work rea-sonably well. I think he found some clear seasonal effects."

Discussion questions:
- What sort of model would you recommend to predict the demand for blood? What would you do with your predictions?
- Why would the presence of seasonal effects be important?
- Taylor suggested using a statistical model to forecast demand. What judgment does a statistical model require?
- What sorts of changes in the environment would you need to account for in your forecasting model?

9.5 Conclusion

Making and interpreting forecasts are important tasks for healthcare manag-ers. Not only are most crucial decisions based on sales forecasts, but also the consequences of overestimating or underestimating demand can be cata-strophic. Overestimating demand can put the financial future of an organiza-tion at risk, whereas underestimating demand can compromise the care of patients and harm the organization's reputation.

Analysts should apply demand theory to their sales forecasts to better recognize changes. Demand theory limits what analysts need to consider: the price of the product, the price of substitutes, and the price of complements. The key idea of demand theory is that the out-of-pocket price drives most consumer demand. The amount the consumer has to pay depends largely on the terms of his or her insurance contract. Is the product covered? What is the required copayment? Changes in the answers to these two questions can shift sales sharply. The same concerns affect the prices of substitutes. The most important substitutes are similar products offered by rivals, but other products that meet some of the same needs should also be considered.

Demographic factors are important. Population size, income per capita, the age distribution of the population, the ethnic makeup of the population, and the insurance coverage of the population are some examples. Although vital, demographic factors tend to be stable in the short term. Demographics are much more important in long-range forecasts.

"Forecasting is hard, especially when it involves the future." This old saying reveals a core truth about forecasting: You often will be wrong. Knowing that, a shrewd manager will make decisions that can be modified as conditions change. The shrewd manager will also know which data are likely to be the most problematic or most variable and will monitor those data carefully.

Management decisions require sales forecasts. Off-the-cuff forecasts often fail to consider key factors and can lead to risky decisions. Imperfect forecasts can be used to make decisions as long as you recognize that your predictions will sometimes be wrong and you structure your decisions accordingly.

Exercises

9.1 The table lists visits for the four clinics operated by your system. You anticipate that volumes will increase by 4 percent next year. Forecast the number of visits for each clinic, and explain what assumptions underlie your forecasts. For example, are you sure that all of the clinics can serve additional clients?

Period	Clinic 1	Clinic 2	Clinic 3	Clinic 4	Total
This year	16,640	41,600	24,960	33,280	116,480
Next year	?	?	?	?	121,139

9.2 Your data for the clinics in Exercise 9.1 suggest that Clinic 2 is operating at capacity and is highly efficient. Its output is unlikely to increase. Furthermore, Clinic 4 has unused capacity but is unlikely to attract additional patients. How would these facts change your answer to Exercise 9.1? Continue to assume that overall volume will rise to 121,139.

9.3 You estimate that the price elasticity of demand for clinic visits is –0.25. You anticipate that a major insurer will increase the copayment from $20 to $25. This insurer covers 40,000 of your patients, and those patients average 2.5 visits per year. What is your forecast of the change in the number of visits?

9.4 A major employer has just added health insurance coverage for its employees. Consequently, 5,000 of your patients will pay a $30 copayment rather than the list price of $100 per visit. These patients average 2.2 visits per year. You believe the price elasticity of demand is between –0.15 and –0.35. What is your forecast of the change in the number of visits?

9.5 The table shows data on asthma-related visits. Is there evidence that these visits vary by quarter? Can you detect a trend? A powerful test would be to run a multiple regression in Excel. If the function is already loaded, you will find it in Data > Data Analysis > Regression. If not, get help in adding the Analysis Tool Pak. To test for quarterly differences, create a variable called Q1 that equals 1 if the data are for the first quarter and 0 otherwise, a variable called Q2 that equals 1 if the data are for the second quarter and 0 otherwise, and a variable called Q4 that equals 1 if the data are for the fourth quarter and 0 otherwise. (Because you will accept the default, which is to have a constant term in your regression equation, do not include an indicator variable for quarter 3.) Also create a variable called Trend that increases by 1 each quarter.

Year	Q1	Q2	Q3	Q4
2001			1,513	1,060
2002	1,431	1,123	994	679
2003	1,485	886	1,256	975
2004	1,256	1,156	1,163	1,062
2005	1,200	1,072	1,563	531
2006	1,022	1,169		

9.6 Your marketing department estimates that Medicare urology visits equal $5 - (1.0 \times C) + (-6.5 \times T_O) + (5 \times T_R) + (0.01 \times Y)$. Here, C denotes the Medicare copayment (now $20), T_O is waiting time in your clinic (now 30 minutes), T_R is waiting time in your competitor's clinic (now 40 minutes), and Y is per capita income (now $40,000).

a. How many visits do you anticipate?

b. Medicare's allowed fee is $120. What revenue do you anticipate?

c. What might change your forecast of visits and revenue?

9.7 Because of fluctuations in insurance coverage, the average price paid out of pocket (P) by patients of an urgent care center varied, as the table shows. The number of visits per month (Q) also varied, and an analyst believes the two are related. The analyst also thinks the data show a trend. Run a regression of Q on P and *Period* to test these hypotheses. Then use the estimated parameters a, b, and c and the values of *Month* and P to predict Q (number of visits). The prediction equation is $Q = a + (b \times Month) + (c \times P)$.

Month	1	2	3	4	5	6	7	8	9	10	11	12
P	$21	$18	$15	$24	$18	$21	$18	$15	$20	$19	$24	$20
Q	193	197	256	179	231	214	247	273	223	225	198	211

9.8 Use the data in Exercise 9.7 to answer these questions:

a. Calculate the naïve estimator, which is $Q_t = Q_{t-1}$.

b. Calculate the two-period moving-average forecast.

c. Calculate the mean absolute deviation for the regression forecast, the naïve forecast, and the two-period moving-average forecast.

d. Which forecast seems to perform the best? Why?

9.9 Sales data are displayed in the table.

Month	Sales	Month	Sales
February	224	January	260
March	217	February	284
April	211	March	280
May	239	April	271
June	234	May	302
July	243	June	286
August	238	July	297
September	243	August	301
October	251	September	309
November	259	October	314
December	270		

    a. Calculate the naïve estimator, which is $Sales_t = Sales_{t-1}$.

    b. Calculate the two-period and three-period moving averages.

    c. Calculate the mean absolute deviation for each of the forecasting methods.

9.10 A pharmaceutical company produces a sinus medicine. Monthly sales (in thousands of doses) for the past three years are shown in the table.

Jan	Feb	Mar	Apr	May	June	July	Aug	Sept	Oct	Nov	Dec
6,788	8,020	1,848	410	586	2,260	2,232	8,018	9,384	6,916	5,698	6,940
9,136	7,420	3,350	1,998	1,972	3,572	4,506	10,474	13,358	8,232	8,218	10,248
9,628	7,826	3,528	2,126	2,070	3,762	4,754	11,010	14,040	8,646	8,634	10,782

    a. Develop a regression model that allows for trend and seasonal components. Obtain the Excel output for this model.

    b. Calculate a two-period moving-average forecast.

    c. Compare the mean absolute deviations for these approaches.

    d. Use one of these models to forecast sales for each month of year 3.

References

Aven, T. 2013. "On How to Deal with Deep Uncertainties in a Risk Assessment and Management Context." *Risk Analysis* 33 (12): 2082–91.

Beech, A. J. 2001. "Market-Based Demand Forecasting Promotes Informed Strategic Financial Planning." *Healthcare Financial Management* 55 (11): 46–56.

Pereira, A. 2004. "Performance of Time-Series Methods in Forecasting the Demand for Red Blood Cell Transfusion." *Transfusion* 44 (5): 739–46.

SUPPLY AND DEMAND ANALYSIS

Learning Objectives

After reading this chapter, students will be able to

- define demand and supply curves,
- interpret demand and supply curves,
- use demand and supply analysis to make simple forecasts, and
- identify factors that shift demand and supply curves.

Key Concepts

- A *supply curve* describes how much producers are willing to sell at different prices.
- A *demand curve* describes how much consumers are willing to buy at different prices.
- A demand curve describes how much consumers are willing to pay at different levels of output.
- At the *equilibrium price*, producers want to sell the amount that consumers want to buy.
- Markets generally move toward equilibrium outcomes.
- Expansion of insurance usually makes the equilibrium price and quantity rise.
- Insurance and professional advice influence the demand for medical goods and services.
- Regulation and technology influence the supply of medical goods and services.
- Demand and supply curves shift when a factor other than the product price changes.

10.1 Introduction

Healthcare markets are in a constant state of flux. Prices rise and fall. Volumes rise and fall. New products succeed at first and then fall by the wayside. Familiar products falter and revive. Economics teaches us that, underneath the seemingly random fluctuations of healthcare markets, systematic patterns can be detected. Understanding these systematic patterns requires an understanding of supply and demand. Even though healthcare managers need to focus on the details of day-to-day operations, they also need an appreciation of the overview that supply and demand analysis can give them.

The basics of supply and demand illustrate the usefulness of economics. Even with little data, managers can forecast the effects of changes in policy or demographics using a supply and demand analysis. For example, the impact of added taxes on hospitals' prices, the impact of increased insurance coverage on the output mix of physicians, and the impact of higher electricity prices on pharmacies' prices can be analyzed. Supply and demand analysis is a powerful tool that managers can use to make broad strategic decisions or detailed pricing decisions.

10.1.1 Supply Curves

Exhibit 10.1 is a basic supply and demand diagram. The vertical axis shows the price of the good or service. In this simple case, the price sellers receive is the same price buyers pay. (Insurance and taxes complicate matters because the price the buyer pays is different from the price the seller receives.) The horizontal axis shows the quantity customers bought and producers sold.

EXHIBIT 10.1
Equilibrium

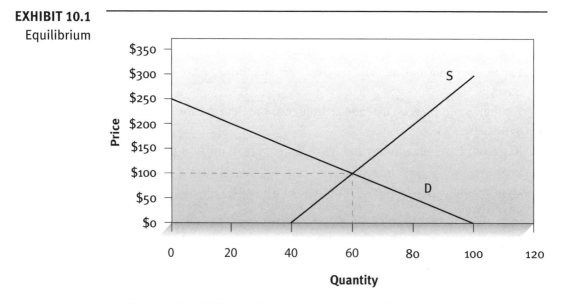

The **supply curve** (labeled S) describes how much producers are willing to sell at different prices. From another perspective, it describes what the price must be to induce producers to sell different quantities. The supply curve in Exhibit 10.1 slopes up, as do most supply curves. This upward slope means that, when the price is higher, producers are willing to sell *more of a good or service* or *more producers* are willing to sell a good or service. When the price is higher, producers are more willing to add workers, equipment, and other resources to sell more. In addition, higher prices allow firms to enter a market they could not enter at lower prices. When prices are low, only the most efficient firms can profitably participate in a market. When prices are higher, firms with higher costs can also earn acceptable profits.

Supply curve
A graphic depiction of how much producers are willing to sell at different prices

10.1.2 Demand Curves

The **demand curve** (labeled D) describes how much consumers are willing to buy at different prices. From another perspective, it describes how much the marginal consumer (the one who would not make a purchase at a higher price) is willing to pay at different levels of output. The demand curve in Exhibit 10.1 slopes down, meaning that, for producers to sell more of a product, its price must be cut. Such a sales increase might be the result of an increase in the share of the population that buys a good or service, an increase in consumption per purchaser, or some mix of the two.

Demand curve
A graphic depiction of how much consumers are willing to buy at different prices

10.1.3 Equilibrium

The demand and supply curves intersect at the **equilibrium price** and quantity. At the equilibrium price, the amount producers want to sell equals the amount consumers want to buy. In Exhibit 10.1, consumers want to buy 60 units and producers want to sell 60 units when the price is $100.

Markets tend to move toward equilibrium points. If the price is above the equilibrium price, producers will not meet their sales forecasts. Sometimes producers cut prices to sell more. Sometimes producers cut production. Either strategy tends to equate supply and demand. Alternatively, if the price is below the equilibrium price, consumers will quickly buy up the available stock. To meet this **shortage**, producers may raise prices or produce more. Either strategy tends to equate supply and demand.

Markets will not always be in equilibrium, especially if conditions change quickly, but the incentive to move toward equilibrium is strong. Producers typically can change prices faster than they can increase or decrease production. A high price today does not mean a high price tomorrow. Prices are likely to fall as additional capacity becomes available. Likewise, a low price today does not mean a low price tomorrow. Prices are likely to rise as capacity decreases. We will explore this concept in more detail in our examination of the effects of managed care on the incomes of primary care physicians.

Equilibrium price
Price at which the quantity demanded equals the quantity supplied (There is no shortage or surplus.)

Shortage
Situation in which the quantity demanded at the prevailing price exceeds the quantity supplied (The best indication of a shortage is that prices are rising.)

10.1.4 Professional Advice and Imperfect Competition

Healthcare markets are complex. The influence of professional advice on consumer choices is a complication of particular concern. The assumption that changes in supply will not affect consumers' choices (i.e., demand) can be misleading. If changes in factors that ought not to affect consumers' choices (such as providers' financial arrangements with insurers) influence providers' recommendations, a supply and demand analysis that does not take this effect into account could be equally misleading. Even more important, few healthcare markets fit the model of a competitive market (i.e., a market with many competitors who perceive they have little influence on the market price). We must condition any analysis on the judgment that healthcare markets are competitive enough that conventional supply curves are useful guides. In markets that are not competitive enough, producers' responses to changes in market conditions are likely to be more complex than supply curves suggest. This text focuses on applications of demand and supply analysis in which neither providers' influence on demand nor imperfect competition is likely to be a problem.

10.2 Demand and Supply Shifts

A movement along a demand curve is called a *change in the quantity demanded*. In other words, a movement along a demand curve traces the link between the price consumers are willing to pay and the quantity they demand. Demand and supply analysis is most useful to healthcare managers in understanding how the equilibrium price and quantity will change in response to shifts in demand or supply. With limited information, a working manager can sketch the impact of a change in policy on the markets of most concern.

What factors might cause the demand curve to shift to the right (greater demand at every price or higher prices for every quantity)? We need detailed empirical work to verify the responses of demand to market conditions, but the list of standard responses is short. Typically, a shift to the right results from an increase in income, an increase in the price of a substitute (a good or service used instead of the product in question), a decrease in the price of a complement (a good or service used along with the product in question), or a change in tastes.

Economists often use mathematical notation to describe demand. $Q = D(P,Y)$ is an example of this notation. It says that the quantity demanded varies with prices (represented by P) and income (represented by Y), which means that quantity, the relevant prices, and income are systematically related. A demand curve traces this relationship when income and all prices other than the price of the product itself do not change.

What factors might cause the supply curve to shift to the right (greater supply at every price or lower prices at every quantity)? Typically, a shift to the right results from a reduction in the price of an input, an improvement in technology, or an easing of regulations. In mathematical notation, we can describe supply as $Q = S(P, W)$. Here, W represents the prices of inputs (the factors such as labor, land, equipment, buildings, and supplies that a business uses to produce its product). Unless technology or regulations are the focus of an analysis, we do not make their role explicit.

CASE 10.1   Worrying About Demand Shifts

"You know, this business is changing," said Terry, the business manager. "It used to be that an administrator like me had to worry only about running a good nursing home and keeping an eye on the other nursing homes in town, but these days we have more competitors than I can shake a stick at. Some of the folks at Sunshine Assisted Living would have been residents in our nursing home a few years ago. Not today, though. We admit their residents only when they are getting close to needing total care. Without changing offices, I feel like I switched from running a nursing home to running a hospice. The thing that has me spooked, though, is this new home health agency. It has billboards out on the interstate with a picture of a senior citizen and a slogan that says, 'Stay healthy. Stay active. Stay home.' I'm worried that it will siphon off a significant part of our residents. It's just supply and demand."

With that Terry jumped up, went over to the whiteboard, and drew a simple graph (Exhibit 10.2). "Here's where we are today. We have a

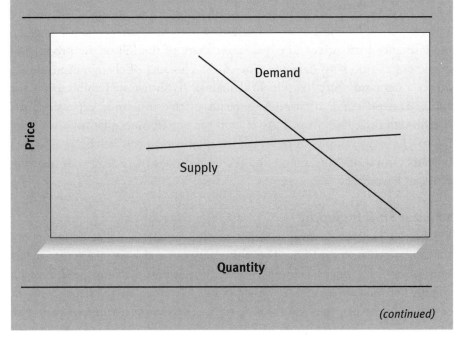

EXHIBIT 10.2
Terry's Supply and Demand Graph

(continued)

CASE 10.1
(continued)

census of about 150, and we're doing fine. But when those home health folks are done with us, we'll be lucky to have a census of 100. I'm worried."

"Whoa, partner," interrupted Tracey, who handled marketing. "I like the graph, but I don't think a home health agency is going to have that sort of impact on us. A 2007 study out of Brown University by Gruneir and colleagues did not find the impact you are describing. I just don't think many of our residents are candidates for home health services. By the time we see them, they need more care than most home health agencies can offer."

Discussion questions:

- Exhibit 10.2 shows the current situation. What did Terry think the graph would look like after the home health care agency entered the market? What did Tracey think the new graph would look like?
- Over the next few years, what demographic changes seem likely to shift the demand for nursing home care?
- What changes in the local market might cause the sort of shift in demand that Terry is concerned about?

10.2.1 A Shift in Demand

We begin our demand and supply analyses by looking at a classical problem in health economics: What will happen to the equilibrium price and quantity of a product used by consumers if insurance expands? Insurance expands when the insurance plan agrees to pay a larger share of the bill or the proportion of the population with insurance increases. This sort of change in insurance causes a **demand shift** (or shift in demand). As shown in Exhibit 10.3, the entire demand curve rotates. As a result of this insurance expansion, the equilibrium price rises from P_1 to P_2 and the equilibrium quantity rises from Q_1 to Q_2. For example, as coverage for pharmaceuticals has become a part of more Americans' insurance, the prices and sales of prescription pharmaceuticals have risen.

Demand shift
A shift that occurs when a factor other than the price of the product itself (e.g., consumer incomes) changes

10.2.2 A Shift in Supply

Exhibit 10.4 depicts a **supply shift** (or shift in supply). The supply curve has contracted from S_1 to S_2. This shift means that at every price, producers want to supply a smaller volume. Alternatively, it means that to produce each volume, producers require a higher price. A change in regulations might result in a shift like the one from S_1 to S_2. For example, suppose that state

Supply shift
Shift that occurs when a factor (e.g., an input price) other than the price of the product changes

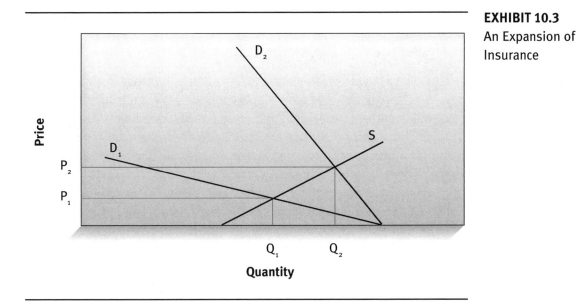

EXHIBIT 10.3
An Expansion of
Insurance

regulations mandated improved care planning and record keeping for nursing homes. Some nursing homes might close down, but the majority would raise prices for private-pay patients to cover the increased cost of care. The net effect would be an increase in the equilibrium price from P_1 to P_2 and a reduction in the equilibrium quantity from Q_1 to Q_2. A manager should be able to forecast this effect with no information other than the realization that the demand for nursing home care is relatively inelastic (meaning that the slope of the demand curve is steep) and that the regulation would shift the supply curve inward.

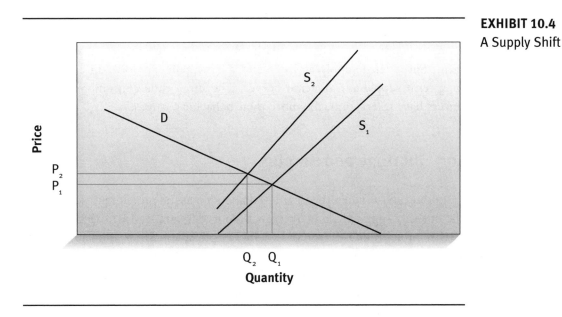

EXHIBIT 10.4
A Supply Shift

The Supply of Physicians' Services

Empirical analyses of supply usually find that an increase in earnings results in higher volume (i.e., supply curves usually slope up). Rizzo and Blumenthal (1994) found that young, male, self-employed physicians fit this pattern. A 1 percent increase in hourly earnings increased annual practice hours by 0.23 percent. One reason that the response was so muted is that an increase in hourly earnings also increases total income, and having a higher income usually leads to a reduction in hours. Confirming this supposition, these authors found that a 1 percent increase in income from all sources reduced annual hours by 0.26 percent. Many young physicians have spouses with high earning potential, which also tends to reduce hours. A 1 percent increase in a physician's spouse's income reduced annual hours by 0.02 percent. In other words, the study found that change in either nonpractice income or in a spouse's earnings shifts the supply curve. So, both practice and nonpractice earnings affected annual hours of work. As is usually the case in labor supply analyses, both effects were relatively small.

The implication for managers is that financial incentives may have modest effects on the decisions of higher-income workers. Managers may need to emphasize the intrinsic rewards of work (or pay a lot to change behavior).

Responses to changing market conditions depend on how much time passes. A change in technology, such as the development of a new surgical technique, initially will have little effect on supply. Over time, however, as more surgeons become familiar with the technique, its impact on supply will grow. Short-term supply and demand curves generally look different from long-term supply and demand curves. The more time consumers and producers have to respond, the more their behavior changes.

10.3 Shortage and Surplus

A shortage exists when the quantity demanded at the prevailing price exceeds the quantity supplied. In markets that are free to adjust, the price should rise so that equilibrium is restored. At a higher price, less will be demanded, leaving a greater supply.

In some markets, though, prices cannot adjust, often because a public or private insurer sets prices too low and consumers demand more than producers are willing to supply. Exhibit 10.5 depicts a shortage situation. The

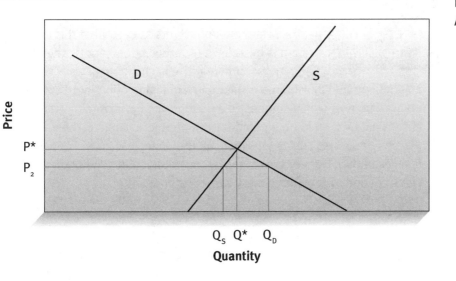

EXHIBIT 10.5
A Shortage

equilibrium price is P* and the equilibrium quantity is Q*, but the insurer has set a price of P_2, so consumers demand Q_D and producers supply Q_S. Because the price cannot adjust, a shortage equal to $Q_D - Q_S$ exists.

A **surplus** exists when the quantity supplied at the prevailing price exceeds the quantity demanded. In markets that are free to adjust, the price should fall so that equilibrium is restored. In some markets, prices are free to fall but do so slowly. For example, in the 1990s, many hospitals had unfilled hospital beds because the combination of managed care and new technology reduced the demand for inpatient care. Over time, insurance companies used this excess capacity to secure much lower rates (even though Medicare and Medicaid rates remained unchanged), and enough hospitals closed or downsized to eliminate the excess capacity.

Surplus
Situation in which the quantity supplied at the prevailing price exceeds the quantity demanded (The best indication of a surplus is that prices are falling.)

CASE 10.2	How Large Will the Shortage of Primary Care Physicians Be?

The Affordable Care Act (ACA) has increased the share of the population with health insurance. Most of the newly insured were reasonably healthy and viewed health insurance as too expensive, given its likely benefits. As a result, the ACA will primarily affect the demand for primary care services, and many anticipate a shortage of primary care physicians (Robeznieks 2013).

(continued)

CASE 10.2
(continued)

Some other observers suggest that this concern is overblown (Auerbach et al. 2013). The production of primary care is changing in ways that shift its supply. One change is the rapid expansion of patient-centered medical homes, which emphasize a greater role for technology, physician assistants, and nurse practitioners. Another change is the growth of nurse-managed clinics (of which MinuteClinic, discussed in Case 7.1, is an example). Both of these innovations reduce the number of physicians needed to provide primary care for a population.

Discussion questions:
- Set up a model of the demand and supply for primary care physicians. (It should have salary on the vertical axis and number of primary care physicians on the horizontal axis.) Assuming that the production of primary care does not change (i.e., the supply curve does not shift), how do you expect the market equilibrium to change?
- How have the incomes of primary care physicians changed in the last few years? Are these changes consistent with your prediction? (You can get income data from Medscape Physician Compensation Reports.)
- Are the changes in the incomes of primary care physicians consistent with the prediction of a shortage? That is, have they risen rapidly?
- If retail clinics and patient-centered medical homes continue to expand, how will they affect the market equilibrium? Which curve would shift as a result—demand or supply?

10.4 Analyses of Multiple Markets

Demand and supply models can also be helpful in forecasting the effects of shifts in one market on the equilibrium in another. Such forecasts can be made only if the markets are related—that is, the products need to be complements or substitutes.

Spetz and colleagues (2006) provided an example of this effect. They showed that the demand for licensed practical nurses (LPNs) increased as the wages of registered nurses (RNs) rose (as a result of the shortage of RNs) (see Exhibit 10.6). Increases in the wages of RNs shifted the demand curve for LPNs from D_1 to D_2. As a result, employment of LPNs rose from Q_1 to Q_2 and wages rose from W_1 to W_2.

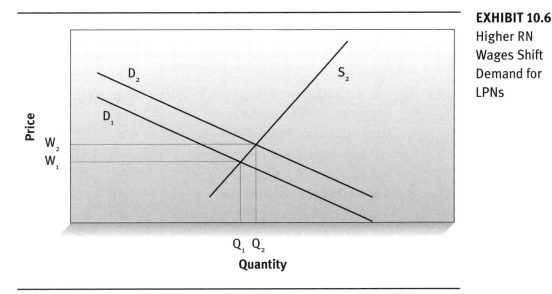

EXHIBIT 10.6
Higher RN
Wages Shift
Demand for
LPNs

Source: Data from Spetz et al. (2006).

10.5 Conclusion

Supply and demand analysis can help managers anticipate the effects of changes in policy, technology, or prices. Supply and demand analysis is a valuable tool that managers can use to quickly anticipate the effects of shifts in demand or supply curves. Short-term shifts in demand are likely to result from one of two factors: changes in insurance or shifts in the prices or characteristics of substitutes or complements. Short-term shifts in supply are likely to result from one of three factors: changes in regulations, shifts in the prices or characteristics of inputs, or changes in technology.

Most demand curves slope down, which means that consumers will buy more if prices are lower. It also means that consumers who are willing to purchase a product only at a low price do not place a high value on it. In contrast, most supply curves slope up, which means that higher prices will motivate producers to sell additional output (or motivate more producers to sell the same output).

Exercises

10.1 Physicians' offices supply some urgent care services (i.e., services patients seek for prompt attention but not for preservation of life or limb).

a. Name three other providers of urgent care services.

b. What sort of shift in supply or demand would result in a market equilibrium with higher prices and sales volume?

c. What might cause such a shift?

d. What sort of shift in supply or demand would result in a market equilibrium with higher prices but lower sales volume?

e. What might cause such a shift?

10.2 Suppose the market equilibrium price for immunizations is $40 and the volume is 25,000.

a. Identify three providers of immunization services.

b. What sort of shift in supply or demand would reduce both prices and sales volume?

c. What might cause such a shift?

d. What sort of shift in supply or demand would result in a market equilibrium with a price above $40 and a volume below 25,000?

e. What might cause such a shift?

10.3 The table contains data on the number of doses of an antihistamine sold per month in a small town.

Price	Demand	Supply
$10	185	208
$9	187	205
$8	188	202
$7	190	199
$6	191	196
$5	193	193
$4	194	190
$3	196	187
$2	197	184
$1	199	181

a. To sell 196 doses to customers, what will the price need to be?

b. For stores to be willing to sell 196 doses, what will the price need to be?

c. How many doses will customers want to buy if the price is $2?

d. How many doses will suppliers want to sell if the price is $2?

e. Is there excess supply or excess demand at $2?

f. What is the equilibrium price? How can you tell?

10.4 The table contains demand and supply data for eyeglasses in a local market.

Price	Demand	Supply
$300	7,400	8,320
$290	7,480	8,200
$280	7,520	8,080
$270	7,600	7,960
$260	7,640	7,840
$250	7,720	7,720
$240	7,760	7,600
$230	7,840	7,480
$220	7,880	7,360

a. At $280, how many pairs will consumers want to buy?
b. How many pairs will consumers want to buy if the price is $290?
c. How many pairs will stores want to sell at $290?
d. Is $290 the equilibrium price?
e. Is there excess supply or excess demand at $290?
f. What is the equilibrium price? How can you tell?

10.5 The exhibit shows a basic demand and supply graph for home care services. Identify the equilibrium price and quantity. Label them P* and Q*.

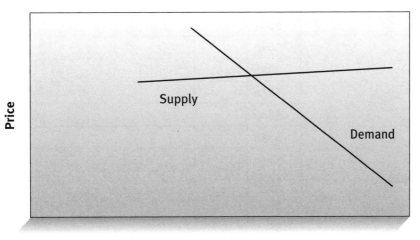

   a. Retirements drive up the wages of home care workers. How would the graph change? How would P* and Q* change?

   b. Improved technology lets home care workers monitor use of medications without going to clients' homes. How would the graph change? How would P* and Q* change?

   c. The number of people needing home care services increases. How would the graph change? How would P* and Q* change?

   d. A change in Medicare rules expands coverage for home care services. How would the graph change? How would P* and Q* change?

10.6 The demand function is $Q = 600 - P$, with P being the price paid by consumers. Put a list of prices ranging from $400 to $0 in a column labeled P. (Use intervals of $50.)

   a. Consumers have insurance with 40 percent coinsurance. For each price, calculate the amount that consumers pay. (Put this figure in a column labeled P_{Net}.)

   b. Calculate the quantity demanded when there is insurance. (Put this figure in a column labeled D_I.)

   c. Plot the demand curve, putting P (not P_{Net}) on the vertical axis.

   d. The quantity supplied equals $2 \times P$. Put these values in a column labeled S.

   e. What is the equilibrium price?

   f. How much do consumers spend?

   g. How much does the insurer spend?

10.7 The demand function is $Q = 1,000 - (0.5 \times P)$. P is the price paid by consumers. Calculate the quantity demanded when there is no insurance. (Put these values in column D_U of the table.)

P	D_U	P_{Net}	D_I	S
$1,000				
$960				
$920				
$880	560	$176	912	952
$840				
$800				
$760				
$720				
$680				
$640				
$600				
$560				

a. The state mandates coverage with 20 percent coinsurance, meaning that the demand function becomes $1,000 - (0.5 \times 0.2 \times P)$.

b. For each price, calculate the amount consumers pay. (Put this figure in column P_{Net}.)

c. Calculate the quantity demanded when there is insurance. (Put this figure in column D_I.)

d. Plot the two demand curves, putting P (not P_{Net}) on the vertical axis.

e. How do D_U and D_I differ? Which is more elastic?

10.8 The supply function for the product in Exercise 10.7 is $160 + (0.9 \times P)$. *P* is the price received by the seller. At the equilibrium price, the quantity demanded will equal the quantity supplied.

f. What was the equilibrium price before coverage? After?

g. After coverage begins, how much will the product cost insurers? How much will the product cost patients? How much did patients pay for the product before coverage started?

10.9 Consumers who can buy health insurance through an employer get a tax subsidy. Use demand and supply analysis to assess how this subsidy affects consumers who cannot buy insurance through an employer.

10.10 Why are price controls unlikely to make consumers better off if a market is reasonably competitive?

10.11 Make the business case why healthcare providers should advocate for expansion of insurance coverage for the poor.

References

Auerbach, D. I., P. G. Chen, M. W. Friedberg, R. Reid, C. Lau, P. I. Buerhaus, and A. Mehrotra. 2013. "Nurse-Managed Health Centers and Patient-Centered Medical Homes Could Mitigate Expected Primary Care Physician Shortage." *Health Affairs* 32 (11): 1933–41.

Gruneir, A., K. L. Lapane, S. C. Miller, and V. Mor. 2007. "Long-Term Care Market Competition and Nursing Home Dementia Special Care Units." *Medical Care* 45 (8): 739–45.

Rizzo, J. A., and D. Blumenthal. 1994. "Physician Labor Supply: Do Income Effects Matter?" *Journal of Health Economics* 13 (4): 433–53.

Robeznieks, A. 2013. "What Doctor Shortage? Some Experts Say Changes in Delivery Will Erase Need for More Physicians." *Modern Healthcare* 43 (45): 14–15.

Spetz, J., W. T. Dyer, S. Chapman, and J. A. Seago. 2006. "Hospital Demand for Licensed Practical Nurses." *Western Journal of Nursing Research* 28 (6): 726–39.

MAXIMIZING PROFITS

After reading this chapter, students will be able to

- define measures of profitability,
- describe two strategies for increasing profits,
- explain why a firm should expand if marginal revenue exceeds marginal cost,
- use a model to choose the profit-maximizing level of output, and
- discuss differences between for-profit and not-for-profit providers.

- All healthcare managers need to understand how to maximize profits.
- Most healthcare organizations are inefficient, so cost reductions can increase profits.
- To maximize profits, organizations should expand as long as marginal revenue exceeds marginal cost.
- *Marginal cost* is the change in total cost associated with a change in output.
- *Marginal revenue* is the change in total revenue associated with a change in output.
- Managers need to understand their costs and not confuse incremental cost with average cost.
- The agency problem arises because the goals of stakeholders may not coincide.

11.1 Introduction

Substantial numbers of healthcare managers serve firms that seek to maximize **profits**. For example, for-profit hospitals, most insurance firms, most physician groups, and a broad range of other organizations explicitly seek

Profits
Total revenue minus total cost

maximum profits. In addition, recognizing that "with no margin, there is no mission," many not-for-profit healthcare organizations act like profit-maximizing firms. And even organizations that are not exclusively focused on the bottom line must balance financial and other goals. Bankrupt organizations accomplish nothing. As a result, even healthcare managers with objectives other than maximizing profits need to understand how to maximize profits. A manager who does not understand the opportunity cost (in terms of forgone profits) of a strategic decision cannot lead effectively. All healthcare managers need to understand how to maximize profits. Finally, as markets become more competitive, the differences between for-profit and not-for-profit firms are likely to narrow.

Profits are the difference between total revenue and total cost. To maximize profits, you must identify the strategy that makes this difference the largest. In other words, identify the product price (or quantity) and characteristics that maximize the difference between total revenue and total cost.

11.2 Cutting Costs to Increase Profits

An obvious way to increase profits is to cut costs. Most healthcare organizations are inefficient, meaning that they could produce the same output at less cost or produce higher-quality output for the same cost. The inference that healthcare organizations are inefficient is based on two types of evidence. First, studies by quality management and reengineering teams have identified that costs can be reduced by increasing the quality of care. For example, a project at Appleton Medical Center reduced cost per case by 21 percent while increasing patient satisfaction by 30 percent (Toussaint, Gerard, and Adams 2010). The second type of evidence results from statistical studies. For example, a sophisticated study of hospital efficiency concluded that inefficiency represented more than 15 percent of costs (Zhivan and Diana 2012).

As Exhibit 11.1 illustrates, the payoff from cost reductions can be substantial. The organization in the exhibit earns $40,000 on revenue of $2.4 million. This operating margin (profits divided by revenue) of 1.7 percent

EXHIBIT 11.1
The Effects of
Cost Reductions
on Profits

	Status Quo	2% Cost Reduction
Quantity	24,000	24,000
Revenue	$2,400,000	$2,400,000
Cost	$2,360,000	$2,312,800
Profit	$40,000	$87,200

suggests that the organization is not very profitable. Reducing costs by only 2 percent changes this picture entirely. As long as the cost cuts represent more efficient operations, all of the cost reductions will increase profits, in this case by 118 percent.

CASE 11.1   Perfecting Patient Care

"I recommend we take the Lean production approach and apply process redesign to our nursing home," said Jamie. "This approach will help us reduce costs, improve employee satisfaction, and attract more residents."

"Thanks, Jamie," said Reilly, the system vice president for finance. "I appreciate your enthusiasm, but my experience has been that cost cutting always involves reducing the quality of care or increasing the pressure on employees. Our strategic vision is not consistent with either of those directions."

"Reilly, I'm going to have to disagree," interjected Logan, the chief operating officer. "My reading of the management literature on the Toyota Production System in healthcare confirms that Jamie is onto something. Waste pervades this place. We are doing things that residents don't want, and we are doing them inefficiently and unsafely. Eliminating wasted time and wasted materials will make life better for everyone. By teaching our managers how to help workers create safe, efficient work processes, we can transform this facility from a very good nursing home to a superb nursing home that makes lots of money. Lee and colleagues (2009) demonstrated that nursing homes are not efficient, and Graban (2012) showed that the approach that Jamie is recommending has worked in hospitals."

Discussion questions:

- Why is inefficiency common in healthcare? Doesn't competition force organizations to be efficient?
- What evidence do we have that process redesign can improve efficiency? Isn't process redesign just another name for making employees work harder? Is there evidence that employees will accept the redesign?
- Plenty of evidence indicates that problems with the quality of care harm patients, but won't improving quality cost more? How could better quality not cost more?

11.2.1 Cost Reduction Through Improved Clinical Management

Cost reductions often require improvements in clinical management because differences in costs are primarily driven by differences in resource use, not differences in the cost per unit of resource. (An organization cannot maximize profits if it overpays for the resources it uses.) In turn, differences in resource use are driven by differences in how clinical plans are designed and executed. Improvements in clinical management require physician cooperation and, more typically, physician involvement. Even though many healthcare professionals make clinical decisions, physicians in most settings have a primary role in decision making.

Having recognized the importance of physicians in increasing efficiency, managers need to ask whether the interests of the organization and its physicians are aligned. In other words, will changes that benefit the organization also benefit its physicians? If not, physicians cannot be expected to be enthusiastic participants in these activities, especially if the advantages for patients are not clear.

Managers are responsible for ensuring that the interests of individual physicians are aligned with the organization or for changing the environment. For example, physicians usually benefit from changes in clinical processes that improve the quality of care or make care more attractive to patients. If managers present the change proposal in this fashion, physicians may understand how they will benefit from the improvements. In other cases, however, physicians cannot be expected to participate in quality improvement activities without compensation. For independent physicians, explicit payments for participation may be required. The same may be true for employee physicians, or participation may be a part of their contractual obligations. In both cases, managers must be aware of the high opportunity cost of time spent away from clinical practice.

Where feasible, physicians' compensation can incorporate bonuses based on how well they meet or exceed clinical expectations. This system helps align the incentives of the organization and its physicians and provides a continuing reminder to improve clinical management.

Profiting from Clinical Improvement

Hospitals usually are paid more when patients experience complications (although Medicare has ended reimbursement for some clinical shortcomings). Because incremental revenues are highly visible and incremental costs are not, hospital administrators may think that

(continued)

(continued)

clinical shortcomings are not eroding margins. An analysis of surgical complications should help dispel that notion (Dimick et al. 2006). Colon resection without complications resulted in costs of $15,464 and a profit margin of 31 percent. When complications occurred, costs more than doubled and the profit turned into a 4 percent loss. Abdominal aortic aneurysm repair without complications entailed costs of $22,822 and a profit margin of 26 percent. With complications, costs nearly tripled and the margin fell to 11 percent. Ventral incisional hernia repair without complications cost $6,321 and produced a profit margin of 19 percent. If complications occurred, costs nearly doubled and the margin fell to 6 percent.

Poor quality reduces hospital profits, even if it substantially increases payments by insurers. And poor quality is a terrible strategy in both the short run and the long run. Poor quality leads to market share losses (Epstein 2010), and this effect is likely to become larger as insurers increasingly use cost and quality data to try to steer patients to efficient, effective, safe providers (Raths 2012).

11.2.2 Reengineering

Reengineering and quality improvement initiatives can increase profits, but that does not mean they will or that they will do so easily. Nothing guarantees that costs will fall, and nothing guarantees that revenues will not fall faster than costs. Especially in hospitals, improvement initiatives often coincide with downsizing efforts, making the staff wary (and sometimes causing the organization to lose the employees it most wants to keep).

Skilled leadership does not guarantee success but is essential to improvement initiatives. For example, a focused effort to improve inpatient quality and reduce costs required a major effort by senior management (Bielaszka-DuVernay 2011). Reengineering and quality management initiatives demand the time and attention of everyone in the organization, meaning that other things are left undone or are done less well. If not done skillfully, reengineering and quality management initiatives can make things worse.

Marginal or **incremental revenue**
The revenue from selling an additional unit of output

11.3 Maximizing Profits

Organizations can also increase profits by expanding or contracting output. The basic rules of profit maximization are to expand as long as **marginal revenue** (or **incremental revenue**) exceeds **marginal cost** (or **incremental cost**),

Marginal or **incremental cost**
The cost of producing an additional unit of output

to shrink as long as marginal cost exceeds marginal revenue, and to shut down if the return on investment is not adequate. If increasing output increases revenue more than costs, profits rise. If reducing output reduces costs more than it reduces revenue, profits rise.

Marginal cost (or incremental cost) is the change in total cost associated with a change in output. Marginal revenue (or incremental revenue) is the change in total revenue associated with a change in output. The challenges lie in forecasting revenues and estimating costs.

As shown in Exhibit 11.2, increasing output from 100 to 120 increases profits because the marginal revenue is greater than the marginal cost. Revenue increases from $2,000 to $2,400 as sales increase from 100 to 120 units, so marginal revenue equals $20 ($400 ÷ 20). Costs increase from $1,500 to $1,600, so marginal cost equals $5 ($100 ÷ 20). The same is true for the expansion from 120 to 140. Marginal revenue falls because the firm has to cut prices to increase sales, and marginal cost rises because the firm is approaching capacity. Even though marginal revenue is nearly equal to marginal cost, profits still rise. Expanding from 140 to 160 reduces profits. Further price cuts push marginal revenue below marginal cost.

Managers need to understand what their costs are and must not confuse incremental costs with average costs. Average costs may be higher or lower than incremental costs. As long as the organization operates well below capacity, average costs usually will exceed incremental costs because of fixed costs. As the firm approaches capacity, however, incremental costs can rise quickly. If the firm needs to add personnel, acquire new equipment, or lease new offices to serve additional customers, incremental cost may well exceed average costs.

The following example illustrates why managers need to understand marginal costs and compare them to marginal revenues. A clinic is operating near capacity when a small PPO (preferred provider organization) approaches it. The PPO wants to bring 100 additional patient visits to the clinic and pay $50 per visit. The manager accepts the deal, even though $50 is less than the clinic's average cost or average revenue. Shortly thereafter, another PPO approaches the clinic. It too wants to bring 100 additional patient visits to

EXHIBIT 11.2
Marginal Cost, Marginal Revenue, and Profits

Quantity	Revenue	Cost	Profit	Marginal Revenue	Marginal Cost
100	$2,000	$1,500	$500		
120	$2,400	$1,600	$800	$20	$5
140	$2,660	$1,840	$820	$13	$12
160	$2,880	$2,120	$760	$11	$14

the clinic and pay $50 per visit. The manager turns down the offer. When criticized for this apparent inconsistency, the manager defends the decision, explaining that the clinic had excess capacity when the first PPO contacted it. The marginal cost for those additional visits was only $10 (see Exhibit 11.3). Signing the first contract increased profits by $4,000 because the marginal revenue was $50 for those visits. When the second PPO contacted the clinic, it no longer had excess capacity and would have had to add staff to handle the additional visits. As a result, marginal costs for the second set of visits would have been $510, and profits would have plummeted.

11.4 Return on Investment

When examining an entire organization rather than a well-defined project, most analysts focus on **return on equity** rather than return on investment. *Equity* is an organization's total assets minus outside claims on those assets. Equity also can be defined as the initial investments of stakeholders (donors or investors) plus the organization's retained earnings.

Return on equity
Profits divided by shareholder equity

What is an adequate return on investment? The answer to this question depends primarily on three factors: what low-risk investments (such as short-term US Treasury securities) are yielding, the riskiness of the enterprise, and the objectives of the organization.

All business investments entail some risk. Those risks may be high, as they are for a pharmaceutical company considering allocating research and development funds to a new drug, or they may be low, as they are for a primary care physician purchasing an established practice in a small town. In any case, a profit-seeking investor will be reluctant to commit funds to a project

	Status Quo	Adding the First PPO	Adding the Second PPO
Quantity	24,000	24,100	24,200
Revenue	$2,400,000	$2,405,000	$2,410,000
Average revenue	$100.00	$99.79	$99.59
Marginal revenue		$50.00	$50.00
Cost	$2,040,000	$2,041,000	$2,092,000
Average cost	$85.00	$84.69	$86.45
Marginal cost		$10.00	$510.00
Profit	$360,000	$364,000	$318,000

EXHIBIT 11.3
Marginal Cost and Profits

that promises a rate of return similar to the yield of low-risk securities. Consequently, when rates of return on low-risk investments are high, investors will demand high yields on higher-risk investments. The size of this risk premium will usually depend on a project's perceived risk. An investor may be content with the prospect of a 9 percent return on investment from a relatively low-risk enterprise but will not find this yield adequate for a high-risk venture.

Because managers must be responsive to the organization's stakeholders, they must also avoid high-risk investments that do not offer at least a chance of high rates of return. What constitutes a high rate of return depends on the goals of the organization and the nonfinancial attributes of an investment. In some cases, an organization that is genuinely committed to nonprofit objectives will be willing to accept a low return (or even a negative return) on a project that furthers those goals.

11.5 Producing to Stock or to Order

Producing to stock
Producing output and then adjusting prices to sell what has been produced

Producing to order
Setting prices and then filling customers' orders

Organizations can **produce to stock** or **produce to order**. One that produces to stock forecasts its demand and cost and produces output to store in inventory. Medical supply manufacturers are an example of this sort of organization. More commonly in the healthcare sector, firms produce to order. They also forecast demand and cost, but they do not produce anything up front. Instead, they set prices designed to maximize profits and wait to see how many customers they attract. Hospitals are an example of this type of organization. This distinction is important because discussions of profit maximization are usually framed in terms of choosing quantities or choosing prices.

Thus far, the content of this chapter has been largely framed in terms of firms that produce to stock; however, its implications apply to healthcare organizations that produce to order. Only by setting prices based on their expectations about demand and cost do they discover whether they have set prices too high or too low. An organization has set prices too high if its marginal revenue is greater than its marginal cost, because that means additional profitable sales at a lower price were missed. An organization has set prices too low if its marginal revenue is less than its marginal cost. Organizations that produce to order must also make the same decisions about rates of return on equity discussed earlier. Is a 5 percent return on investment large enough to justify operating an organ transplant unit? How important is the unit to the organization's educational goals? What are the alternatives?

When organizations contract with insurers or employers, estimates of marginal revenue should be easy to develop. To estimate marginal revenue for a new contract, calculate projected revenue under the new contract, subtract revenue under the old contract, and divide by the change in volume. For sales to the general public, economics gives managers a tool: marginal revenue equals $p \times (1 + 1/\varepsilon)$, where p is the product price and ε is the price elasticity of demand. (See Chapter 8 for more information about elasticity.) Most healthcare organizations face price elasticities in the range of –3.00 to –6.00, so marginal revenue can be much less than the price. For example, if a product sells for \$1,000 and the price elasticity of demand is –3.00, its marginal revenue will equal \$1,000 × (1 – 1/3.00), or \$667. In contrast, if the price elasticity of demand is –6.00, its marginal revenue will equal \$1,000 × (1 – 1/6.00), or \$833. As demand becomes more elastic, marginal revenue and price become more alike. Unless the elasticity becomes infinite, though, marginal revenue will be less than price.

11.6 Not-for-Profit Organizations

The strategies of not-for-profit organizations may differ from those of for-profit organizations because of more severe **agency** problems, differences in goals, and differences in costs. These forces have multiple effects.

Agency
An arrangement in which one person (the agent) takes actions on behalf of another (the principal)

11.6.1 Agency Problems

All organizations have agency problems. Agency problems are conflicts between the interests of managers (the agents) and the goals of other stakeholders. For example, a higher salary benefits a manager, but it benefits stakeholders only if it enhances performance or keeps the manager from leaving (when a comparable replacement could not be attracted for less). Not-for-profit firms face three added challenges. They cannot turn managers into owners by requiring them to own company stock (which helps to align the interests of managers and other owners). In addition, no one owns the organization, so no one may be policing the behavior of its managers to ensure that they are serving stakeholders well. Furthermore, assessing the performance of managers in not-for-profit organizations is a challenge. A not-for-profit organization may earn less than a for-profit competitor for many reasons. Is it earning less because of its focus on other goals, because of management's incompetence, or because the firm's managers are using the firm's resources to live well? Often the cause is difficult to pinpoint.

11.6.2 Differences in Goals

Goals other than profits can influence an organization's behavior, though they need not. Not-for-profit firms gain benefits from the pursuit of goals other than profit. Managers should consider how their decisions affect the benefits derived from these other goals. To best realize its goals, a not-for-profit organization should strive to make marginal revenue plus marginal benefit equal to marginal cost. Marginal benefit is the net marginal benefit to the firm from expanding a line of business. Three cases are possible:

1. If the marginal benefit is greater than 0, the not-for-profit will produce more than a for-profit.
2. If the marginal benefit equals 0, the not-for-profit will produce as much as a for-profit.
3. If the marginal benefit is less than 0, the not-for-profit will produce less than a for-profit.

A further complication is that the marginal benefit may depend on other income. A struggling not-for-profit may act like a for-profit, but a highly profitable not-for-profit may not.

11.6.3 Differences in Costs

Not-for-profit organizations' costs also may differ. First, the not-for-profit may not have to pay taxes (especially property taxes), which tends to make the not-for-profit's average costs lower. On the other hand, the not-for-profit firm's greater agency problems may result in less efficiency and higher average and marginal costs.

The fundamental problem is that we cannot predict how not-for-profit organizations will differ from for-profit firms. This lack of forecast is frustrating for analysts and raises a question for policymakers: If we do not know how not-for-profit organizations benefit the community, why are they given tax breaks?

11.7 Conclusion

Even managers of not-for-profit organizations need to know how to maximize profits. They must identify appropriate product lines, price and promote those product lines to realize an adequate return on investment, and produce those product lines efficiently. Most healthcare organizations are less profitable than they could be because they are less efficient than they could be. Leadership must be effective for efficiency to increase. Cost reductions and quality improvements are easier to talk about than to realize, especially where clinical plans (i.e., physician practices) must change to improve efficiency.

Decisions to expand or contract should be based on incremental costs and revenues. Few healthcare managers know what their costs are, so they often have difficulty forecasting revenues and estimating costs to be able to make these decisions.

Not-for-profit organizations may or may not resemble for-profit organizations. In some cases, their goals and performance are similar. Managers need to understand why the goals of not-for-profit organizations are worthy of tax preferences and be able to make that case to donors and regulators.

CASE 11.2   Tax Exemption for Not-for-Profit Hospitals

"Tax exemption for not-for-profit hospitals is a historical relic," said Tyler at a hospital board meeting. "When income tax started in 1894, there was no Medicare, no Medicaid, and no insurance. People with money got care at home. The role of hospitals was to care for the poor. These days, hospitals are profitable businesses that serve paying customers. Even lobbyists for the industry concede that that exemption from federal, state, and local taxes almost certainly costs more than the care not-for-profit hospitals provide for free to the poor. For-profits, which pay income and property taxes, provide about as much uncompensated care as not-for-profits. Plus, a lot of free care is mandatory. Federal and state laws require all hospitals to provide emergency care without regard for ability to pay.

"Look, well-run 'not-for-profit' hospitals make plenty of money, and their managers get paid very well. I have no problem with that, but they shouldn't get a tax break, too." With that, Tyler sat down.

Corey then approached the microphone, saying, "I know that we provide charity care. But Suburban Clinic, which is for-profit and pays local property taxes, does too. And it provides only a little less than we do. A first guess at our property value would be $60 million. The local taxes on that would be about $1.8 million. Even using the inflated estimates that we float, which are based on list prices, there's no way that its community benefit approaches that amount of money. Have you seen the roads in this town? We could really use the tax revenue. And I wouldn't mind a tax cut. My taxes help pay for our nonpayment of taxes. You know, we bought three for-profit physician practices, and I see no difference in the way they are run. I think this is just a scam to avoid paying taxes."

After Corey sat down, Lee, the hospital's CEO, took the floor. "We provide a broad array of benefits to this community. We provide charity care, our prices are lower than our competitors, we operate a nursing school, we operate asthma and heart failure programs that consistently lose money, and we operate a number of community outreach programs. I think this community is well served by its recognition of our charitable mission. Yes, we are profitable, but we need to stay in business. I look forward to working with the board of assessors to

(continued)

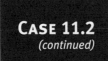

CASE 11.2
(continued)

clear up any questions about the merits of our not-for-profit status. I am confident that they are based on a misunderstanding of the situation."

Several more speakers came to the microphone, but none brought a lot of new information. Next, the board of assessors had to make a decision about the status of the hospital.

Discussion questions:
- What evidence about the level of community benefit provided by not-for-profit and for-profit hospitals is available?
- Why does using list prices tend to inflate estimates of community benefit?
- Are there other important differences between not-for-profit and for-profit hospitals?
- Would the city be better off if it taxed the hospital and paid for charity care?
- More broadly, is tax exemption a good way to encourage private organizations to serve the public interest?
- What should the board of assessors do? What are its options?

Exercises

11.1 A clinic has $1 million in revenues and $950,000 in costs. What is its operating margin?

11.2 The owners of the clinic in Exercise 11.1 invested $400,000. What is the return on investment? Is it adequate?

11.3 A laboratory has $4.2 million in revenues and $3.85 million in costs. What is its operating margin?

11.4 The owners of the laboratory in Exercise 11.3 invested $6 million. What is the return on investment?

11.5 Go to the website of the Board of Governors of the Federal Reserve System (www.federalreserve.gov). What is the current annual yield for one-year Treasury securities?

11.6 Go to the Yahoo! Finance website (http://finance.yahoo.com) and look up the operating margin and return on equity for Community Health Systems (symbol CYH). How does this company compare to Aetna (AET), Amgen (AMGN), Laboratory Corporation of America (LH), and Tenet Healthcare Corporation (THC)?

11.7 A not-for-profit hospital realizes a 3 percent return on its $200,000 investment in its home health unit. Its current revenue after discounts and allowances is $382,000. Administrative costs are $119,000, clinical personnel costs are $210,000, and supply costs are $47,000. Providing home health care is not a core goal of the hospital, and it will sell the home health unit if it cannot realize a return of at least 12 percent. A process improvement team has recommended significant changes to the home health unit's billing processes. The team has concluded that these changes could reduce costs by $20,000 and increase revenues by $5,000. Analyze the data that follows and assess whether the changes would make the home health unit profitable enough to keep.

	Old	New
Revenue	$382,000	$387,000
Cost	$376,000	$356,000
Profit	$6,000	$31,000
Return on investment	3%	16%

11.8 The table shows cost and revenue data for an outpatient surgery clinic. Calculate the clinic's marginal cost, marginal revenue, and profits at each level of output. Which price maximizes its profits?

Surgeries	250	300	350	400	450
Price	$2,000	$1,920	$1,800	$1,675	$1,550
Revenue	$500,000	$576,000	$630,000	$670,000	$697,500
Cost	$516,000	$538,500	$563,500	$591,000	$621,000

11.9 The price–quantity relationship has been estimated for a new prostate cancer blood test: $Q = 4,000 - (20 \times P)$. Use a spreadsheet to calculate the quantity demanded and total spending for prices ranging from $200 to $0, using $50 increments. For each $50 drop in price, calculate the change in revenue, the change in volume, and the additional revenue per unit. (Call the additional revenue per unit *marginal revenue*.)

11.10 The table shows output and cost data. Calculate the average total cost, average fixed cost, average variable cost, and marginal cost schedules. If the market price were $500, should the firm shut down in the short run? In the long run?

Quantity	0	5	10	15	20	25	30	35
Total cost	$20,000	$20,500	$20,975	$21,425	$21,850	$22,300	$22,775	$23,275

11.11 A clinic's average and marginal cost per case is $400. It charges $600 per case and serves 1,000 customers. Its marketing team predicts that it will expand its sales to 1,250 customers if it cuts its price to $550. How do profits change if it cuts prices? What is the firm's marginal revenue? Why is marginal revenue not equal to $550?

11.12 A clinic's average and marginal cost per case is $400. It charges $600 per case and serves 1,000 customers. Its marketing team predicts that it will expand its sales to 1,250 if it signs a contract for a price of $550 with a local health maintenance organization. How do profits change if it signs the contract? What is the firm's marginal revenue? Why is its marginal revenue different from the marginal revenue in the previous exercise?

11.13 Why would a for-profit organization that incurs losses choose to operate?

11.14 Why would a for-profit organization that is earning profits choose to exit a line of business?

References

Bielaszka-DuVernay, C. 2011. "Redesigning Acute Care Processes in Wisconsin." *Health Affairs* 30 (3): 422–25.

Dimick, J. B., W. B. Weeks, R. J. Karia, S. Das, and D. A. Campbell Jr. 2006. "Who Pays for Poor Surgical Quality? Building a Business Case for Quality Improvement." *Journal of the American College of Surgeons* 202 (6): 933–37.

Epstein, A. J. 2010. "Effects of Report Cards on Referral Patterns to Cardiac Surgeons." *Journal of Health Economics* 29 (5): 718–31.

Graban, M. 2012. *Lean Hospitals.* New York: CRC Press.

Lee, R. H., M. J. Bott, B. Gajewski, and R. L. Taunton. 2009. "Modeling Efficiency at the Process Level: An Examination of the Care Planning Process in Nursing Homes." *Health Services Research* 44 (1): 15–32.

Raths, D. 2012. "Targeting Chronic Illness Together: Health Plans Support Providers Through Predictive Analytics." *Healthcare Informatics* 29 (5): 25–27.

Toussaint, J., R. A. Gerard, and E. Adams. 2010. *On the Mend: Revolutionizing Healthcare to Save Lives and Transform the Industry.* Cambridge, MA: Lean Enterprise Institute.

Zhivan, N. A., and M. L. Diana. 2012. "U.S. Hospital Efficiency and Adoption of Health Information Technology." *Health Care Management Science* 15 (1): 37–47.

CHAPTER

12

PRICING

Learning Objectives

After reading this chapter, students will be able to

- apply the standard marginal cost pricing model,
- explain why price discrimination can increase profits,
- explain the link between pricing and profits, and
- discuss the importance of price setting.

Key Concepts

- Pricing is important.
- *Marginal cost pricing* maximizes profits in most cases.
- Marginal cost pricing uses estimates of the price elasticity of demand and incremental costs to set the profit-maximizing price.
- The consequences of setting prices incorrectly can be substantial.
- *Price discrimination* is common in healthcare and other industries.
- Price discrimination can substantially increase profits.
- Contracting demands the same information as pricing.

12.1 Introduction

Pricing is important. Prices set too low or too high will drag down profits. The trick is to set prices so that your organization captures profitable business and discourages unprofitable business. To maximize profits, marginal revenue should just equal marginal cost (assuming the product line is profitable). To maximize other objectives, organizations should start with profit-maximizing prices.

Pricing is a continuing challenge for healthcare organizations for three reasons. First, many managers do not have a clear pricing strategy. They lack the necessary data to make good decisions and may be mispricing their products or selling the wrong product lines. Second, many managers lack skills and experience in setting prices and negotiating contracts. Third, the pricing strategy that is best for the organization may not be the pricing strategy various departments or clinics prefer. Managers of these units may have incentives to price products too high or too low. In the absence of a clear strategy and good data, how prices are actually set will be up for grabs.

12.2 The Economic Model of Pricing

Marginal cost pricing
Using information about marginal costs and the price elasticity of demand to set profit-maximizing prices

The economic model of pricing, **marginal cost pricing**, clearly identifies a pricing strategy that will maximize profits. This strategy also identifies the information needed to set prices.

The economic model of pricing is simple. First, find out what your incremental costs are. (Remember, incremental costs are the same as marginal costs.) Second, estimate the price elasticity of demand facing *your organization's product*. (Demand for the products of your organization will usually be much more elastic than the overall demand for the product. See Chapter 8 for more information about elasticity.) Third, calculate the appropriate markup, which will equal $\varepsilon/(1 + \varepsilon)$. (Here, ε represents the price elasticity of demand for your organization's product.) Multiplying this markup times your organization's incremental cost gives you the profit-maximizing price. The profit-maximizing price will equal $[\varepsilon/(1 + \varepsilon)] \times MC$, where MC represents the incremental cost. So, if the price elasticity of demand is -2.5 and the incremental cost is 3.00, the profit-maximizing price would be $[-2.5/(1 - 2.5)] \times 3.00$, or 5.00.

By now you may have noted that the pricing rule is just a restatement of the profit maximization rule from Chapter 11, which states that marginal revenue equals marginal cost. The formula for marginal revenue is $Price \times (1 + \varepsilon)/\varepsilon$, so $MC = Price \times (1 + \varepsilon)/\varepsilon$. Solve this formula for *Price* by dividing both sides by $(1 + \varepsilon)/\varepsilon$, and you end up with $Price = MC/[(1 + \varepsilon)/\varepsilon]$, which is the same as $[\varepsilon/(1 + \varepsilon)] \times MC$.

Data on incremental costs are important for a wide range of management decisions. Pricing is one more reason to estimate incremental costs. Estimating the right price elasticity of demand can be more of a challenge. Three strategies can provide you with this information. One would be to hire a marketing consultant. Depending on how much your organization is willing to spend, the consultant can provide you with a rough or fairly detailed estimate. Another strategy would be to combine information on overall market price elasticities of demand with information on your market share for this product line. (Chapter 8 lists a number of market price elasticities.) Dividing the overall price elasticity of demand by your market share gives an estimate of the price elasticity your organization faces. For example, if the overall price elasticity is -0.3 and your organization commands an eighth of the market, you would estimate that your organization faces a price elasticity of demand of –0.3/0.125, or –2.4. The third strategy would be to experiment. For example, raise a product's price by 5 percent and see how much demand falls. Because the price elasticity of demand equals the percentage change in quantity sold divided by the percentage change in price, this calculation is straightforward.

Exhibit 12.1 illustrates how different profit-maximizing markups can be. An organization facing a price elasticity of demand of –2.5 and an incremental cost of $10.00 should have a markup of $6.67. In contrast, a similar organization facing a price elasticity of demand of –5.5 should set a markup of $2.22. Each of these choices maximizes profits, given the market environment each firm faces. Clearly, organizations that face less elastic demand enjoy larger markups. The payoffs of differentiating your products can be substantial because these products face less elastic demand.

12.3 Pricing and Profits

What should you do if the rate of return from a line of business is inadequate? The obvious solution is to raise prices. Unfortunately, like many obvious strategies, this one will often be wrong. If a product line yields an inadequate return on investment, four strategies should be explored.

1. Make sure your price is not too high or too low. Return to the maximum pricing formula and see if you calculated incorrectly, or whether your estimate of the price elasticity of demand was inaccurate.

Elasticity	Price
−1.5	$30.00
−2.5	$16.67
−3.5	$14.00
−4.5	$12.86
−5.5	$12.22
−6.5	$11.82
−7.5	$11.54
−8.5	$11.33
−9.5	$11.18

EXHIBIT 12.1
Profit-Maximizing Prices When Incremental Costs Equal $10

2. Reassess your estimate of incremental costs. If it is too high, your prices will also be too high, and vice versa.

3. See how much you can cut your costs. Most healthcare firms should be able to reduce costs substantially. To see whether yours can be brought down, take a look at costs and business practices in firms you think are efficient.

4. If all else fails, exit the line of business.

The consequences of setting price incorrectly can be substantial. In Exhibit 12.2 the profit-maximizing price should be $15.00. Setting a price much lower or much higher than $15.00 reduces profits significantly. Note, though, that being a bit too high or a bit too low is not disastrous. Being a little off in your estimates of incremental cost or the price elasticity of demand will usually mean your profits will be a little smaller than they could have been.

Pricing is an important component of marketing. How is the marginal cost pricing model too simple? The main concern is that it does not account for strategy. For example, demand for an innovative product will typically be quite inelastic. The resulting high margins, unfortunately, will attract a host of rivals. Your organization may want to forgo some immediate profits to discourage entry by competitors. Alternatively, aggressive price cutting in mature markets is likely to encourage price cutting by your competitors. In markets with relatively few competitors, not rocking the boat by cutting prices may allow everyone to enjoy stable, high prices and high profits. These factors demand careful study, but even if you do not follow the marginal cost pricing scenario, it should be your starting point.

EXHIBIT 12.2
Profits When Incremental and Average Costs Equal $10 and the Price Elasticity of Demand Equals −3.0

Price	Profits
$5.00	($881,059)
$7.50	($130,527)
$10.00	$0
$12.50	$28,194
$15.00	$32,632
$17.50	$30,824
$20.00	$27,533
$22.50	$24,172
$25.00	$21,145

12.4 Price Discrimination

Price discrimination is common in healthcare, as it is in other industries. It refers to charging different customers different prices for the same product. Price discrimination makes sense if different customers have different price elasticities of demand and if resale of the product by customers is not possible. Most healthcare providers and their products meet these criteria. Healthcare providers contract with an array of individuals and insurance plans. The price sensitivities of those purchasers differ widely, and services can seldom be resold. So, profit-maximizing healthcare firms will want to explore opportunities for price discrimination (or more politely, different discounts for different customers).

Price discrimination
Selling similar products to different individuals at different prices

Price discrimination can increase profits. Suppose half your customers (group A) have price elasticities of –3.00 and half (group B) have price elasticities of –6.00. The demand curve for group A is 16,000 – 800 × *Price*, and the demand curve for group B is 16,000 – 1,045 × *Price*. (You can verify that the group A elasticity is –3.00 at a price of $15.00 and the group B elasticity is –6.00 at a price of $12.00.) Your average and incremental costs are $10. In setting prices you could use the average price elasticity of demand (–4.50) and charge everyone $12.86. Or you could charge group A $12.00 and charge group B $15.00 (which is what the marginal cost pricing model tells us to do). As Exhibit 12.3 illustrates, not employing price discrimination leaves a substantial amount on the table.

So, aside from managers (who are eager to learn new ways to improve profits) and consumers (who are eager to learn new ways to get discounts), why should price discrimination matter to anyone? Some observers think the different prices reflect **cost shifting**, not price discrimination. According to the cost shifting hypothesis, price reductions negotiated by PPOs or imposed by Medicaid will raise costs for everybody else. The cost shifting hypothesis is widely believed. For example, in 2013 the *Dallas Morning News* argued that employers and consumers were paying billions more each year because Medicare and Medicaid payments were too low (Landers 2013).

Cost shifting
The hypothesis that price differences are due to efforts by providers to make up for losses in some lines of business by charging higher prices in other lines of business

The cost shifting hypothesis might be true but probably is not. Most of the empirical evidence from the contemporary marketplace is inconsistent with

Group	Without Price Discrimination			With Price Discrimination		
	Price	Quantity	Profit	Price	Quantity	Profit
A	$12.86	5,712	$16,336	$15.00	4,000	$20,000
B	$12.86	2,561	$7,324	$12.00	3,460	$6,920
		8,273	$23,660		7,460	$26,920

EXHIBIT 12.3 Profits With and Without Price Discrimination

the cost shifting hypothesis (White 2013). Why does the hypothesis persist? There are three possibilities. First, the cost shifting hypothesis may be a rationalization for widespread discounting. No customer likes getting the smallest discount, so perhaps healthcare firms lead the customer to believe a small discount is due to cost shifting ("We could give you a better price if it weren't for the big discount we're forced to give Medicare!"). This scenario is the most likely. Second, cost shifting might be real, reflecting poor management on the part of profit-seeking organizations. If a firm raised prices for some customers because other customers negotiated a discount, either prices were too low to begin with or the firm was acting imprudently in raising prices. Third, cost shifting might be real, reflecting responses of not-for-profit firms that had set prices lower than a well-managed, for-profit firm would have. However, pressure on the bottom lines of healthcare organizations— profit and nonprofit— means that, if it existed, cost shifting is probably a thing of the past.

CASE 12.1   Price Discrimination in Practice

What do American Airlines, Walgreens, Staples, Stanford University, AT&T, the Mayo Clinic, and Safeway have in common? They all price discriminate (Valentino-Devries, Singer-Vine, and Soltani 2012). They charge different customers different amounts for the same product.

Pharmaceutical discounts are the clearest examples of healthcare price discrimination because the products are identical. Only the prices differ. A cash customer (e.g., someone without insurance coverage) would pay the highest price, the list price.

Most customers pay much less than list price. Insurers negotiate discounts with manufacturers and pharmacies. These discounts are typically about 30 percent (Herper 2012). Some hospitals and HMOs have their own pharmacies and can negotiate even better deals with manufacturers. These organizations sometimes pay as little as 40 percent of list price. Most discounts come in the form of rebates, meaning that a purchaser pays the list price up front but gets a payment from the seller later. This process makes resale more difficult and limits price transparency (Morgan, Daw, and Thomson 2013).

The federal government has multiple discount programs. The largest is the Medicaid rebate program, which requires manufacturers to pay a rebate that varies by the type of drug. Prices, formularies, and copayments vary from state to state, so whether the Medicaid rebate

(continued)

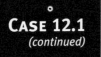

CASE 12.1
(continued)

program covers the most effective medications or gets the best prices is not clear (Millar et al. 2011).

Many federally funded clinics and hospitals are eligible for the Medicaid discount. However, these agencies can often negotiate better deals because they can buy wholesale and because they can choose drugs for their formularies.

Tribal and territorial governments can use the prices on the Federal Supply Schedule, which federal agencies use to buy common supplies and services. The Department of Defense, the Department of Veterans Affairs (VA), the Public Health Service, and the Coast Guard may get prices that are slightly lower than the Federal Supply Schedule because of a provision called the *federal ceiling price*. This provision caps the price using a formula based on private-sector transactions. Finally, these agencies can try to negotiate prices below the federal ceiling price. The VA, which uses a national formulary, has used its bargaining power to get substantially better prices. Frakt, Pizer, and Feldman (2012) report that the VA's prices are 37 to 44 percent lower than Medicare prices.

Discussion questions:

- Why do drug firms give discounts voluntarily?
- Do other healthcare providers routinely give discounts to some customers?
- Why do the uninsured typically pay the highest prices?
- Why would a hospital usually get a better price for a drug than an insurance company?
- Why does the VA get such low prices?
- Suppose a law was enacted that required drug manufacturers to give state Medicaid agencies the same price they negotiated with the VA. How would Medicaid and VA prices change?
- Should Medicare adopt the VA formulary?

Similar price differences are common in other industries with similar characteristics. Have you ever wondered why it makes sense for one passenger to have paid $340 for a flight and another passenger in the same row to have paid $99? Why does it make sense for a matinee to cost half as much as the same movie shown two hours later?

When the incremental cost of production is small, when buyers can be separated into groups that have very different price elasticities of demand, and when resale is not possible, price discrimination is usually profitable.

Most healthcare firms, both not-for-profit and for-profit, fit this profile, so their managers need to know how to price discriminate. With no margin, there is no mission. Price discrimination helps increase margins.

12.5 Multipart Pricing

Thus far we have focused on simple pricing models. In fact, a wide range of pricing models may be applicable. One is the multipart pricing model, in which customers pay a fee to be eligible to use a service and separate additional fees as they use the services. An obvious example would be a managed care plan. The trade-off is that a low entry fee (premium) yields more customers. High copayments reduce costs (either increasing profit margins or reducing premiums), but at some point high copayments will drive away customers. The right combination is always a balancing act. A related pricing strategy is tying. Tying links the prices of multiple products. Again, the goal is to balance multiple prices so as to maximize profits.

CASE 12.2	**What Should You Charge?**

Suppose that Exhibit 12.4 is your practice's marketing forecast.

EXHIBIT 12.4
Marketing
Forecast

Price	Low-Income Clients	High-Income Clients	Total
$35.75	2,125	14,250	16,375
$35.25	2,375	14,750	17,125
$34.75	2,625	15,250	17,875
$34.25	2,875	15,750	18,625
$33.75	3,125	16,250	19,375
$33.25	3,375	16,750	20,125
$32.75	3,625	17,250	20,875
$32.25	3,875	17,750	21,625
$31.75	4,125	18,250	22,375
$31.25	4,375	18,750	23,125

(continued)

CASE 12.2
(continued)

EXHIBIT 12.4
Marketing
Forecast
(continued)

Price	Low-Income Clients	High-Income Clients	Total
$30.75	4,625	19,250	23,875
$30.25	4,875	19,750	24,625
$29.75	5,125	20,250	25,375
$29.25	5,375	20,750	26,125
$28.75	5,625	21,250	26,875
$28.25	5,875	21,750	27,625
$27.75	6,125	22,250	28,375
$27.25	6,375	22,750	29,125

Discussion questions:
- By law, you must charge everyone the same price. What do you charge?
- Your costs equal $100,000 plus $20 per visit. What are your revenues, costs, and profits?
- If you could charge low-income and high-income customers different prices, what prices would you charge each group? What would your revenues, costs, and profits be? Would this scenario be ethical? How would you try to identify the two groups? (You cannot do income surveys of your patients.)

12.6 Pricing and Managed Care

Are these issues relevant in markets dominated by managed care? Yes. One needs the same information to set a price or to evaluate a contract. Accepting a contract in which marginal revenue is less than incremental cost almost never makes sense because such a situation reduces profits. Such contracts make sense only when these losses are really marketing expenses, and even in these cases the money probably could be better spent elsewhere. Similarly, giving a large discount to a buyer who is not sensitive to price almost never makes sense. For example, a managed care plan that needs your organization's participation to offer a competitive network is not in a good bargaining position and should not get the best discount.

The flip side of the pricing problem, contracting, is even tougher. Economic models of pricing tell us that managers need to know what their incremental costs are, what markup over incremental costs they should expect, and what their rivals will bid. Each of these will be uncertain to some degree, and many healthcare firms have only sketchy cost data. This fact is especially true for incremental costs, which many firms are not prepared to track. Without good data on incremental costs, managers will be flying blind and may be tempted to base their bids on average costs. This reaction usually costs some profitable business opportunities.

CASE 12.3   Should My Firm Accept This Contract?

You are the manager of a 20-physician cardiology practice. You are getting ready to advise your board about a proposal for capitated specialty care from a local HMO. Data from your fee-for-service practice show billings per member per month of $100 for visits, $80 for catheterizations, and $115 for lab. The practice owns the labs, and the profits are shared among the partners. Your estimate is that costs (aside from physician income) equal 25 percent of charges.

The proposal from the HMO is for a rate of $275 per member per month. Your immediate reaction is to reject it. Your CFO makes two comments that give you pause: "Our overhead will drop significantly if we accept this proposal and convert 25 percent of our business to capitation. In addition, we should anticipate that our rates for visits, catheterizations, and tests will drop significantly once we convert."

In this case the town has only two other cardiology groups. You are not sure whether they have been asked to bid or not. Your legal counsel has warned you that direct discussions with your rivals might leave you open to an antitrust suit.

Discussion questions:
- Why is your initial response to reject the offer?
- Why might overhead go down if you accept the contract?
- Why might utilization rates go down?
- What are the risks of accepting or refusing?
- What should you do next? Should you accept the proposal? Should you make a counteroffer?

12.7 Conclusion

Pricing is important, but many healthcare firms lack direction. Without a clear model of pricing, managers are unable to realize their firm's goals. They do not know what their incremental costs are or what sort of price elasticity of demand their organization faces. As a result, they do not know what prices to charge. This lack of knowledge reduces profits in two ways. The organization may set its prices too high or too low. Alternatively, the organization may participate in the wrong markets. It may accept contracts it should refuse or refuse contracts it should accept.

The economic model of pricing tells managers what they should do. Its implications apply to both pricing and contracting, so it remains an important part of every healthcare manager's tool kit. Actually applying this model will not always be easy, but not knowing what to do is harder still.

Price discrimination is everywhere in healthcare, and many organizations rely on it to remain profitable. Profitable price discrimination requires a little more information than setting a single price, so effective price discrimination is challenging. In addition, many healthcare managers are mesmerized by tales of cost shifting. Cost shifting is unlikely to be responsible for differences in price. If managers genuinely believe cost shifting is occurring, the belief steers them in the wrong direction.

Exercises

12.1 The marginal cost pricing model calculates a markup over marginal costs using estimates of the price elasticity of demand. Will any other pricing strategy result in higher profits?

12.2 If cost shifting is just a useful public relations ploy, why does it get so much attention?

12.3 Will raising prices increase the rate of return from a line of business?

12.4 Can you think of a healthcare firm that does not price discriminate (i.e., charge different customers different amounts for the same product)?

12.5 Price discrimination requires the ability to distinguish customers who are the most price sensitive and the ability to prevent arbitrage (resale of your products by customers who buy at low prices). What attributes of healthcare products make these tasks easy to do?

12.6 Your pharmacy provides services to Medicare and PPO patients. You estimate a price elasticity of demand of –2.2 for Medicare patients and –5.3 for PPO patients. Your marginal and average cost for dispensing a prescription is $2. What is the profit-maximizing dispensing fee for Medicare and PPO patients? Why might the price elasticities of demand differ?

12.7 Your dental clinic provides 3,000 exams for private pay patients and 1,000 exams for members of a union. Your fixed costs are $50,000 and your incremental cost is $40.

    a. Private pay patients have a price elasticity of demand of –3. What do you charge them?

    b. The union has negotiated a fee of $50. Is it profitable to treat members of the union?

    c. What would happen to your profits if you stopped treating members of the union?

    d. If the union negotiated a fee of $45 instead, what would you charge private pay patients?

    e. What does this tell you about cost shifting versus price discrimination?

12.8 You provide therapeutic massage services, focusing on stress reduction services that are not covered by insurance. Your monthly overhead is $2,000. You value your time at $20 per half hour (how long a therapeutic massage takes). Supplies per massage cost $4. You currently charge $75 per massage and have a volume of 100 clients per month. Your trade journal says that a 5 percent reduction in prices typically results in a 7.5 percent increase in volume. What would happen to your volume, revenues, and profits if you cut your price to $70? If you raised your price to $80?

12.9 The table shows case-mix-adjusted price and volume data for Dunes Hospital. Calculate its marginal cost, marginal revenue, and profits at each level of output. What price should it choose?

Admissions	6,552	9,048	9,672	9,984	10,296
Revenue	$52,416,000	$70,574,400	$73,507,200	$73,881,600	$74,131,200
Cost	$42,588,000	$59,264,400	$63,835,200	$66,393,600	$68,983,200
Price	$8,000	$7,800	$7,600	$7,400	$7,200

12.10 Your firm spent $100 million developing a new drug. It has now been approved for sale, and each pill costs $1 to manufacture. Your market research suggests that the price elasticity of demand in the general public is –1.1.

a. What price do you charge the public?

b. What would happen to profits if you charged twice as much?

c. What role does the $100 million in development costs play in your pricing decision?

d. The Medicaid agency has made a take-it-or-leave-it offer of $2 per pill. Do you accept? Why or why not?

12.11 Why are most healthcare providers able to charge different groups of purchasers different prices for the same products?

12.12 A clinic has incremental costs per case of $10 and overhead costs of $100,000. It faces a price elasticity of demand of –2.

a. What is the clinic's profit-maximizing price?

b. How would the profit-maximizing price change if overhead costs doubled?

c. With excess capacity, would serving Medicaid customers for a fee of $16 make sense?

d. How would the profit-maximizing price change if Medicaid raised its fee to $18?

12.13 You manage a not-for-profit hospital in a competitive market. Suppose you decide to charge less than the profit-maximizing price to your customers.

a. What effect would that decision have on profits?

b. What effect would that decision have on you and your career?

12.14 Assume the price elasticity of demand for physicians' services is –0.2. If your marginal cost per visit is $20, what is your profit-maximizing price if you control 5 percent of the market? What is your profit-maximizing price if you control 15 percent of the market? What lessons do you draw from this information?

12.15 A busy urgent care clinic has average costs of $40 and incremental costs of $60.

a. How could incremental costs be higher than average costs?

b. The clinic charges $80 for a visit. What price elasticity of demand does this information imply?

c. Volume is currently 200 visits per week. What are the clinic's profits?

d. An HMO guarantees at least 10 patients per week. It proposes a fee of $55. Should the clinic accept the contract?

e. What happens to profits if it accepts the contract?

References

Frakt, A. B., S. D. Pizer, and R. Feldman. 2012. "Should Medicare Adopt the Veterans Health Administration Formulary?" *Health Economics* 21 (5): 485–95.

Herper, M. 2012. "Inside the Secret World of Drug Company Rebates." *Forbes.* Published May 10. www.forbes.com/sites/matthewherper/2012/05/10/why-astrazeneca-gives-insurers-60-discounts-on-nexiums-list-price/.

Landers, J. 2013. "What Is Cost-Shifting? Why Do Hospitals Do It?" *Dallas Morning News Biz Beat Blog*, May 7. http://bizbeatblog.dallasnews.com/2013/05/what-is-cost-shifting-why-do-hospitals-do-it.html/.

Millar, T. P., S. Wong, D. H. Odierna, and L. A. Bero. 2011. "Applying the Essential Medicines Concept to US Preferred Drug Lists." *American Journal of Public Health* 101 (8): 1444–48.

Morgan, S., J. Daw, and P. Thomson. 2013. "International Best Practices for Negotiating 'Reimbursement Contracts' with Price Rebates from Pharmaceutical Companies." *Health Affairs* 32 (4): 771–77.

Valentino-Devries, J., J. Singer-Vine, and A. Soltani. 2012. "Websites Vary Prices, Deals Based on Users' Information." *Wall Street Journal.* Published December 24. http://online.wsj.com/news/articles/SB10001424127887323777204578189391813881534.

White, C. 2013. "Contrary to Cost-Shift Theory, Lower Medicare Hospital Payment Rates for Inpatient Care Lead to Lower Private Payment Rates." *Health Affairs* 32 (5): 935–43.

13

ASYMMETRIC INFORMATION AND INCENTIVES

Learning Objectives

After reading this chapter, students will be able to

- define asymmetric information and opportunism,
- describe two strategies for aligning incentives,
- explain why opportunism is a special management challenge in healthcare, and
- discuss challenges in limiting opportunism.

Key Concepts

- *Asymmetric information* is a situation in which one party to a transaction has better information about it than another.
- Asymmetric information allows the better informed party to act opportunistically.
- Asymmetric information is a common problem for managers.
- Aligning incentives helps reduce the problems associated with asymmetric information.
- Concerns about risk, complexity, measurement, strategic responses, and team production limit the extent of incentive-based payments.
- Only a few forms of incentive-based contracts are common in healthcare.

13.1 Asymmetric Information

Asymmetric information confronts healthcare managers in most of their professional roles. Vendors typically know more about the strengths and weaknesses of their products than do purchasers. Employees typically know more about their health problems than do human resource or health plan managers. Subordinates typically know more about the effort they have put into their

Asymmetric information
Information known to one party in a transaction but not another

Agent
A person who takes actions on behalf of another person (the principal)

Principal
The organization or individual represented by an agent

Opportunism
Taking advantage of a situation without regard for the interests of others

assignments than do their superiors. Providers typically know more about treatment options than do their patients. In all of these examples, one party, commonly called an **agent**, has better information than another party, commonly called a **principal**. Unless the principal is careful, the agent may take advantage of this information asymmetry—in other words, engage in **opportunism**.

Asymmetric information can result in two types of problems. One is that mutually beneficial transactions may not take place if concern about asymmetric information is too great. The other is that resources may be wasted because of agents' opportunism or principals' costly precautions. For example, an insurer cannot easily discern whether a treatment is really needed (Arrow 1963). In response, an insurer may not cover services thought likely to be abused, may require substantial consumer payments to restrain demand, or may require prior authorization before providing coverage. As a result, consumers may not use helpful services because the services cost too much. Alternatively, the plan, providers, and consumers may experience increased costs due to the requirement for prior authorization. (The insurer must staff the authorization office, the provider must spend time and money getting authorizations, and the consumer is likely to experience delays and repeat visits.) Asymmetric information also affects managers directly. Managers are often poorly informed about the quality, efficiency, and customer satisfaction issues that their subordinates face. But managers are also often poorly informed about whether costs are padded, whether quality problems are avoidable, or whether staffing is adequate. Fearing that subordinates will take advantage of them, managers may require reviews or audits. Both increase costs without directly adding to the output of the organization.

Asymmetric information is a concern when

1. the interests of the parties diverge in a meaningful way,
2. the parties have an important reason to strike a deal, and
3. determining whether the explicit or implicit terms of the deal have been followed is difficult.

These circumstances are far from rare. Unfortunately, they are an invitation to act opportunistically.

13.2 Opportunism

Opportunism can take many forms. Crime is one form. For example, deliberately billing a health plan for services that were not actually rendered is a form of opportunism more commonly known as *fraud*. The forms of opportunism that managers deal with are not usually so stark. Cruising the Internet rather than making collection calls, using the supplies budget to refurbish your office, scheduling a physical therapy visit of questionable value to meet volume targets, and referring a patient to a specialist for a problem you could easily handle are also examples of opportunism.

From experience, we know that some individuals are opportunistic some of the time. Some individuals seldom act opportunistically, whereas others often do. As a first step, we try to avoid dealing with those who are the most opportunistic. We then try to set up systems to restrain those who may be tempted. These systems will be imperfect because our ability to anticipate what may happen and how individuals may react is imperfect.

13.2.1 Remedies for Asymmetric Information

Remedies for asymmetric information focus on aligning the interests of the parties or monitoring the behavior of the agent. Changes in incentives are usually part of the preferred strategy because monitoring is usually expensive and nonproductive. For example, healthcare plans are commonly subject to utilization review designed to control use of services. Utilization review rarely changes recommended therapies, however, despite its cost and annoyance. Health plans would love to eliminate utilization review. Without it, a plan would rapidly gain market share because it could increase consumer satisfaction, increase provider satisfaction, and reduce premiums. In addition to being costly, monitoring may be difficult. For example, a product that a vendor honestly recommended may fail or may not meet your needs, or it may work but have features you don't need and cost more than a more suitable product. Monitoring is likely to be only part of the remedy for asymmetric information.

13.2.2 The Special Challenges for Healthcare

The challenges posed by asymmetric information are not unique to healthcare, although their extent poses special problems for healthcare managers. Three features make asymmetric information especially troublesome in the healthcare sector:

1. By paying the bills of healthcare providers, insurance creates a principal–agent relationship not found in most fields.
2. Insurance reduces the patient's incentive to monitor the performance of healthcare providers because it limits the patient's exposure to financial opportunism.
3. Asymmetric information is intrinsic to most provider–patient relationships. Patients typically seek providers' services because they want information, so the threat of opportunism is always present.

Opportunism is such an obvious risk that institutions appear to have developed behaviors to limit it (Arrow 1963). One of the most obvious is our preference for dealing with those who have proven themselves. For example, primary care physicians tend to refer patients to physicians who have served them and their patients well. For fear of losing this business, specialists who might be tempted to provide unnecessary services will be reluctant to do so. These sorts of ongoing relationships—between buyer and seller, patient and provider, and supervisor and subordinate—tend to deter observable opportunism. Much of the regulation of the healthcare sector also serves to deter opportunism. The problem is that these mechanisms work only when opportunism is detectable. In many cases, it is not.

13.2.3 Signaling

Signaling
Sending messages
that reveal
information
another party does
not observe

When differences in quality or other attributes of care are hard to observe, agents may use **signaling** to reassure principals. Signals should tell prospective clients about the agent, should be hard to counterfeit, and should be relatively inexpensive. Brand names are classic signals. Including a Pfizer label on a new drug costs little and reassures consumers that the drug meets stringent quality standards because substandard quality would hurt Pfizer's sales. The challenge is to prevent others from counterfeiting the labels. Surprisingly, branding in the healthcare market, especially branding of healthcare services, is not common. Quality certification is another strategy for dealing with asymmetric information. For example, hospital accreditation by The Joint Commission is a signal of quality that is difficult to counterfeit. Unfortunately, the process is so expensive that many smaller hospitals do not seek accreditation.

Other signals may be useful but are likely to be less credible. For example, high prices and high levels of advertising also serve as quality signals because low-cost, low-quality providers could not afford to advertise frequently or raise prices (Wang 2011). In markets with standardized products, poorly informed agents can buy information (e.g., by subscribing to *Consumer Reports*) or copy well-informed agents. The more individualized products are, the less this strategy works, so its value in the healthcare market is unclear. Although we can identify healthcare cases in which signaling reduces the problems associated with asymmetric information, it is far from a comprehensive solution.

13.3 Incentive Design for Providers

Recognition that the insurance system of the United States created multiple incentives for inefficiency triggered the growth of managed care. Providers were faced with strong incentives to deliver care as long as the benefits exceeded their patients' costs, and costly care was often free for insured patients. Neither party had a compelling reason for taking the true cost of care into account. We have already discussed redesign of consumer payments, so let's consider how incentives relate to provider payments.

CASE 13.1   Improving Safety

"Our first priority is improving safety. Some of our nursing homes have very high workers' compensation costs, which just kills the bottom line. Plus, it really gets in the way of providing high-quality care. If workers are shuttling in and out of the nursing home, they cannot build relationships with residents and they will have trouble working together," said Rowan, the CEO, looking around the table.

Braver than most of the employees, Dominique homed in on the complex issues this simple idea raised. "Right now we give administrators bonuses and promotions based on profitability. We have to recognize that unsafe work practices may boost productivity; for example, it may take longer to lift patients the safe way. In addition, managers who are working on promoting safety will not be doing the marketing or process improvement work that could boost their facility's profits. It is absolutely true that poor worker safety hurts the system's profits, but it may not hurt the nursing home's profits. After all, the system, not the individual nursing home, pays the workers' compensation premium."

"We have to be smart about this," Casey interjected. "A 1997 article by Puelz and Snow described a restaurant chain that began paying managers a fixed wage plus a share of the restaurant's profits plus a bonus for reducing workers' compensation claims. Some managers improved safety, but some apparently stopped reporting minor accidents (which could get them and us in real trouble). We have to make sure that we get managers to focus on making nursing homes safer places to work, not on convincing workers not to file claims."

Discussion questions:
- Who is the principal and who is the agent in this scenario?
- How is the agent better informed than the principal?
- How do poorly aligned incentives affect the system and individual administrators?
- What could the system do to convince nursing home administrators to improve safety?
- Are financial incentives a part of the action plan? Why or why not?
- How could nursing home administrators signal to the company that they are improving safety?

Incentives are implicit in the four most common methods of paying providers: fee-for-service payments, salaries, capitation, and case-based payment. Each of these methods has some advantages and disadvantages.

Exhibit 13.1 contrasts the incentives created by different payment systems. Note that fee-for-service and salary compensation systems incorporate opposite incentives. The incentive structures of capitation and case-based payment systems are similar and fall between these opposite cases. Fee-for-service, case-based, and capitation payment systems immediately reward providers who have large numbers of clients. Having more clients means higher revenues in all of these systems. In contrast, unless other incentive systems are in place (such as review by superiors or the possibility of promotion), salary and budget payment systems do not reward providers according to the number of clients they serve.

The only form of payment that rewards providers who provide a large volume of services per client is fee-for-service payment. In case-based and capitation systems, the disincentive for high volumes of service per client is tempered by the rewards for attracting additional clients. Just as they do not reward for large numbers of clients, salary and budget systems also deter providers from delivering high volumes of service per client.

All of the payment systems except fee-for-service encourage providers to avoid clients with complicated, expensive problems (or at least encourage them to prefer clients with simple, inexpensive problems). Expensive clients, when combined with fixed payments per case or per period, are financially unrewarding for providers. Likewise, all of the payment systems except fee-for-service motivate providers to refer patients to external services (such as church-sponsored organizations or services provided by friends), as long as they are cost-effective from the provider's perspective. From society's

EXHIBIT 13.1
Financial Incentives of Alternative Compensation Systems

	Fee-for-Service	Case-Based	Capitation	Salary or Budget
Number of clients	+	+	+	–
Services per client	+	–	–	–
Client acuity[a]	+	–	–	–
Unbillable services[b]	–	+	+	+

Note: A "+" indicates that the compensation system rewards producing more of an output or using more of an input. A "–" indicates that the compensation system rewards producing less of an output or using less of an input.
[a] In this context, client acuity refers to the amount of services that a client is likely to need. Higher acuity means that a client is likely to need more services.
[b] Unbillable services include both services for which the provider cannot bill because of the provisions of the insurance plan and services provided by others.

perspective, patients should be referred elsewhere as long as the marginal benefit of doing so exceeds the marginal cost. Providers who are paid on the basis of cases, capitation, or salary may refer patients too often, especially if the provider does not bear the full cost of the services of community organizations or other external services. In contrast, only billable services can be profitable in fee-for-service systems. Fee-for-service creates an incentive not to use external resources (or at least not to use the organization's resources to improve clients' access to them) and typically rewards providers who refer patients too infrequently, from society's perspective.

None of these payment systems solves the asymmetric information problem. Providers still usually know more about appropriate treatment options than do patients or insurers. Fee-for-service providers inclined toward opportunism are still able to recommend additional billable services, case-based providers are still able to avoid unprofitable cases, capitated providers are still able to recommend limited treatment plans, and salaried providers are still able to limit how much they do.

This discussion should not be construed as an assertion that only financial incentives matter. Such an assertion would be inconsistent with basic economic theory, which postulates that principals and agents balance alternative objectives. Only some of these goals will be financial. For example, some physicians may offer extensive patient education programs because of their commitment to the health of their patients or because the programs are an effective marketing tool, even if the fee-for-service payment system does not treat these programs as a billable service. Nonetheless, economics anticipates an aggregate response to financial incentives and predicts that physicians will offer more of such services if the fee-for-service payment system offers compensation for them or if they are profitable under case-based or capitation arrangements.

Suppose that a physician schedules four patients per hour for 30 hours per week and works 48 weeks per year (see Exhibit 13.2). Under plan A, the physician earns $20 per patient and has a total income of $115,200. (This example bases compensation on visits to simplify the discussion, not to define an attractive fee-for-service compensation plan. More sensible fee-for-service

Plan	Base Salary	Marginal Compensation	Volume Payments	Total Income
A	$0	$20	$115,200	$115,200
B	$80,000	$20	$35,200	$115,200
C	$100,000	$20	$35,200	$135,200
D	$57,600	$10	$57,600	$115,200

EXHIBIT 13.2
An Illustrative Model of Incentives

systems base compensation on billings, relative value units, and so forth.) Plan B provides a base salary of $80,000 plus $20 per patient for visits in excess of 4,000. At the margin, plans A and B have the same incentives, even though plan B combines salary- and volume-based payments. Each plan pays $20 per patient and provides the same total income. This example illustrates that blended compensation systems can give agents similar incentives with less risk than pure compensation systems.

The incentives of plan C are subtly different from the incentives of plans A and B. Plan C offers a $100,000 base salary plus $20 per patient for visits in excess of 4,000. Although plan C pays $20 per visit at the margin like plans A and B, the physician's income will be higher under plan C than it would be with the same number of patients under plan A or B. Consequently, the physician may feel less need to add an additional patient at the end of the day or double book to squeeze in an acutely ill patient. In this case, **income effects** are the effects incentive systems have on physicians' decisions about the number of patients they will treat (Rizzo and Blumenthal 1994).

Plan D offers a base salary of $57,600 plus $10 for each patient visit. Even though the physician's income will be the same with 5,760 patients per year under plans A, B, and D, the physician may choose to see fewer patients under plan D because the marginal reward is smaller.

Income effects
Effects of income shifts on amounts demanded or supplied (Shifts may be due to changes in income or due to changes in purchasing power caused by price changes.)

13.4 Insurance and Incentives

How much have compensation systems changed since 2010, given the importance of how providers are paid? Less than you might suspect. For example, even in areas in which managed care is pervasive, most physicians continue to be paid on the basis of their productivity (typically measured by billings, visits, or net revenue), just as they were at the turn of the twenty-first century (Landon and Roberts 2013). In addition, even though hospital outpatient services represent one of the fastest growing components of medical spending, many health plans continue to pay hospital outpatient departments on the basis of discounted charges (Crosson et al. 2009). Charges, however, seldom reflect costs accurately (Rich et al. 2013). As a result, charge-based payments can make some services very profitable and some services very unprofitable, thereby creating powerful incentives to expand production of some services and curtail production of others.

A striking feature of most insurance plans is payment based on the source of the patient's treatment. Reflecting their historical development, most payment systems are designed to compensate providers. Few are designed to encourage provision of efficient, patient-centered care. Some traditional HMOs might profit by enhancing and integrating care, but most Americans are covered by insurance products that pay individual providers on a fee-for-service basis (Rich et al. 2013). For this reason, Medicare's Physician Group Practice Demonstration, launched in 2005, was an innovation. This project rewarded ten large practices for improving the quality and efficiency of care delivered to Medicare fee-for-service beneficiaries. The demonstration sought to encourage coordination of care, more efficient delivery of services, improved processes, and better outcomes. Thus far it has been more successful in improving processes of care than in increasing efficiency (Colla et al. 2012).

13.5 Limits on Incentive-Based Payments

A number of factors limit how complete incentive-based payments can be. Concerns about risk, complexity, and team production make agents reluctant to enter into incentive-based compensation arrangements. Likewise, concerns about opportunism make principals reluctant because a high-powered incentive system may leave them worse off if agents respond in unanticipated ways.

13.5.1 Risk

Capitation, utilization withholding, and case-based payment systems are often referred to as *risk-sharing systems*. This term is somewhat misleading. The goal of these systems is incentive alignment; risk sharing is a side effect. For example, capitation gives physicians incentives to use resources wisely, so capitation succeeds if physicians do not run unnecessary tests or if they avoid hospitalizing patients when better community treatment options are available. Full-risk capitation, in which physicians are responsible for all of their patients' costs, gives physicians incentives to take such steps. Unfortunately, the financial risks associated with full-risk capitation can be substantial. One patient with a rare, expensive illness can bankrupt a solo practice; an unexpected jump in pharmaceutical prices can bankrupt a small provider-owned HMO. These risks are one reason capitation's growth has stalled and many organizations are avoiding full-risk capitation (Mechanic and Zinner 2012).

13.5.2 Complexity

Providers and employees are more likely to respond to simple, comprehensible systems than to complex, confusing systems. Simple systems limit the use of incentives and the problems they create. If you want the payment system to reward physicians for keeping customer satisfaction high, MMR (measles, mumps, and rubella) vaccination rates high, out-of-formulary drug use low, hospitalization rates low, hospital lengths of stay short, after-hours response times prompt, record updates prompt, and asthma follow-up appointments timely, the system is likely to be unwieldy. Moreover, the reward associated with each component of the system is likely to be small.

13.5.3 Opportunism

Managers must anticipate opportunistic responses to incentive systems. An agent with better information can harm the principal. In many cases, whether an agent has lived up to contract requirements is difficult to ascertain. In other cases, the agent may act in ways the principal did not anticipate. Some responses will necessitate system redesign; some will have to be tolerated to prevent the system from becoming excessively complex. For example, one response to the price reductions introduced by PPOs was to unbundle services. Physicians and other providers began to bill separately for services once included in the standard office visit. While insurers attempted to limit unbundling in a variety of ways, the fundamental problem remained that the incentives of physicians and insurers were misaligned (Goldfield et al. 2008). Physicians' profits would be higher when they billed for more services, but insurers' profits would be higher when physicians billed for fewer services.

13.5.4 Team Production

Team production also limits the use of incentives. Production of healthcare products usually involves a number of people, and the shortcomings of one person can undermine the efforts of the entire team. For example, rudeness by one disaffected team member can negate the efforts of others to provide exemplary customer service. This interdependency can also weaken the effects of individual incentives. Workers who try hard to do a good job or physicians who are conscientious about reducing length of stay are likely to feel that their efforts are not appreciated if the shortcomings of others deny them bonuses. Building and maintaining effective teams are important tasks for managers. Unless carefully structured, financial incentives tend to reward individualistic behavior, which usually weakens teams. Equally problematic, team financial incentives (i.e., every member of the team receives a bonus when the team reaches its goals) often fail to motivate workers.

13.6 Incentive Design for Managers

Incentives for managers can be financial or nonfinancial. If both types are used, the two incentive systems should operate in tandem. Otherwise, they may worsen the problems created by asymmetric information (Baker, Jensen, and Murphy 1988).

Incentive pay for managers is a partial response to the asymmetric information problem. It usually takes the form of bonus payments, profit sharing, or stock options. In most cases, it is a modest part of total compensation and is only loosely tied to managers' performance.

How Much Do Physician Incentives Affect the Use of Expensive Services?

According to a classic study of alternative managed care plans (Josephson and Karcz 1997), incentives have a considerable effect on physicians' use of expensive services. One of the most interesting features of this study is its delineation of how incentives differed for two cohorts of HMO physicians. One cohort of primary care physicians were partners in a capitated, multispecialty group practice that served 22,136 beneficiaries of a large New England HMO. Aside from stop-loss insurance, the physician owners of the practice were at full risk for these beneficiaries' use of services. Unspent capitation funds were distributed to the physicians at the end of the year, so the incentive to keep costs down was significant.

The other cohort of physicians included solo practice physicians who were members of three independent practice association (IPA) HMOs. These physicians were paid on a fee-for-service basis with 10 to 20 percent of the payment withheld. At the end of the year, the with-holdings were split equally among the physicians, the hospital, and the HMO. The only risk that these IPA physicians faced was that higher than expected volumes of service per patient would reduce their shares of the withholdings. They also had limited motivation to keep costs down. Fee-for-service payments provided significant incentives to keep volumes (hence costs) up, and the split of the withholding pool weakened their incentives to limit the use of costly services.

The patients of the capitated physicians used fewer emergency department services. They averaged only 70 visits per thousand members per year. In contrast, the patients of the IPA physicians averaged more than five times as many emergency department visits per year. One reason for this differential was that physicians in the capitated practice operated an after-hours urgent care center to accommodate more than 4,000 patient visits. In addition, the physicians in the capitated practice made a concerted effort to serve walk-in patients during office hours to ensure that they were not diverted to the emergency department. In contrast, the IPA physicians, who bore little of the high cost of emergency department care, often referred patients to the emergency department for treatment of unexpected minor illnesses.

(continued)

(continued)

Patient incentives, which the study did not consider, may have accounted for some of the difference between the groups. The IPA HMOs may have incorporated weaker incentives for patients to avoid using the emergency department. Although likely to have an impact, differences in patients' incentives do not explain why the prepaid group practice provided comprehensive urgent care services and the IPA practices did not; the physicians decided to provide these services. Capitation aligned the incentives of the physicians and the health plan because both of them benefited by reducing the use of high-cost emergency department services.

In this case, saving money probably improves the quality of care. In addition to being expensive, care in the emergency department tends to be poorly integrated with other outpatient care. Emergency department physicians may lack timely access to patients' records, and communication with patients' primary care physicians tends to be problematic.

Four concepts underlie incentive pay for managers:

1. Financial incentives can strongly motivate people to perform in ways the organization desires, yet organizations seldom want managers to focus only on duties that will increase their pay. (Fee-for-service compensation presents the same problem.)
2. Managers' goals are often not fully defined. Managers need to respond creatively to problems or, better yet, position the organization to respond to problems that are not yet evident. Performance assessment based on intangibles would be difficult, if not impossible.
3. Most managers' performance is hard to measure. When an individual's productivity becomes hard to measure, compensation based on individual productivity ceases to make sense.
4. What is measurable and what is desired are unlikely to coincide. Compensation based on measurable outputs is likely to increase opportunism as managers react to what is rewarded rather than to what is sought.

Gainsharing
A strategy for rewarding those who contribute to an organization's success

For these reasons, incentive pay for those with significant management roles generally needs to reflect the success of the overall organization. The dilution of incentives that results from using profit sharing or **gainsharing** is a reasonable price to pay for promoting team-oriented behavior. Gainsharing is like profit sharing but can base bonuses on a broader array of outcomes.

Members of a group can earn bonuses for hitting production, customer satisfaction, profit, quality, or cost targets. As individual contributions become less discernible, the more effective group incentives are likely to be. Members of the group will be able to monitor each other more easily, alignment of the group's and the organization's incentives will become more important, and the group will more easily alter how it does its work. For example, hospital care is produced by teams, but pay for many physicians depends on their personal billings. To encourage physicians to participate in hospital performance improvement activities, implementing payments to physicians that are based on the performance of the hospital is often helpful. (Chapter 6 discussed gainsharing in not-for-profit hospitals, where profit sharing is not permitted.)

Incentive pay is only part of an effective incentive system. Economic theory does not imply that individuals will not respond to opportunities to do challenging work, public celebrations of their accomplishments, or a positive review by a trusted mentor. An effective manager will consider these tools as well. Successful organizations require cooperation in management and production, so a nonfinancial system that rewards cooperation is a sensible option for aligning incentives. Promotions typically combine financial and nonfinancial rewards.

CASE 13.2 Improving Total Knee Replacement at Brigham and Women's Hospital

In 2007 John Wright gathered a group of people from all of the professions involved in total knee replacement at Brigham and Women's Hospital—surgery, anesthesia, nursing, physical therapy—to formulate a single standard way of doing knee replacements (Gawande 2012). The team carefully studied the medical literature, conducted some small-scale trials, worked together to develop a standard protocol, and tried to get everyone to follow suit. The new protocol involved changes in anesthesia, changes in the prostheses used, changes in medications, changes in postoperative activities for patients, and changes in physical therapy. The new protocol reduced costs, improved pain control, improved the mobility of patients, and shortened length of stay. Lowe (2011) quotes Wright as saying, "Our primary goal is to improve the outcome and the process of care for the patient. Invariably when we pay attention to these concerns, we find that we achieve the secondary goals of efficiency and cost savings."

(continued)

CASE 13.2
(continued)

One of the most controversial changes involved limiting the prostheses that surgeons could use.

Even minor differences in prostheses can result in changes to the operation, and surgeons have strong preferences about prostheses. But some prostheses cost far more than others, and little evidence indicated that the more expensive prostheses were better. The surgeons now use a single source for 75 percent of their prostheses, sharply improving the hospital's bargaining power (Gawande 2012).

Discussion questions:
- Why would standardization reduce costs? How could it improve quality?
- How could the hospital reward physicians for helping standardize prostheses?
- How would this reward system help align incentives?
- Are any strategies less likely to cause problems with the Medicare Inspector General?
- Why would choosing a standard prosthesis improve the hospital's bargaining position?

13.7 Conclusion

Incentive restructuring is an imperfect response to the problem of asymmetric information, as are all responses to this problem. The rewards of incentive systems are usually based on results, not what agents actually do, and agents can respond opportunistically to virtually any incentive system. The challenge is to align the incentives of all the individuals in a system with the interests of its stakeholders. Because good incentive systems must balance competing objectives, no magic formula exists. In addition, managers must anticipate that incentives may have multiple effects and that designing incentive systems and keeping them up to date will be expensive.

Exercises

13.1 Describe some healthcare situations in which an agent has taken advantage of a principal. Then describe some healthcare transactions that have not taken place because of fears about asymmetric information.

13.2 Identify some ways that nursing homes can signal high quality to consumers. Which of these signals are most apt to be reliable?

13.3 Provide an example of costly monitoring in the healthcare workplace. Can you think of an employment contract that would allow a reduction in monitoring without a reduction in quality?

13.4 What are some strategies for reducing adverse selection in insurance markets? What sorts of problems do these solutions cause?

13.5 One physical therapist is paid $20 per session. Another is paid $400 per week plus $20 per session in excess of 20 sessions per week. A third is paid $400 per week, plus $200 per week for having all paperwork complete and filed within 48 hours, plus $20 per session in excess of 30 sessions per week. How do the therapists' incentives to produce sessions compare? How do their incentives to complete paperwork differ?

13.6 One physician is paid $100 per visit. Another is paid $2,500 per week plus $100 per session in excess of 20 sessions per week. A third is paid $2,000 per week plus $100 per session in excess of 20 sessions per week. The third physician is also paid a weekly bonus of $500 for being in the top quartile in management of common chronic diseases, appropriate antibiotic use, preventive counseling, screening tests, and appropriate prescribing in elderly patients. How do the physicians' incentives compare?

13.7 The Federal Trade Commission requires that firms advertise truthfully. Why does this requirement promote competition? Would firms be better or worse off if the Federal Trade Commission adopted a "let the buyer beware" policy?

13.8 Your firm sells backup generators to hospitals and clinics. The generators are guaranteed to operate on demand for two years. Your data show that the generators run an average of 42 hours per year. Your firm offers an extended warranty that covers the next three years. Your data show that repairs are needed for 2 percent of units during this three-year period. When repairs are needed, the average cost is $4,000. You charge $400 for the extended warranty, and about 20 percent of your clients buy it.

a. The extended warranty has been a consistent money loser. Claims average $1,000 per customer. How could this situation happen, given the data above?

b. Would raising the premium to $1,000 solve this problem?

c. What would you recommend that your company do to solve this problem?

13.9 For the population as a whole, average healthcare spending is $1,190 per year. Those with a family history of cancer (5 percent of the population) spend $20,000 on average, and those with no family history (95 percent of the population) spend $200. An insurer is offering first-dollar coverage for $1,200.

a. You are not risk averse and do not have a family history of cancer. Do you buy coverage?

b. You are not risk averse and have a family history of cancer. Do you buy coverage?

c. If you were risk averse, how would your answers to the two previous questions change?

d. What could an insurer do to prevent this sort of adverse selection?

e. What would be wrong with having everyone undergo a physical exam to qualify for coverage?

13.10 You want to hire a new laboratory technician. Excellent technicians generate $1,000 in value-added service each week. Adequate technicians generate $500 in value-added service each week. Half of the graduates are excellent, and half are adequate.

a. You cannot tell who is highly capable and who is adequate. You are prepared to pay each technician according to the value he or she adds. What salary do you offer?

b. Who will accept this offer?

c. Is there any way that excellent technicians could communicate their productivity?

d. Propose a compensation system that will attract both types of technicians and pay no one more than the value he or she adds.

13.11 A new test identifies individuals with a genetic predisposition to develop heart disease before age 70. People who are predisposed to heart disease cost twice as much to insure as those who are not.

a. Can you make a case that a law prohibiting this test would be a good idea?

b. The test is not expensive. Would you prefer to skip the test and buy insurance at a premium that covers everyone or take the test and buy insurance at a premium that covers your group?

13.12 Your hospital wants to buy practices to expand its primary care networks. You are aware that physicians who want to sell their practices differ. Some love to practice medicine and love seeing patients. They want to sell their practices to focus on patient care 50 hours per week. Some physicians love to play golf and want to provide patient care no more than 35 hours per week. Propose a compensation plan that will allow you to hire only physicians who love to practice.

13.13 Having access to the books and understanding local markets better than new owners, the owners of medical practices generally understand their finances better than prospective buyers do. What sorts of transactions tend to take place as a result of this information asymmetry? What sorts of transactions tend not to take place? What can buyers and sellers do to offset this information asymmetry?

13.14 You are considering acquiring a firm rumored to have developed an effective gene therapy for diabetes. The value of the firm depends on this therapy. If the therapy is effective, the firm is worth $100 per share; otherwise, the firm is worth no more than $20 per share. Your company's management and marketing strengths should increase the share price by at least 50 percent in either case. You must make an offer for the firm now, before the results of clinical trials are in. The current owner of the firm will sell for the right price. Make an offer for the firm. Explain why you think your offer makes sense.

References

Arrow, K. J. 1963. "Uncertainty and the Welfare Economics of Medical Care." *American Economic Review* 53 (5): 941–73.

Baker, G. P., M. C. Jensen, and K. J. Murphy. 1988. "Compensation and Incentives: Practice vs. Theory." *Journal of Finance* 43 (3): 593–616.

Colla, C. H., D. E. Wennberg, E. Meara, J. S. Skinner, D. Gottlieb, V. A. Lewis, C. M. Snyder, and E. S. Fisher. 2012. "Spending Differences Associated with the Medicare Physician Group Practice Demonstration." *Journal of the American Medical Association* 308 (10): 1015–23.

Crosson, F. J., S. Guterman, N. Taylor, R. Young, and L. Tollen. 2009. *How Can Medicare Lead Delivery System Reform?* The Commonwealth Fund Issue Brief. Published November. www.commonwealthfund.org/Publications/Issue-Briefs/2009/Nov/How-Can-Medicare-Lead-Delivery-System-Reform.aspx.

Gawande, A. 2012. "Big Med." *The New Yorker.* Published August 13. www.newyorker.com/reporting/2012/08/13/120813fa_fact_gawande.

Goldfield, N., R. Averill, J. Vertrees, R. Fuller, D. Mesches, G. Moore, J. H. Wasson, and W. Kelly. 2008. "Reforming the Primary Care Physician Payment System." *Journal of Ambulatory Care Management* 31 (1): 24–31.

Josephson, G., and A. Karcz. 1997. "The Impact of Physician Economic Incentives on Admission Rates." *American Journal of Managed Care* 3 (1): 49–56.

Landon, B. E., and D. H. Roberts. 2013. "Reenvisioning Specialty Care and Payment Under Global Payment Systems." *Journal of the American Medical Association* 310 (4): 371–72.

Lowe, C. 2011. "Champions in Health Care: John Wright, Physician." *Boston Business Journal*. Published August 26. www.bizjournals.com/boston/print-edition/2011/08/26/champions-in-health-care-john-wright.html.

Mechanic, R., and D. E. Zinner. 2012. "Many Large Medical Groups Will Need to Acquire New Skills and Tools to Be Ready for Payment Reform." *Health Affairs* 31 (9): 1984–92.

Puelz, R., and A. Snow. 1997. "Optimal Incentive Contracting with *Ex Ante* and *Ex Post* Moral Hazards: Theory and Evidence." *Journal of Risk and Uncertainty* 14 (2): 169–88.

Rich, E. C., T. K. Lake, C. S. Valenzano, and M. M. Maxfield. 2013. "Paying the Doctor: Evidence-Based Decisions at the Point-of-Care and the Role of Fee-for-Service Incentives." *Journal of Comparative Effectiveness Research* 2 (3): 235–47.

Rizzo, J. A., and D. Blumenthal. 1994. "Physician Labor Supply: Do Income Effects Matter?" *Journal of Health Economics* 13 (4): 433–53.

Wang, R. 2011. "Listing Prices as Signals of Quality in Markets with Negotiation." *Journal of Industrial Economics* 59 (2): 321–41.

ECONOMIC ANALYSIS OF CLINICAL AND MANAGERIAL INTERVENTIONS

After reading this chapter, students will be able to

- identify when a cost-minimization analysis is appropriate,
- distinguish between cost–benefit analysis and cost–utility analysis,
- explain why economic evaluation is necessary in healthcare, and
- discuss the importance of comparing the best alternatives.

- Analyses of interventions are designed to support decisions, not make them.
- Comparing the most plausible alternatives is vital. Well-done analyses will not be enlightening if we consider the wrong choices.
- Four types of analysis are common: cost-minimization analysis (CMA), cost-effectiveness analysis (CEA), cost–utility analysis (CUA), and cost–benefit analysis (CBA).
- The simplest and most productive type of analysis is CMA.
- CBA and CUA are potentially more powerful but pose many questions.
- Modeling costs entails identifying the perspective involved, the resources used, and the opportunity costs of those resources.
- Focusing on the direct costs of interventions is best.
- Modeling benefits is the most difficult part of economic evaluation of clinical interventions.

14.1 Introduction

Until recently, economic analyses of clinical interventions were uncommon. Healthcare decision makers had little or no incentive to assess whether procedures were worth their costs, or even whether those procedures could be done more efficiently. A fee-for-service payment system tells decision makers what procedures are worth. Practical managers in a fee-for-service environment will not worry about genuinely balancing value and cost.

The emergence of bundled payment systems and the growth of capitation have made economic analyses of clinical interventions more relevant. In a bundled payment system, getting the same outcome at lower cost directly increases profits. In a capitated system, the options are even greater: Getting the same outcome more cheaply still increases profits, but strategies such as increasing prevention, self-care, or adherence to clinically effective protocols can also have a significant payoff. In short, the value of analyzing clinical interventions has risen sharply.

Analyses of clinical interventions ask deceptively simple questions, such as "Are the benefits of this intervention greater than its costs?" and "Is this intervention better than the alternatives?" Such questions are often difficult to answer because assessing the benefits of clinical interventions is difficult. While the second question may sound much like the first, it is easier to answer because it does not require assigning the benefits an explicit value.

These questions must be asked because even in a wealthy society, resources are limited. When an individual chooses to purchase a drug or be screened for a condition, he or she cannot use those resources for other purposes. The same is true for society. If money spent on an electrocardiogram could be used to greater benefit elsewhere, the resources should be reallocated to those other uses. Ideally, we would like to use resources to maximum benefit. Practically, we seek to avoid pure waste and interventions in which the benefits are smaller than the costs.

Why are economic analyses of clinical interventions needed? Public and private insurers need information on which to base coverage decisions. Most patients lack opportunities to become familiar with all the potential outcomes of therapy. In addition, healthcare providers often need information to make the case for a new form of treatment. Because the stakes can be high, patients and providers are reluctant to innovate without evidence.

Analyses of clinical interventions are designed to support decision making, not to make decisions. By providing a framework for synthesizing and understanding information, economic analyses can help decision makers avoid bad decisions.

Four types of analysis are common. **Cost-minimization analysis** (CMA), **cost-effectiveness analysis** (CEA), **cost–utility analysis** (CUA), and **cost–benefit analysis** (CBA) all compare the costs and benefits of alternative interventions. All four use the same methods to measure costs, but they use different strategies for assessing benefits.

Cost-minimization analysis
An analysis that measures the cost of two or more innovations with the same patient outcomes

Cost-effectiveness analysis
An analysis that measures the cost of an innovation per unit of change in a single outcome

Cost–utility analysis
An analysis that measures the cost of an innovation per quality-adjusted life year

Cost–benefit analysis
An analysis that compares the value of an innovation with its costs (Value is measured as willingness to pay for the innovation or willingness to accept compensation to allow it to be implemented.)

CMA is the most useful for managers. Although it is more limited in scope than the others, it is simpler to apply. CMA answers our second question, "Is this intervention better than the alternatives?" Unfortunately, it cannot answer it in every case. If the better alternative also costs more or if the least expensive alternative does not work as well, CMA is not helpful.

CEA extends CMA somewhat. When the better strategy costs more, CEA answers the question "What is the cost per unit of this gain?" This simple piece of information is likely to be of genuine value to managers because it will validate strategies with a small cost per unit and negate those with a large cost per unit. CEA does not, however, directly compare the costs and benefits of a strategy as CUA and CBA do.

14.2 Cost Analysis

Before examining these four types of analysis in more detail, we will briefly review the basics of cost analysis. Measuring costs involves three tasks:

1. identifying the perspective involved,
2. identifying the resources used, and
3. identifying the opportunity costs of those resources.

Costs are often poorly understood (and poorly measured), even though the issues are seldom very complex.

14.2.1 Identifying Cost Perspective
Identifying a cost perspective is an essential first step. Confusion about costs usually arises because the analyst has not been clear about the perspective. Decision makers usually respond to the costs they see, and different decision makers typically see different portions of the cost. This notion may seem abstract, so here is a simple example. An insurance plan (an HMO) wishes to increase use of a generic drug in place of the brand-name equivalent. The generic product costs $50, of which $4 is paid by the patient and $46 is paid by the plan. The branded product costs $100, of which $5 is paid by the patient and $95 is paid by the plan. From the plan's perspective, switching to the generic saves $49. From the consumer's perspective, switching to the generic saves $1. From the perspective of society as a whole, switching to the generic saves $50. These different perspectives are all valid, yet they may lead to very different choices.

Another example shows how differences in cost perspectives can lead to different perceptions of the cost of a good or service. Suppose the same

HMO encourages use of an over-the-counter drug because the drug is not a covered benefit. The over-the-counter product costs $10, of which $0 is paid by the plan. The prescription product costs $15, of which $5 is paid by the patient and $10 is paid by the plan. From the consumer's perspective, the switch increases costs from $5 to $10. Because consumers share the costs of covered medications with many other beneficiaries, they will want to switch to over-the-counter medications only if those medications are more effective or more convenient than prescription medications. From the insurer's perspective, the switch reduces costs from $10 to $0. The switch makes sense for the insurer as long as the prescription medication is not "too much better" than the over-the-counter medication. From the perspective of society, the switch reduces costs from $15 to $10 and makes sense only if the over-the-counter medication is "nearly as good" as the prescription medication.

Societal perspective
A perspective that takes account of all costs and benefits, no matter to whom they accrue

A **societal perspective** on costs is usually the right perspective for two reasons. The societal perspective recognizes all costs, no matter to whom they accrue. Other perspectives typically fail to consider important costs, which is seldom a good long-run strategy. Those to whom costs have been shifted try to avoid them and try to avoid contracting with organizations that shift costs to them.

14.2.2 Identifying Resources and Opportunity Costs

Cost equals the volume of resources used in an activity multiplied by the opportunity cost of those resources. Keeping these two components of cost separate is useful because either can vary. A clinical understanding of a process helps a manager to identify the resources used in an intervention; a well-documented clinical pathway is even more helpful.

Most of the time the opportunity cost of a resource simply equals what you paid for it. The opportunity cost of $100 in supplies is $100. The opportunity cost of an hour of nursing time is $27 if the total compensation of a nurse is $27 per hour. Calculating the opportunity cost is more complex when the cost of a resource has changed since you bought it and you would not buy it at its current price. In these cases you have to calculate the value of the resource in its best alternative use.

Economic theory provides a powerful tool for simplifying cost analyses. It says to focus on the resources you add (or do not need) as a result of an intervention. In other words, focus on incremental costs. This task can be difficult but is less complex than pondering, for example, exactly what proportion of the CFO's compensation should be allocated to a triage process in the emergency room.

14.2.3 Direct and Indirect Costs

Implicit in this advice is a recommendation to focus on the direct costs of interventions, or those costs that result because an intervention has been tried. For example, the costs of a drug and its administration are direct costs of drug therapy. The costs of associated inpatient and outpatient care are also direct costs. If healthcare costs associated with ineffectiveness or adverse outcomes are present, those should be counted as well. By the same token, costs the patient incurs because he or she undertakes the treatment are direct costs. Added childcare, transportation, and dietary costs that result directly from therapy should be counted from a societal cost perspective. From the perspective of the healthcare system, however, these added costs for patients would not be counted. (Of course, as noted above, a cost perspective that ignores the effects on customers is likely to result in poor decisions.)

Most "indirect" costs represent a confusion of costs with benefits. Healthier people typically spend more on food, recreation, entertainment, and other joys of life, but this additional spending is not a part of the costs of interventions that restored health. (Individuals have independently made the judgment that this additional spending is worthwhile.) By the same token, we should not treat a recovered patient's future spending as a cost of the intervention that permitted the recovery—unless, as with transplant patients' immunosuppressive drugs, these costs are an integral part of the intervention. That a transplant patient feels healthy enough to play tennis certainly signals that the operation was a success, but the cost of knee surgery for this overenthusiastic athlete should not be considered a cost of the transplant.

14.3 Types of Analysis

We have identified four types of analysis: CBA, CEA, CUA, and CMA. Be aware that mislabeling is the norm, not the exception. A "cost–benefit analysis" could be anything, and the meaning of "cost-effectiveness analysis" has changed over the years. Exhibit 14.1 shows when each type of analysis is needed.

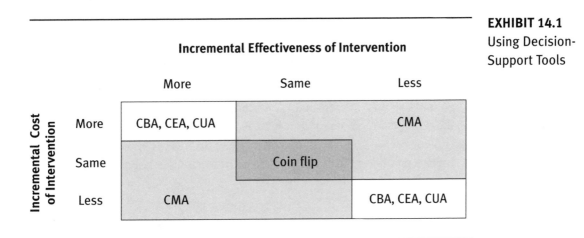

EXHIBIT 14.1
Using Decision-Support Tools

If deciding which strategy is best is very difficult, the choice of strategy shouldn't matter because they all support decision making. If the options look so similar that choosing the best one is difficult, do not perform a detailed analysis. A coin flip will suffice. Of course, when populations are large, even small differences in cost or benefit per case can result in significant differences from society's perspective. However, for working managers, small differences are not worthy of attention.

CASE 14.1 Teledermatology

"Well, this analysis does not suggest to me that it makes sense to push ahead with fancy telemedicine equipment for our practice. As I read the data, it costs us $280 to provide a consult to a patient via telemedicine and $320 to do it face-to-face. Telemedicine might boost our profits a little, but I can't imagine too many patients will want to give up meeting their dermatologist in person. So," Reese, the practice's CFO, summed up, "I recommend against this project."

"If that were the whole story," said Carroll, the director of marketing, "I would agree with you. But this looks only at our costs. We need to think about the costs patients bear. Many of our patients are children, so they have to be driven across town by a parent. By the time you figure in the travel costs and time costs parents incur to bring their children here, a face-to-face visit could easily cost $100 more than a telemedicine visit. And that back-of-the-envelope calculation just looks at people in the local area. We know children in the western half of the state are not getting the care they should. There are very few dermatologists out there, and there are no dermatologists who specialize in treating pediatric skin cancer. The time and travel costs for those patients could easily be $200 per visit. We can't just look at our own costs."

"I hadn't thought of that," said Reese. "I was focusing on these cost estimates, not taking into account the opportunity to do group visits—which our patients have been asking about—very inexpensively. This technology will let one of our doctors or nurses talk to eight patients at once in their homes. It's mostly teaching and coaching, so the patients do not need ultra-high-resolution monitors on their home computers. We could even do some follow-up visits that way, so I think there are options this analysis of $280 per visit does not consider."

(continued)

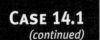

CASE 14.1
(continued)

Discussion questions:
- Does Shea's point about patients' costs make sense?
- Which perspective on costs looks more like a societal perspective to you?
- Would using telemedicine equipment mean giving up face-to-face dermatologist visits?
- What would be the advantage, if any, of being able to serve patients in the western half of the state?
- What would be the advantage, if any, of being able to offer telemedicine group visits?
- What is your assessment of the promise of telemedicine for this practice?

14.4 Cost-Minimization Analysis

The simplest and most productive type of analysis is CMA, which identifies the intervention with the lowest costs. As long as the intervention has outcomes at least as good as those of the alternatives, CMA is the analysis of choice. While CMA avoids most of the problems associated with measuring benefits, it does not escape them entirely. The most common problem in CMA is a lack of evidence that the least-cost option has outcomes at least as good as the other choices.

Steps in Cost-Minimization Analysis

1. Estimate the expected costs for each option.
2. Show that the least-cost option has outcomes at least as good as higher-cost alternatives.

An Example of Cost-Minimization Analysis

Treatment guidelines for patients hospitalized with community-acquired pneumonia recommend antibiotic therapy for eight days. The scientific

(continued)

(continued)

basis for eight days of antibiotics is limited, and some researchers have suggested that briefer treatments may be appropriate. Because community-acquired pneumonia is a common problem, substantial savings might be possible with briefer treatments (Scalera and File 2013).

Opmeer and colleagues (2007) conducted a randomized controlled trial to compare three-day and eight-day antibiotic therapies. At day three of treatment, patients with community-acquired pneumonia who had significantly improved were randomly assigned to five days of placebo or five days of antibiotics. Patients were then followed for 28 days.

Although patients who received three-day treatment had shorter hospital stays and missed less work, none of the clinical outcomes was significantly different from the outcomes for eight-day treatment. Costs for the three-day treatment were about 4 percent lower.

14.5 Cost-Effectiveness Analysis

CEA recognizes that measuring the incremental cost of improving outcomes may be useful when a more effective intervention costs more. In at least some cases, the incremental cost will be so high or so low that a decision can be based on it.

Steps in Cost-Effectiveness Analysis

1. Estimate the expected costs for each option.
2. Establish how much the higher-cost option improves outcomes.
3. Calculate the cost per unit of improvement in outcome (e.g., the cost per life year gained or the cost per infection avoided).

An Example of Cost-Effectiveness Analysis

Pregnant women should stop smoking for many reasons, but more than 25 percent of low-income women smoke during pregnancy (Ruger et al. 2008). Trying to increase quit rates, Ruger and colleagues (2008) conducted a randomized control trial of motivational interviewing by public health nurses for low-income pregnant women.

(continued)

> *(continued)*
>
> Motivational interviewing is a type of counseling that helps clients explore why they want to stop smoking, what problems smoking causes for them, why they are ambivalent about quitting, and how life as a nonsmoker would be different. Motivational interviewing did not appear to increase the number of women who quit smoking, but it appeared to help those who had already quit avoid a relapse. Among patients who had recently quit smoking when they entered the study, 82.1 percent of usual care patients and 57.1 percent of motivational interview patients resumed smoking during the six months of follow-up.
>
> Adding motivational interviewing increased costs by $304. It also reduced the probability of a relapse by 25 percentage points and added 0.36 life years, so the incremental cost per relapse prevented was $1,217 and the incremental cost per life year gained was $851. The low cost per life year gained suggests that using motivational interviewing to reduce relapse rates is sensible.

In some cases, CEA is not helpful. If the cost per life year saved is $35,000 or if the cost per injury prevented is $10,000, the answer will not seem obvious. In these cases CBA or CUA may be needed.

14.6 Cost–Benefit Analysis

CBA is also relatively simple, but its validity is unknown. CBA is appropriate when the option with the best outcomes costs more. CBA begins with a comparison of two or more options to find out how their costs differ, then attempts to estimate the difference in benefits directly. Two very different strategies are used for estimating benefits. One uses statistical techniques to infer how much consumers are willing to pay to avoid risks. The other uses surveys of the relevant population to determine whether the added benefits are worth the cost.

Neither method's validity has been clearly established. The fundamental challenge arises from concerns about consumers' abilities to make decisions involving small probabilities of harm. If consumers do not assess these probabilities accurately, their life choices and their responses to surveys will not be reliable. In addition, multiple challenges to the validity of statistical inferences are always present, and statistical estimates of benefits are imprecise. Surveys may not give us valid measures of willingness to pay or willingness to accept compensation. First, they ask consumers to make complex assessments of services they have not yet used. Answers to hypothetical, complex questions are suspect. Second, consumers may misrepresent their preferences, believing they will have to pay more out of pocket if they answer willingness-to-pay questions accurately. Therefore, even though CBA can provide invaluable information to decision makers, its accuracy can be suspect.

Two other criticisms are worth noting. Early CBA studies based estimates of benefits on estimates of increases in labor market earnings. A few minutes of reflection will reveal problems with this approach. Is improved health for retired persons of no value? If people are willing to pay out of pocket for the care of their pets (who have no earning power), aren't changes in earnings a poor guide to the value of medical interventions? Earnings-based estimates of benefits have left a legacy of skepticism of CBA among healthcare analysts. A second complaint is that willingness to pay usually rises with income. This finding is profoundly troubling to analysts who would prefer a healthcare system that is more egalitarian than the current system in the United States. (While this complaint is not really a criticism of CBA, it is sometimes presented as such.)

For an illustration of how CBA works, return to the example of the switch from a branded product to a generic one. Recall that the branded drug costs $100 and the generic drug costs $50. Uninsured consumers would buy the branded product only if its benefits were large enough for them to be willing to pay $100. Few consumers would be willing to pay this much to get the branded product because branded and generic drugs seldom differ. Current users of a branded drug, however, face both real and perceived risks to switching, such as the risk of an allergic reaction to different inert ingredients. Remember, from the insured consumer's perspective, the cost differential is only $1, from $5 for the branded product to $4 for the generic. Current users of the drug may be willing to pay $75, in which case the marginal benefit of the branded drug will appear larger than its marginal cost. Current users have an incentive to make sure others bear the financial risk of higher costs. Asking people who are not current users is also problematic. The opinion of someone who does not have a disease the drug is intended to treat or who has not used both drugs is not likely to hold much value.

Steps in Cost–Benefit Analysis

1. Estimate the expected incremental costs of the more expensive option.
2. Survey consumers to find out whether they would be (a) willing to pay enough to cover the added costs of an option with better outcomes or (b) willing to accept compensation that would be

(continued)

(continued)

> less than the cost savings of an option with worse outcomes. Alternatively, use market data to estimate how much consumers are willing to pay to avoid risks or willing to accept to take on risks.
>
> 3. Compare the incremental benefits and costs.

An Example of Cost–Benefit Analysis

Implantable cardioverter-defibrillators reduce the risk of cardiac arrest and save lives. Unfortunately, this treatment remains expensive; typically costing more than $60,000. In addition, many implantable cardioverter-defibrillators never fire, they must be replaced every few years, and having one implanted often results in increased anxiety and depression. Cost-effectiveness studies yield ambiguous results, so a group of researchers sought to assess how patients valued implantable cardioverter-defibrillators (Nowakowska et al. 2011). To do so, they asked patients if they would be willing to pay one of seven different prices to have their implantable cardioverter-defibrillator replaced. The prices ranged from $5,000 to $35,000.

Three-quarters of the patients were unwilling to pay the price they were asked about, and the median willingness to pay was less than $5,000. As is typical in cost-benefit analyses, the amount that patients were willing to pay rose with family income.

An alternative (and probably preferable) approach to this analysis would be to ask a random sample of adults if they would prefer a less expensive insurance plan that did not cover implantable cardioverter-defibrillators. This approach would be more compelling because most insurance plans currently cover implantable cardioverter-defibrillators. Only a few people could afford an implantable cardioverter-defibrillator if they had to rely solely on their own resources.

14.7 Cost–Utility Analysis

CUA rivals CBA as a complete comparison of alternative interventions. (Note that a number of analysts do not distinguish between CEA and CUA.) CUA seeks to measure consumer values by eliciting valuations of health states. This information is then used to "quality adjust" health gains, so that decision makers can consider the cost per quality-adjusted life year (QALY) saved. (We will explain how QALYs are calculated later.)

CUA is complex, and its validity is unknown. It is appropriate whenever CBA is, and at a formal level the two are essentially equivalent. At a practical level, however, the process of calculating benefits is different. CUA measures how alternative interventions change the health status of patients and how patients evaluate those changes.

Exhibit 14.2 walks through the calculations for a CUA. Suppose 215 people each get treatments A and B. At the end of one year the number of survivors differs for the two treatments (N_A and N_B), as does the average utility level (U_A and U_B). We use these data to calculate how many additional QALYs we get as a result of using treatment B. We then calculate the cost per QALY if we switch to treatment B.

Four uncertainties are associated with this calculation, aside from the usual problems of assessing the clinical effectiveness of treatments. First, should we limit our questions to patients? Family, friends, and strangers are sometimes willing to help patients afford care. Second, can patients answer questions about satisfaction adequately and accurately? Third, what discount rate should we use? While the example uses 3 percent, another rate might give us different answers, and we do not know what the right rate is. Fourth, assuming all other calculations are correct, at what cost per QALY should we draw the line? At the risk of sounding unduly negative, the validity of CUA hinges on finding satisfactory answers to these questions, which is not likely.

Unlike CMA or CBA, CUA requires that the analyst explicitly discount future QALYs. A technique commonly used in banking and finance, **discounting** reflects that benefits we realize far in the future are worth less than benefits we realize now. Discounting is valid because money can earn interest. To pay a bill that will come due in the future, one can set aside a

Discounting
Adjusting the value of future costs and benefits to reflect the willingness of consumers to trade current consumption for future consumption

EXHIBIT 14.2
A Cost–Utility Analysis

	$QALY_A$					$QALY_B$	$QALY_B - QALY_A$	
							Discounted	
	N_A	U_A	$N_A \times U_A$	N_B	U_B	$N_B \times U_B$	0%	3%
Year 1 outcomes	200	0.95	190.00	210	0.96	201.60	11.60	11.26
Year 2 outcomes	195	0.94	183.30	199	0.93	185.07	1.77	1.67
							13.37	12.93
Cost per QALY (with a $300,000 cost difference between A and B)							$22,438	$23,201

Note: N_A and N_B refer to the number of participants. U_A and U_B refer to the average utility score of participants.

smaller amount today. For example, if we invest \$100 at an interest rate of 7 percent, we will have \$160.58 at the end of ten years. We can reverse this calculation to show that the value of a guaranteed payment of \$160.58 that we will get in ten years is \$100. (Usually future values are discounted by $1/(1 + r)^n$, with r the discount rate and n the number of periods in the future the cost or benefit will be realized.)

As long as the interest rate is fixed, discounting is easy to figure on a spreadsheet. A single formula, $PV \times (1 + r)^n = FV$, lets us do all the necessary calculations. In this formula, PV refers to the present value of future costs or benefits, or the amount we are investing today; r refers to the interest rate; n refers to the number of time periods involved; and FV refers to the future value of future costs or benefits, or the amount we will have at the end of the investment period. We use the same formula to calculate the present value of future costs and benefits. The formula becomes $PV = FV/(1 + r)^n$. If we knew the size and timing of an intervention's costs and benefits and the right discount rate, calculating the present value of the QALYs associated with it would be a simple matter. In fact, we don't know the right discount rate and are not sure that the discount rate is constant for a given individual, let alone for different individuals. Sensitivity analysis is the best we can do in this regard. This analysis entails varying the discount rate over a reasonable range (typically 0 to 10 percent) and seeing if the answer changes. If not, the result is insensitive to the value of the discount rate. But if the answer does change, we have to use our judgment.

Steps in Cost–Utility Analysis

1. Estimate the expected costs for each option.
2. Estimate the number of people alive in each year in each cohort.
3. Using a survey of consumers, estimate the average utility score for each option for each person who is alive in each year.
4. Multiply the utility score (which will range from zero to one) by the number of people alive in each year for all the cohorts being compared. The product is the number of quality-adjusted life years (QALYs) for each cohort.
5. Discount the QALYs using rates of 2 to 5 percent.
6. Add the QALYs for each option, then find the difference.
7. Divide the difference in cost between options by the difference in QALYs.
8. Decide whether the cost per QALY is too high.

An Example of Cost–Utility Analysis

Are stents cost-effective for patients with stable angina (chest pain resulting from an inadequate supply of blood to the heart)? Stents come in two forms: bare metal and drug eluting. A bare-metal stent is a mesh tube of thin stainless steel or cobalt chromium alloy wire. A drug-eluting stent has a coating that slowly releases a medication that slows the rate of restenosis (the blood vessels narrowing again after the treatment). Since their introduction in the late 1970s, stents have been shown to be highly effective in treating angina. During this same period, however, medical therapy has also improved dramatically. Hence a team of researchers asked which approach was best given the options available as of 2011 (Wijeysundera et al. 2013).

The lifetime cost for medical therapy averaged $22,952, the lifetime cost for a bare metal stent averaged $25,952, and the lifetime cost for a drug-eluting stent averaged $25,536. Patients who got medical therapy were forecast to have a quality-adjusted life expectancy of 10.10 years. The forecast was 10.26 years for patients who got a bare metal stent and 10.20 years for patients who got a drug-eluting stent. Because the bare metal stent cost less and led to a longer quality-adjusted life expectancy, it dominated the drug-eluting stent. Compared to medical therapy, a bare metal stent cost a little more than $13,000 per QALY. This calculation, which is called the *incremental cost-effectiveness ratio*, divides the cost difference by the QALY difference. On the basis of this calculation, the team concluded that bare metal stents were cost-effective for most patients. The team also concluded that drug-eluting stents were cost-effective only for certain patients with diabetes, who were at very high risk of restenosis.

This analysis used data from multiple sources. The analysis also had to rely on a number of assumptions. In recognition of these factors, the team conducted a wide array of sensitivity analyses, which entailed redoing their calculations using different data or assumptions. Not surprisingly, their forecasts of how long patients survived were the key factors in their conclusions. Modest changes in costs, quality of life, or survival could change the conclusions. And such changes are likely, meaning that any conclusion is likely to change as technology changes.

In addition, many technical issues remain to be resolved in CUA. In particular, the validity of the quality adjustment that underlies QALYs is unknown. Of course, the core idea of CUA—that what happens to an individual patient is the only source of value for medical interventions—will not always be correct.

14.8 Conclusion

Except for CMA or possibly CEA, our advice is "Don't try this at home." When you need evidence to make a decision, turn to the literature. If no guidance is to be found there, do CMA or CEA (or modify existing studies using your costs). If these tools do not provide a clear direction, use clinical judgment. CBA and CUA are research tools, not management tools. Still, these techniques can help make your organization more efficient. Applied judiciously, they will help your organization identify and provide the most efficient therapies, which will reduce your costs and increase your options.

The importance of comparing the right options is often lost in the discussion of these analyses. Failing to compare reasonable alternatives renders CMA, CEA, CBA, and CUA useless. The best choice will usually be clear if the most plausible alternatives are compared. And if the best choice is not clear, either choice may be appropriate.

Exercises

14.1 Why have economic analyses of clinical and administrative innovations become more important?

14.2 Why is cost-minimization analysis most likely to be useful for managers?

14.3 Why would an economist object to including overhead costs in CMA analysis?

14.4 A clinic finds that it can reduce costs by eliminating appointments. The clinic is able to eliminate some telephone staff, and physicians become more productive. Patients wait until the physician is available, so the physician has virtually no downtime. Does this analysis adopt a societal view of costs? Why might this analysis result in a bad managerial decision?

14.5 Treating a patient with congestive heart failure with tPlex rather than Isother increases average life expectancy to 12.3 years from 11.5 years. The added cost of therapy is $14,000. What is the cost per life year? Should you choose tPlex or Isother?

14.6 Compared with a drip system, a new type of infusion pump reduces the cost of administering chemotherapy from $25 per dose to $20 per dose. The complication rate of each system is 2 percent. Which should you choose? What sort of analysis should you do?

14.7 After choosing between the options in Exercise 14.6, you discover that an infusion pump with a dosage monitoring system costs $15 per dose. Its monitoring functions reduce the complication rate to

1 percent. Which of the three options do you prefer? What principle does this illustrate?

14.8 Switching from one anesthesia drug to another reduces costs by $100 per patient. What additional information do you need to do a cost-minimization analysis?

14.9 A vaccine costs $200 per patient. Administration of the vaccine to 1,000 people is expected to increase the number of pain-free days for this population from 360,000 to 362,000. Calculate the cost per additional pain-free day due to vaccination. Is vaccination a good investment?

14.10 An acute care hospital has found that having geriatric nurse specialists take charge of discharge planning for stroke patients reduces length of stay from 5.4 days to 5.2 days. On average the geriatric nurse specialist (who earns $27 per hour including fringe benefits) spends 3.3 hours on discharge planning per patient. Supply and telephone costs are less than $10 per discharge plan. Your accounting staff tell you the average cost per day is $860 and the incremental cost per day is about $340. Is this innovation financially attractive? Whether it is or not, what alternatives should the hospital consider?

14.11 The current cost function for a lab that evaluates Pap smears is $C = 200{,}000 + 25 \times Q$. Q, the annual volume of tests, is forecast to be 30,000. The incremental cost is $25 because each evaluation requires $20 worth of a technician's time and $5 worth of supplies. Calculate the average cost of an evaluation.

14.12 You are comparing replacement of the current lab, which has a cost function of $C = 200{,}000 + 25 \times Q$, with an automated lab that has a cost function of $C = 300{,}000 + 20 \times Q$. Doing so would reduce the error rate from 1.5 percent to 1 percent. Your volume is expected to be 18,000 tests per year. Should you choose the automated lab? Briefly explain your logic.

14.13 The expected cost of Betazine therapy is $544. It is effective 57 percent of the time, with a 6 percent chance of an adverse drug reaction. The following table shows data for Alphazine, a new treatment. Estimate the rate of adverse drug reaction and the expected cost of treatment. Use Excel to construct a decision tree for this problem. Should you choose Alphazine or Betazine?

			Probability	Cost
Effective	63%	Adverse drug reaction	5%	$700
		No adverse drug reaction	95%	$500
Ineffective	37%	Adverse drug reaction	5%	$800
		No adverse drug reaction	95%	$600

References

Nowakowska, D., J. R. Guertin, A. Liu, M. Abrahamowicz, J. Lelorier, F. Lesperance, J. M. Brophy, and S. Rinfret. 2011. "Analysis of Willingness to Pay for Implantable Cardioverter-Defibrillator Therapy." *American Journal of Cardiology* 107 (3): 423–27.

Opmeer, B. C., R. el Moussaoui, P. M. M. Bossuyt, P. Speelman, J. M. Prins, and C. A. de Borgie. 2007. "Costs Associated with Shorter Duration of Antibiotic Therapy in Hospitalized Patients with Mild-to-Moderate Severe Community-Acquired Pneumonia." *Journal of Antimicrobial Chemotherapy* 60 (5): 1131–36.

Ruger, J. P., M. C. Weinstein, S. K. Hammond, M. H. Kearney, and K. M. Emmons. 2008. "Cost-Effectiveness of Motivational Interviewing for Smoking Cessation and Relapse Prevention Among Low-Income Pregnant Women: A Randomized Controlled Trial." *Value in Health* 11 (2): 191–98.

Scalera, N. M., and T. M. File Jr. 2013. "Determining the Duration of Therapy for Patients with Community-Acquired Pneumonia." *Current Infectious Disease Reports* 15 (2): 191–95.

Wijeysundera, H. C., G. Tomlinson, D. T. Ko, V. Dzavik, and M. D. Krahn. 2013. "Medical Therapy v. PCI in Stable Coronary Artery Disease: A Cost-Effectiveness Analysis." *Medical Decision Making* 33 (7): 891–905.

PROFITS, MARKET STRUCTURE, AND MARKET POWER

Learning Objectives

After reading this chapter, students will be able to

- describe standard models of market structure,
- discuss the importance of market power in healthcare,
- calculate the impact of market share on pricing,
- apply Porter's model to pricing, and
- discuss the determinants of market structure.

Key Concepts

- If the demand for its products is not perfectly elastic, a firm has some market power.
- Most healthcare organizations have some market power because their rivals' products are not perfect substitutes.
- Having fewer rivals increases market power.
- Firms with no rivals are called *monopolists*.
- Firms with only a few rivals are called *oligopolists*.
- More market power allows larger markups over marginal cost.
- Barriers to entry increase market power.
- Regulation is often a source of market power.
- Product differentiation and advertising can be sources of market power.

15.1 Introduction

What distinguishes very competitive markets (those with below-average profit margins) from less competitive markets (those with above-average profit margins)? An influential analysis by Porter (1985) argues that profitability depends on five factors:

1. the nature of rivalry among existing firms,
2. the risk of entry by potential rivals,
3. the bargaining power of customers,
4. the bargaining power of suppliers, and
5. the threat from substitute products.

For the most part, Porter's model explains profit variations in terms of variations in market power. Firms in industries with muted price competition, little risk of entry by rivals, limited customer bargaining power, and few satisfactory substitutes have significant market power. Firms with market power face customer demands that are not particularly price elastic. As a result, markups can be large. We will use the Porter framework to examine the links between profits, market structure, and market power.

Three characteristics of healthcare markets reduce their competitiveness. First, many healthcare markets have only a few competitors, which mutes rivalry among firms. Second, this muted rivalry persists in many healthcare markets because cost and regulatory barriers limit entry. Third, many healthcare products have few close substitutes. The lack of close substitutes makes the market demand less elastic and may make the demand for an individual firm's products less elastic. These factors give healthcare firms market power and allow high markups.

The bargaining power of suppliers varies. A detailed examination of differences in suppliers' bargaining power is beyond the scope of this book, but one change is important to note. Physicians are suppliers to many healthcare organizations, and physicians' incomes have stagnated since the early 1990s, reflecting a deterioration of their bargaining position.

The most significant change in healthcare markets has been the growth of managed care. Managed care dramatically enhances the bargaining power of most healthcare customers. As a result, many healthcare firms face more competitive markets and narrower margins than they previously faced.

Profit-oriented managers will usually seek to gain market power. The most ambitious will try to change the nature of competition. For example, faced with determined managed care negotiators, healthcare providers may merge to reduce costs and improve their bargaining positions, which can improve margins. But even when an organization cannot change a market's competitive structure, it still has two options: It can seek to become the low-cost producer, or it can seek to differentiate its products from those of the competition. Either strategy can boost margins, even in competitive markets.

15.2 Rivalry Among Existing Firms

Most healthcare organizations have some market power. Price elasticities of demand are small enough that an organization will not lose all its business to rivals with slightly lower prices. Market power has several implications. Obviously, it means firms have some discretion in pricing because the market does not dictate what they will charge. Flexibility in pricing and product specifications means managers must consider a broad range of strategies, including how to compete. Some markets have aggressive competition in price and product innovation; other markets do not. Managers have to decide what strategy best fits their circumstances. The prospect of market power also gives healthcare organizations a strong incentive to differentiate their products. The amount of market power an organization has typically depends on how much its products differ from competitors' in terms of quality, convenience, or some other attribute.

Healthcare organizations generally have market power because their competitors' products are imperfect substitutes. Reasons that competitors' products are imperfect substitutes include differences in location or other attributes, or even product familiarity. For example, a pharmacy across town is less convenient than one nearby, even if it has lower prices. Because consumers choose to patronize the more expensive but closer pharmacy, it has market power.

Medical goods and services are typically "experience" products, in that consumers must use a product to ascertain that it offers better value than another. For instance, patients do not know whether a new dentist will meet their needs until the first visit. Likewise, consumers have to try a generic drug to be sure it works as well as the branded version. Because of this need to try out healthcare products, comparison of medical goods and services is costly, and consumers tend not to change products when price differences are small. These factors make it difficult to assess whether competing products are good substitutes, thus increasing market power.

As we will see in Section 15.6, advertising decisions depend on the differences that determine market power. Attribute-based differences usually demand extensive advertising. Information-based differences often reward restrictions on advertising.

Many healthcare providers have few competitors. This is true for hospitals and nursing homes in most markets, and often for rural physicians. Where the market is small, either because the population is small or because the service is highly specialized, competitors will usually be few. And when a firm has few rivals, all have some market power, if only because each controls a significant share of the market. Firms with few competitors recognize that they have flexibility in pricing and that what their rivals do will affect them.

A perfectly competitive market, in which buyers and sellers are price takers (i.e., a market in which both believe that they cannot alter the market price), offers a baseline with which to contrast other market structures. In perfect competition, firms operate under the assumption that demand is very

Do Physicians Really Have Market Power?

Physicians appear to have market power even though most markets have many physicians. Two studies have attempted to calculate the price elasticity of demand faced by individual physicians (Lee and Hadley 1981; McCarthy 1985). One estimated price elasticities from –2.8 to –5.1; another found a very similar range of –3.1 to –3.3. Not surprisingly, demand for the services of individual physicians is much more elastic than the demand for physicians' services as a whole. (After all, other physicians may not be perfect substitutes for your physician, but they are fairly close substitutes.) These estimates suggest markups will be large, meaning physicians have a good deal of market power. Furthermore, by organizing themselves into independent practice associations, which bargain with insurers on behalf of member physicians, physicians effectively increase their market share and market power (Page 2004; Tollen et al. 2011).

price elastic. The only way to realize above-normal profits is to be more efficient than the competition. Firms disregard the actions of their rivals, in part because potential entrants face no barriers and in part because firms have so many rivals. In any other market structure, organizations will produce less and charge higher prices.

Few healthcare markets even remotely resemble perfectly competitive markets. Some have only one supplier and are said to be *monopolistic*. For example, the only pharmacist in town is a **monopolist**. A number of markets have many rivals, all claiming a small share of the market. At first glance these markets may look perfectly competitive, but they have one key difference: Customers do not view the services of one supplier as perfect substitutes for the services of another. Each dentist has a different location, a different personality, or a different treatment style. Firms such as these are said to be **monopolistic competitors**.

Other markets have only a few competitors and are said to be *oligopolistic*. Markets with many competitors can also be oligopolistic if a few competitors have a significant market share. A local market with two hospitals serving the same area is oligopolistic, as is a market with 15 PPOs, the two largest of which have 40 percent of the market. Because the decisions of some competitors determine the strategies of others, oligopolistic markets differ from other markets in an important way. **Oligopolists** must act strategically and recognize their mutual interdependence. We will explore this situation in more detail in Chapter 16.

Monopolist
A firm with no rivals

Monopolistic competitor
A competitor with multiple rivals whose products are imperfect substitutes

Oligopolist
A firm with only a few rivals or a firm with only a few large rivals

15.3 Customers' Bargaining Power

A longtime distinguishing feature of healthcare markets has been that they contain many buyers, all with limited bargaining power. This statement is not true of every market. The emergence of managed care firms, which identify efficient providers and those who will give substantial price concessions, changes the picture. (Of course, Medicare and Medicaid, the original PPOs, have had a major influence on healthcare markets since their inception.) So in addition to the number of sellers, healthcare market structures depend on the market shares of PPOs and HMOs (including Medicare and Medicaid, where appropriate) and the number of each in the market.

15.4 Entry by Potential Rivals

Barriers to entry in healthcare markets may be market based or regulation based. Generally, regulation-based barriers are more effective. Whatever the source, restrictions on entry reduce the number of competing providers and make demand less price elastic. In other words, entry restrictions, whether necessary or not, increase market power.

The best way to erect entry barriers and gain market power is to have the government do it for you. This strategy has two fundamental advantages. First, it is perfectly legal and eliminates public and private suits alleging antitrust violations. Second, the resulting market power is usually more permanent because government-sanctioned entry barriers will not be eroded by market competition.

State licensure forms much of the basis for market power in healthcare. Licensure prevents entry by suppliers with similar qualifications and encroachments by suppliers with lesser qualifications. For example, state licensure laws typically require that pharmacy technicians work under the direct supervision of registered pharmacists and that a registered pharmacist supervise no more than two technicians. These restrictions clearly protect pharmacists' jobs by limiting competition from technicians.

Intellectual property rights can also provide entry barriers. Innovating organizations can establish a monopoly for a limited period by securing patents. A US patent gives the holder a monopoly for 17 years. The patent holder must disclose the details of the new product or process in the application but is free to exploit the patent and sell or license the rights. Patents are vitally important in the pharmaceutical industry because generic products are excluded from the market until the patent expires.

Copyrights create monopolies that protect intellectual property rights. Unlike patents, copyrights protect only a particular expression of an idea, not the idea itself. Copyright monopolies normally last for the life of the author plus 50 years. Trademarks (distinctive visual images that belong to a particular organization) also grant monopoly rights. As long as they are used and defended, trademarks never expire. All these legal monopolies create formidable barriers to entry for potential competitors.

Strategic actions can also prevent or slow entry by rivals. Rivals will not want to launch unprofitable ventures, and firms can try to ensure entrants will lose money. **Preemption**, **limit pricing**, innovation, and mergers are common tactics. Preemption involves moving quickly to build excess capacity in a region or product line and thereby ward off entry. For example, building a hospital with excess capacity means that a second hospital would face formidable barriers. Not only would it exacerbate the capacity surplus, but this excess capacity could cause a price war. Managed care firms would not miss the opportunity to grab larger discounts. Worse still for the prospective entrant, most of the costs of the established firm are fixed. Its best strategy would be to capture as much of the market as it can by aggressive price cutting. In contrast, the rival's costs are all incremental. It can avoid years of losses by building elsewhere.

Preemption
Building excess capacity in a market to discourage potential entrants

Limit pricing
Setting prices low enough to discourage entry into a market

Limit pricing is another tactic established firms or those with established products can use. Limit pricing means setting prices low enough to discourage potential entrants. By giving up some profits now, an organization can avoid the even bigger profit reductions that competition might cause later. In essence, the firm acts as though demand were more elastic than it is. Limit pricing only works if the firm is an aggressive innovator. Otherwise, competitors will eventually enter the market with lower costs or better quality, and the payoff to limit pricing will be minimal.

Innovation by established organizations can deter entry as well. Relentless cost reductions and quality improvement means entrants will always have to play catch-up, which does not promise substantial profits.

Mergers increase market power by changing market structure. A well-conceived, well-executed merger can reduce costs or increase market power, either of which can increase profit margins. The publicized goal of most mergers is cost reductions resulting from consolidation of some functions. The accompanying anticipation of improvement in the firm's bargaining position is usually left unspoken. Customers and suppliers usually must do business with the most powerful firms in a market. For example, failure to contract with a dominant health system will pose problems for customers and suppliers, so the system can anticipate better deals. Whether cost savings or market share gains are the more important goal of a merger is debatable.

15.5 Market Structure and Markups

Having market power does not eliminate the need to set profit-maximizing prices. Organizations should still set prices so that marginal revenue equals

Market Share	Market Elasticity	Firm's Elasticity	Marginal Cost	Profit- Maximizing Price
48%	−0.60	−1.25	$10.00	$50.00
24%	−0.60	−2.50	$10.00	$16.67
7.5%	−0.60	−8.00	$10.00	$11.43
5%	−0.60	−12.00	$10.00	$10.91

EXHIBIT 15.1
Market Share and Markups

marginal cost. If the return on equity is inadequate, the organization should exit the line of business.

15.5.1 Markups

What changes with a gain in market power is markups. A firm with substantial market power will find it profitable to set prices well above marginal cost. Exhibit 15.1 shows that a firm with a substantial amount of market power ($\varepsilon = -2.5$) will have a 67 percent markup. In contrast, a firm with a moderate amount of market power ($\varepsilon = -8.0$) will only have a 14 percent markup. Finally, a firm with very little market power ($\varepsilon = -12.0$) will have a 9 percent markup.

Organizations with market power benefit from markup. However, their customers face higher prices, which results in their using the product less or not at all. As a result, managers' goals depend on whether they are buying or selling. Managers seek to reduce their suppliers' market power while increasing their own. If your suppliers have substantial market power and you have none, your profit margins will suffer.

Mergers Result in Price Increases

In 2012, the number of hospital mergers and acquisitions rose to 352, meaning that the consolidation of hospital markets continues (Barr and Kutscher 2013). In principle, the merger of two hospitals allows cost savings. The merged hospitals would need less excess capacity to cope with spikes in demand, could avoid duplicate services, and could share some overhead expenses. Harrison (2011) estimates that about two-thirds of merging hospitals can anticipate savings and that the average cost reduction is about 2 percent; smaller hospitals are more apt to realize cost reductions (Valdmanis 2010). The challenges of merging two disparate organizations, which can be substantial, suggest that other motives matter as well.

(continued)

(continued)

The other motive for consolidation is to increase market power. A single hospital or a two-hospital system is in a much better bargaining position than two independent hospitals serving the same area. For example, prices for comparable services were 13 to 25 percent higher in **concentrated markets** than in more competitive markets (Robinson 2011).

Recognizing that hospital consolidations could push prices up, federal antitrust authorities have opposed some hospital mergers. The authorities have lost most of these suits. Courts have generally seen the not-for-profit status of merging hospitals as a guarantee of price restraint, although the economics literature provides little support for this expectation.

On the contrary, most studies have found that merging not-for-profit hospitals significantly increases markups (Gaynor and Town 2012). For example, a study of a merger of two not-for-profit California hospitals found that prices increased much faster than average at one, but not at the other (Tenn 2011). Likewise, a study of hospital mergers in Chicago found that one of the mergers led to much higher prices and the other did not (Haas-Wilson and Garmon 2011). The effects of mergers depend on the nature of the hospitals involved and the nature of the competition in their market. The literature suggests that if two small hospitals in a competitive market merge, their ability to negotiate higher prices will be limited. In contrast, if two large hospitals in a smaller market merge, their ability to negotiate can be substantial.

Concentrated market
A market with few competitors or dominant firms

15.5.2 The Impact of Market Structure on Markups

Analyses of the impact of market structure on markups require information on prices and costs, which is typically closely guarded by managers. A few healthcare studies, however, such as Nyman's (1994) study of nursing homes, found higher markups in areas in which there was greater market concentration.

A concentrated market has relatively few competitors or a few dominant firms. Economists often use the Hirschman-Herfindahl Index (HHI) to measure market concentration. The HHI equals the sum of the squared market shares of the competitors in a market. The HHI gets larger as the number of firms gets smaller or as the market shares of the largest firms increase. For example, a market with five firms, each of which claimed 20 percent of the market, would have an HHI of 2,000. In contrast, a market with five firms, four of which each claimed 15 percent of the market while the fifth claimed 40 percent, would have an HHI of 2,500. The study found that a 1 percent increase in the HHI was associated with a 0.13 to 0.15 percent increase in prices. This increase might not seem like much, but prices would be 3 or 4 percent higher in a market with an HHI of 2,500 than in a market with an HHI of 2,000. Such a difference should have a major impact on profits.

Attributes other than market power can also result in high markups. White, Reschovsky, and Bond (2014) point out that, in addition to having a large market share, providing specialized services, having a good reputation, and being a member of a system also result in higher prices.

Insurer Market Structure Affects Prices, Too

Melnick, Shen, and Wu (2011) reported that most hospitals are in markets with many insurers. Most insurers, in contrast, confront markets with only a few competing hospitals. The average HHI for health insurers in metropolitan areas was 1,714; the average for hospitals was 3,361. Not surprisingly, prices were higher in concentrated (high HHI) hospital markets and lower in concentrated insurer markets.

Three changes are underway that may change negotiations between hospitals and insurers (Keckley, Copeland, and Scott 2013). First, insurers are merging, so concentration in the health insurance market is increasing. Second, insurers are offering plans that exclude high-priced hospitals. These plans are called *narrow networks*. Third, insurers anticipate selling many more policies to individuals. They also expect that demand for these individual policies will be much more sensitive to differences in premiums. All of these changes will tend to increase the bargaining power of private insurers relative to hospitals.

15.6 Market Power and Profits

Market power does not guarantee profits. A firm with market power will set prices well above marginal cost but may not earn an adequate return on equity. However, firms with market power can use strategies to boost profits that firms without market power cannot.

Three competitive strategies are common among firms with market power: **price discrimination**, **collusion**, and **product differentiation**. We discussed price discrimination in Chapter 12; in this chapter we will focus on collusion and product differentiation.

15.6.1 Collusion

Collusion, or conspiring to limit competition, has a long history in medicine. As in other industries, the temptation to avoid the rigors of market

Price discrimination
Selling similar products to different individuals at different prices

Collusion
A secret agreement between parties for a fraudulent, illegal, or deceitful purpose

Product differentiation
The process of distinguishing a product from others

competition can be beguiling. Collusion is profitable because demand is less elastic for the profession than for each individual participant. For example, if the price elasticity of demand for physicians' services is about –0.20 and the price elasticity of demand for an individual physician's services is about –3.00, an individual physician can earn a greater income by cutting prices, yet raising prices will increase the income of the profession as a whole.

Exhibit 15.2 shows how a 10 percent price increase would change total revenue for organizations facing different elasticities. (The change in total revenue due to a price cut = [percentage change in price + percentage change in quantity] + [percentage change in price × percentage change in quantity].) For the profession as a whole, raising prices will increase revenues because demand is inelastic. For each individual professional, raising prices will reduce revenues unless other professionals change their prices, which would make demand less elastic. Of course, others are likely to respond to price cuts by cutting their own prices, so revenues will climb far less than a naïve analysis would suggest.

The implication of Exhibit 15.2 is that physicians as a group would increase their incomes if they refused to give discounts to managed care organizations. What is good for the profession, however, is not what is good for its individual members. Individual physicians would be tempted to decry managed care discounts but make private deals with HMOs. From the perspective of the profession, penalizing defectors would prevent this problem.

In the 1930s, Oregon physicians did just that. Faced with an oversupply of physicians, excess capacity in the state's hospitals, and widespread concern about the costs of healthcare, insurance companies in Oregon attempted to restrict use of physicians' services. Medical societies in Oregon responded by threatening to expel physicians who participated in these insurance plans. Because membership in a county medical society was usually a requirement for hospital privileges, this response was a serious threat. This threat and physicians' ultimate refusal to deal with insurance companies led the insurers to abandon efforts to restrict use of physicians' services (Starr 1982).

EXHIBIT 15.2
Elasticity
and Revenue
Changes

Price Increase	Elasticity	Quantity Change	Revenue Change
10%	–0.1	–1%	8.9%
10%	–0.2	–2%	7.8%
10%	–0.3	–3%	6.7%
10%	–3.0	–30%	–23.0%
10%	–3.5	–35%	–28.5%
10%	–4.0	–40%	–34.0%

In most industries these steps would be recognized as illegal, anticompetitive activities. However, the belief that antitrust laws did not apply to the medical profession was widespread until a 1982 Supreme Court decision to the contrary. Since then the Federal Trade Commission has sued to prevent boycotts of insurers, efforts to deny hospital privileges to participants in managed care plans, and attempts to restrict advertising. In short, healthcare professionals and healthcare organizations are treated no differently than other businesses.

The benefits of collusion are clear. By restricting competition, firms can reduce the price elasticity of demand and increase markups. Collusion only increases profits, however, until it is detected.

15.6.2 Product Differentiation and Advertising

Product differentiation takes two forms: attribute based and information based. In **attribute-based differentiation**, customers recognize that two products have different attributes, even though they are fairly close substitutes, and may not respond to small price differences. In **information-based differentiation**, customers have incomplete information about how well products suit their needs. Information is expensive to gather and verify, so customers are reluctant to switch products once they have identified one that is acceptable. Both forms reduce the price elasticity of demand for a product and create market power (Caves and Williamson 1985).

Both attribute-based and information-based product differentiation are common in healthcare. For example, a board-certified pediatrician who practices on the west side of town clearly provides a service that is different from a board-certified pediatrician who practices on the east side of town. If the two practices were closer together, more customers would view them as equivalent. Alternatively, armed only with a sense that the technical skills, interpersonal skills, and prices of surgeons can vary significantly, a potential customer who has found an acceptable surgeon is not likely to switch just because a neighbor was charged a lower fee for the same procedure. Of course, the customer might be more likely to switch if complication rates, patient satisfaction scores, and prices for both surgeons were posted on the Internet for easy comparison.

The role of information differs sharply in attribute-based and information-based product differentiation. Extensive advertising makes sense for products that differ in attributes that matter to consumers. The more clearly customers see the differences, the less elastic demand will be and the higher markups can be for "better" products. In contrast, restrictions on advertising (and even restrictions on disclosure of information) make sense in situations with information-based product differentiation. The harder it is for customers to see that products do not differ in ways that matter to them, the less elastic demand will be and the higher markups can be.

Attribute-based differentiation Making customers aware of differences among products

Information-based differentiation Making customers aware of a product's popularity, reputation, or other signals that suggest high value

The coexistence of attribute-based and information-based product differentiation in healthcare leads to confusing advertising patterns. Attribute-based product differentiation demands advertising. Getting information about product differences into the hands of customers is integral to this type of product differentiation. For example, pharmaceutical manufacturers have launched extensive direct-to-consumer advertising campaigns. On the other hand, better customer information erodes the market power created by information-based product differentiation. Where information-based product differentiation is common, as it is in much of healthcare, a temptation to restrict advertising is present. Because private restrictions on advertising are usually illegal, the most successful limits have been based in state law.

Despite these divergent incentives, advertising has increased in recent years. One reason has been court rulings that professional societies cannot limit advertising. However, advertising has also increased in some sectors—such as inpatient care—where advertising has long been legal. The real driving force seems to be increased competition for patients.

The nature of healthcare products and the nature of healthcare markets combine to make advertising more common. Most healthcare firms have market power and competition to some degree. Advertising helps differentiate one product from another, so it increases margins. In monopoly markets (e.g., the only hospital in an isolated town), product differentiation is not useful. The provider already has high margins, and advertising is unlikely to increase them. In markets with many providers (e.g., retailers of over-the-counter pain medications), margins may be low, but differentiating one seller from another is difficult and advertising expenditures will be unlikely to increase revenues.

Patients cannot easily assess the quality of most healthcare goods and services before using them. Because of this fact, advertising can perform a useful service, that of giving consumers information they would have difficulty getting otherwise. If consumers gained no information from advertising, they would probably ignore it. Having information about a product differentiates it from products about which one does not have information. Providers who offer exceptional values also need to advertise to ensure that consumers are aware of their low prices or high quality. Studies of advertising in healthcare generally find that banning advertising results in higher prices. Indeed, increasing price transparency represents one strategy for reducing healthcare prices (Reinhardt 2013).

The economic logic behind advertising and innovating is simple: Continue as long as the increase in revenue is greater than the increase in cost. Stop when marginal revenue from advertising or product differentiation just equals the marginal costs. This logic differs from the standard rule only in that the cost of differentiation (advertising or innovating) is included in the marginal costs. Exhibit 15.3 shows the calculations organizations need to consider. Suppose the firm starts with profits of $100,000. In case 1 it anticipates

	Incremental Revenue	Incremental Costs		Profit
		Production	**Advertising**	
Baseline				$100,000
Case 1	$50,000	$30,000	$10,000	$110,000
Case 2	$50,000	$30,000	$22,000	$98,000

EXHIBIT 15.3
Advertising and Profits

that incremental advertising costs of $10,000 will allow it to increase revenues by $50,000. Because the incremental costs of production are only $30,000, spending more on advertising makes sense in case 1. In case 2 the firm has the same production cost forecasts but anticipates that it will need to spend $22,000 on advertising to increase revenues by $50,000. The higher advertising costs in case 2 mean that an attempt to increase sales would be unprofitable. As long as the incremental costs of production and advertising are less than incremental revenue, increasing advertising will increase profits. Managers need to take into account both advertising and production costs. Advertising only makes sense for products with significant margins.

The profit-maximizing amount of advertising is determined by consumers' responses to advertising and prices. The profit-maximizing rule is that advertising costs (measured as a percentage of sales) should equal $-\alpha/\varepsilon$. In other words, an organization will maximize profits when its ratio of advertising to sales equals -1 times the ratio of the advertising elasticity of demand, $-\alpha$, to the price elasticity of demand, ε. The advertising elasticity of demand is the percentage increase in the quantity demanded when advertising expenses increase by 1 percent. Obviously, advertising that does not increase sales is not worth doing. Firms with less elastic demand will want to spend more on advertising. A firm with an advertising elasticity of demand of 0.1 should spend 2.5 percent of its revenues on advertising if its price elasticity of demand is -4.00, but another firm with an advertising elasticity of demand of 0.1 should spend 5 percent of revenues on advertising if its price elasticity of demand is -2.00.

CASE 15.1	**Deregulating Pharmaceutical Advertising**

"Direct-to-consumer advertising informs and educates consumers. It lets consumers know their conditions may be treatable, and it informs consumers about the possible risks associated with pharmaceuticals.

(continued)

CASE 15.1
(continued)

It helps them ask their doctors and pharmacists better questions. Consumers are not stupid. They understand that we are trying to sell a product and they will balance our sales pitch with information from other sources. Advertising only makes sense for products that really work. If consumers try an advertised product and it doesn't work, we have shot ourselves in the foot. Consumers won't believe our next pitch. Remember, we have $2 billion in sales, so we have a lot to lose if consumers stop trusting our brand. Advertising is information—information about products that have been rigorously reviewed for safety and effectiveness. Consumers want to know about drugs with more convenient dosing, reduced side effects, and fewer interactions. Direct-to-consumer advertising helps consumers make better choices because, quite frankly, doctors and pharmacists are not educating the public. Deregulating direct-to-consumer advertising would be a progressive step for this country." The vice president for public affairs stopped talking and waited for questions.

"That's a very impressive argument," said the senator. "But aren't firms using advertising to create entry barriers? And don't entry barriers result in higher prices for consumers and their insurance companies? In my view, drug companies are using advertising to differentiate their products and jack up their margins. Furthermore, this strategy seems to be a very haphazard way of educating (and perhaps misinforming) the public. Only drugs with blockbuster potential are going to show up on television, and nobody can afford to promote a cheap, safe, and effective generic product. The drug companies are trying to get consumers to use high-priced branded products, not the inexpensive alternatives. So we wind up spending more without improving the health of the public. The case of Vioxx is instructive. It was heavily promoted, even though it had modest advantages over much less expensive products, and became a $2.5 billion blockbuster. Then we learned Vioxx increased the risks of heart attack and stroke. That was consumer education? I think we should ban direct-to-consumer advertising, not expand it."

Discussion questions:
- How could advertising be a barrier to entry?
- Could advertising reduce barriers to entry for a new product?
- Presumably drug companies are trying to differentiate their products from the competition. Will consumers be better off or worse off if the companies succeed?

(continued)

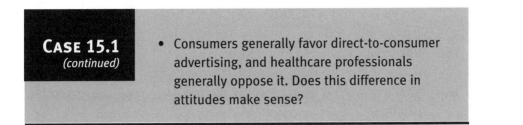

CASE 15.1
(continued)

- Consumers generally favor direct-to-consumer advertising, and healthcare professionals generally oppose it. Does this difference in attitudes make sense?

Product differentiation (through innovation or advertising) is a process, not an outcome. Differentiation, although potentially profitable, tends to erode. Product differentiation can be clear-cut (e.g., an open MRI facility), less distinguishable (e.g., "patient-centered care"), barely noticeable (e.g., "meals that don't taste like hospital food"), emotional (e.g., "doctors who care"), or frivolous (e.g., stripes in tooth gel). In all of these instances, however, successful differentiation asks to be copied and generally is, necessitating ceaseless efforts to differentiate products.

15.7 Conclusion

Most healthcare firms have some market power. Market power allows higher markups and can result in higher profits. As a result, firms try to acquire market power or defend the market power they have. The best way to acquire or defend market power is via regulation. Competitors find it more difficult to erode market power gained as a result of government action.

Organizations can take steps to gain market power without government action. Common strategies include preemption, limit pricing, and innovation, all of which are designed to discourage potential entrants. Mergers can also result in market power, as can collusion with rivals. Unlike other strategies for gaining market power, mergers and collusion often create legal problems. Mergers may result in public or private antitrust lawsuits, as does collusion once it has been discovered.

Firms with market power can compete in a variety of ways. Where feasible, firms seek to gain market power via product differentiation and advertising. This situation makes managers' roles more challenging. Of course, the profit potential of market power creates an incentive to seek it, even without a guarantee of profits.

Exercises

15.1 What does it mean to have market power? Are firms with market power extremely profitable?

15.2 Can you identify a healthcare firm with market power? What characteristics led you to choose the firm that you did?

15.3 Why would a merger reduce costs? Why would a merger increase markups? Why do many mergers fail nonetheless?

15.4 What information would you like to have when planning advertising spending?

15.5 Why might banning advertising drive up prices?

15.6 Offer examples of attribute-based product differentiation and information-based product differentiation.

15.7 Two physical therapy firms want to merge. The price elasticity of demand for physical therapy is –0.40. Firm A has a volume of 10,400, fixed costs of $50,000, marginal costs of $20, and a market share of 8 percent. Firm B has a volume of 15,600, fixed costs of $60,000, marginal costs of $20, and a market share of 12 percent. The merged firm has a volume of 26,000, fixed costs of $100,000, marginal costs of $20, and a market share of 20 percent.

a. What are the total costs, prices, revenues, and profits for each firm and for the merged firm?

b. How does the merger affect markups and profits?

15.8 A local hospital offered to buy Firm A in Exercise 15.7 for $5,000, and the offer was refused. However, many observers now perceive that Firm A is "in play" and may be sold if the right offer comes along.

a. In successful transactions, purchasers have typically paid 10 times current profits. How much would Firm A be worth to a buyer from outside the industry?

b. Would you expect that Firm B would be willing to pay more or less than an outside buyer?

c. What is the most Firm B would be willing to pay for Firm A?

15.9 Two clinics want to merge. The price elasticity of demand is –0.20, and each clinic has fixed costs of $60,000. One clinic has a volume of 7,200, marginal costs of $60, and a market share of 2 percent. The other clinic has a volume of 10,800, marginal costs of $60, and a market share of 4 percent. The merged firm would have a volume of 18,000, fixed costs of $80,000, marginal costs of $60, and a market share of 6 percent.

a. What are the total costs, revenues, and profits for each clinic and for the merged firm?

b. How does the merger affect markups and profits?

15.10 What would each of the clinics in Exercise 15.9 be worth to an outside buyer (using the guideline of 10 times annual profits)? What would each of the clinics be worth to each other?

15.11 A hospital anticipates that spending $100,000 on an advertising campaign will increase bed days by 1,000. The marketing department anticipates that each additional bed day will yield $2,000 in additional revenue and will increase costs by $1,200. Should the hospital proceed with the advertising campaign?

15.12 A clinic is considering reducing its advertising budget by $20,000. The clinic forecasts that visits will drop by 100 as a result. Costs are $140 per visit and revenues are $180 per visit. Should the clinic reduce its advertising budget?

15.13 The price elasticity of demand for dental services is –0.25. In a market with 100 dentists, the local dental society demanded and received an 8 percent increase in prices from the dominant dental insurance company. What should happen to the dentists' revenues and profits? (Assume that average costs equal marginal costs.) Would this agreement be stable? Explain.

15.14 The marginal cost of a physician visit is $40. In a county with 50 physicians, the local medical society negotiated a rate of $90. Previously, any physician who offered discounts to an insurer or a patient could be cited for unethical behavior, be expelled from the medical society, and lose admitting privileges to the county's sole hospital. But having lost an antitrust lawsuit, the medical society has agreed to stop enforcing its prohibitions against discounting, to allow any physician with a valid license to be a member of the medical society, and to stop linking admitting privileges to medical society membership.

   a. The price elasticity of demand for physicians' services is –0.18. What price maximizes profits for the individual physicians in the county?

   b. If all the physicians act independently, will their incomes go up or down?

   c. Is there any way the physicians could legally act to sustain a price of $90?

References

Barr, P., and B. Kutscher. 2013. "Taking a Different Path: Annual M&A Report Shows Year of Strong Growth, Rise of Nontraditional Deals." *Modern Healthcare* 43 (4): S1–S7.

Caves, R. E., and P. J. Williamson. 1985. "What Is Product Differentiation, Really?" *Journal of Industrial Economics* 34 (2): 113–32.

Gaynor, M., and R. Town. 2012. *The Impact of Hospital Consolidation—Update*. Robert Wood Johnson Foundation Synthesis Project Policy Brief No. 9. Published June. www.rwjf.org/content/dam/farm/reports/issue_briefs/2012/rwjf73261.

Haas-Wilson, D., and C. Garmon. 2011. "Hospital Mergers and Competitive Effects: Two Retrospective Analyses." *International Journal of the Economics of Business* 18 (1): 17–32.

Harrison, T. D. 2011. "Do Mergers Really Reduce Costs? Evidence from Hospitals." *Economic Inquiry* 49 (4): 1054–69.

Keckley, P., B. Copeland, and G. Scott. 2013. "The Future of Health Care Insurance: What's Ahead?" *Deloitte Review* 13: 117–31.

Lee, R. H., and J. Hadley. 1981. "Physicians' Fees and Public Medical Care." *Health Services Research* 16 (2): 185–203.

McCarthy, T. R. 1985. "The Competitive Nature of the Primary-Care Physician Services Market." *Journal of Health Economics* 4 (2): 93–117.

Melnick, G. A., Y. Shen, and V. V. Wu. 2011. "The Increased Concentration of Health Plan Markets Can Benefit Consumers Through Lower Hospital Prices." *Health Affairs* 30 (9): 1728–33.

Nyman, J. A. 1994. "The Effects of Market Concentration and Excess Demand on the Price of Nursing Home Care." *Journal of Industrial Economics* 42 (2): 193–204.

Page, S. S. 2004. "How Physicians' Organizations Compete: Protectionism and Efficiency." *Journal of Health Politics, Policy and Law* 29 (1): 75–105.

Porter, M. E. 1985. *Competitive Advantage*. New York: Free Press.

Reinhardt, U. E. 2013. "The Disruptive Innovation of Price Transparency in Health Care." *Journal of the American Medical Association* 310 (18): 1927–28.

Robinson, J. C. 2011. "Hospital Market Concentration, Pricing, and Profitability in Orthopedic Surgery and Interventional Cardiology." *American Journal of Managed Care* 17 (6): e241–e248.

Starr, P. 1982. *The Social Transformation of American Medicine*. New York: Basic Books.

Tenn, S. 2011. "The Price Effects of Hospital Mergers: A Case Study of the Sutter-Summit Transaction." *International Journal of the Economics of Business* 18 (1): 65–82.

Tollen, L., A. Enthoven, F. J. Crosson, N. Taylor, A. M. Audet, C. Schoen, and M. Ross. 2011. *Delivery System Reform Tracking: A Framework for Understanding Change*. The Commonwealth Fund Issue Brief. Published June. www.commonwealthfund.org/Publications/Issue-Briefs/2011/Jun/Delivery-System-Reform-Tracking.aspx.

Valdmanis, V. G. 2010. "Measuring Economies of Scale at the City Market Level." *Journal of Health Care Finance* 37 (1): 78–90.

White, C., J. D. Reschovsky, and A. M. Bond. 2014. "Understanding Differences Between High- and Low-Price Hospitals: Implications for Efforts to Rein in Costs." *Health Affairs* 33 (2): 324–31.

GOVERNMENT INTERVENTION IN HEALTHCARE MARKETS

Learning Objectives

After reading this chapter, students will be able to

- describe the advantages of perfectly competitive markets,
- explain when markets may be inefficient, and
- discuss alternative approaches to market failure.

Key Concepts

- Given the right conditions, competitive markets can produce optimal outcomes.
- Markets organize vast amounts of information about costs and preferences.
- Perfectly competitive markets lead to efficient production and consumption.
- Markets are dynamically efficient.
- Most markets are imperfect.
- Markets may be inefficient when externalities or public goods are present.
- Markets may be inefficient when competition or information is imperfect.
- Efficient market outcomes may not be equitable.
- Clear assignment of property rights may improve market outcomes.
- Taxes or subsidies may improve the efficiency of some markets.
- Public provision of some products may be efficient.

16.1 Government Intervention in Healthcare

Government intervention in healthcare is extensive, even in a market-oriented society like the United States. This chapter explores the rationale for government intervention, assuming that the goal is the promotion of the public well-being. We will begin by looking at the virtues of markets and then examine problems with markets. The chapter concludes by considering ways that governments might intervene.

16.1.1 On the Virtues of Markets

Pareto optimal
An allocation of resources in which no reallocation of resources is possible that will improve the well-being of one person without worsening the well-being of another

Under the right conditions, competitive markets can lead to an allocation of resources that is **Pareto optimal**—that is, no one can be made better off without making someone worse off (Debreu 1959). These conditions are restrictive:

1. Each market should have large numbers of buyers and sellers.
2. Markets involve the sale of undifferentiated products.
3. All buyers and sellers know all of the relevant information about the market.

Markets also require maintenance of law, order, and property rights, so this list of conditions may be incomplete. Nonetheless, these conditions are seldom satisfied, leaving us with questions that are more complex and more difficult. Would relying more on markets to allocate resources make us better or worse off? Would changing the laws and regulations make us better or worse off? The difficulty is that we must choose not between perfect markets and perfect governments but between imperfect versions of each. Much of this chapter focuses on the shortcomings of markets. First, though, let's explore some of the virtues of markets.

16.1.2 Information Processing

What should the price of gasoline be? Is an additional flight between Chicago and Tulsa, Oklahoma, worth enough to consumers to justify the cost of operating it? Are consumers willing to pay for the capabilities of satellite telephones? Is there a shortage of nurses? Markets help us answer such questions.

In an ideal market, goods and services are made, distributed, and used so that the market value of production is as large as possible. The resulting prices spread information throughout the economy, coordinating the decisions of many decentralized producers and consumers. The quest for profits encourages producers to seek low-cost ways of creating the products consumers most want while using resources in the most valuable way possible. Because the decisions made by consumers are designed to maximize satisfaction, maximizing market values results in maximizing well-being. The equilibrium of an ideal market is Pareto optimal. Furthermore, market exchange is voluntary. Individuals can choose to trade or not, affording considerable freedom to participants.

In a planned economy, well-intentioned officials who use their power wisely and justly may find price setting difficult. The planning process does not automatically yield the information needed to set prices. In addition, because price setting is a political act in a planned economy, officials may have difficulty setting prices correctly even when they know the proper levels.

CASE 16.1   Setting Prices for Walkers

Wal-Mart sells a walker called the Carex Explorer for $59.92. Medicare covers the Explorer, but it used to pay more than $100 (Leonhardt 2008). Between 1989 and 2011, Medicare paid for equipment such as walkers using a fee schedule equal to 95 percent of a product's average wholesale price (an unverified number provided by manufacturers). This system kept Medicare fees substantially higher than typical retail prices (US Government Accountability Office 2012).

As a part of the Medicare Modernization Act of 2003, Medicare accepted bids for ten types of equipment in ten metropolitan areas. The median accepted bid was 26 percent lower than the existing Medicare fee. Equipment manufacturers and retailers responded by lobbying Congress to discard the bids and delay the program, and the House of Representatives obliged by passing a bill to ditch the bids. In fact, it was only with the passage of the Affordable Care Act that Medicare was able to launch competitive bidding in 2011 (Japsen 2013). Even though Medicare anticipated savings of 45 percent on competitively bid products and 72 percent for mail-order products, in 2013 more than 200 members of Congress signed a letter asking that the program be delayed (Blum 2013). This example demonstrates three points. First, a well-designed bidding process can result in lower prices for public programs. Second, such programs are expensive and take a long time to set up and implement. Third, efforts to switch to a bidding process will encounter opposition from those whose profits are at risk.

Discussion questions:
- What are the risks of a bidding process like the one described in this case?
- Why would elected representatives side with the manufacturers and retailers on this issue?
- Suppose that Medicare sought bids for enough cardiac care to serve beneficiaries in your hometown. What would happen economically and politically? Could you design a way of insulating Medicare from political pressure? Would you want to?
- What problems other than paying too much might distorted fee schedules cause?

16.1.3 Static Resource Allocation

Perfectly competitive markets allocate products efficiently to the consumers most willing to pay for them. In other words, production and consumption are efficient. Products are produced as inexpensively as possible. No resources are wasted in making goods and providing services. Reorganization of production would increase costs.

Exchanges of goods and services in perfectly competitive markets all take place at the same price. As a result, consumers who value products will buy them. Products are not wasted on consumers who feel they are worth less than the amount spent to produce them.

Perfectly competitive markets result in an optimal mix of output. Their combination of least-cost production and highest-value consumption means that changes would reduce satisfaction. At the competitive optimum, price equals marginal benefit, which in turn equals marginal cost. Shifts in the output of the economy would cause the marginal cost to be higher or lower than the marginal value to consumers, which would not be optimal.

Perfectly competitive markets are not necessarily fair. Different distributions of incomes result in different market outcomes. A perfectly competitive market might lead to an efficient outcome in which most consumers have comparable incomes, or a perfectly competitive market might lead to an efficient outcome in which most consumers are ill-housed and ill-nourished and only a handful live in palaces.

16.1.4 Dynamic Resource Allocation

In a market economy, successful innovations are highly profitable. Unsuccessful innovations and inertia are highly unprofitable. As a result, markets are efficient in a dynamic sense. They respond quickly to changes in economic conditions and encourage innovation.

At the simplest level, markets squelch products that customers do not want. A product that does not create more value for potential buyers than its alternatives will fail quickly. Compounding this effect, those in authority or those with established products have difficulty preventing change; rivals are free to develop new products, and customers are free to buy them.

More important, markets reward innovation that customers want. A product that is as good as its alternatives is not likely to be more profitable than the others, whereas a better product promises high short-term profits. Customers will pay a premium for a better product, and substantial profits will follow if the market is large enough. Before too long, though, competitors will introduce similar products, and profit margins will fall. Producers must innovate continuously to maintain above-average profit margins.

Because innovation is intrinsic to market economies, we often fail to notice it. For most of human history, however, innovation was not routine.

Before 1700, most people used the same technology their grandparents used. Income per capita changed little for hundreds of years (Baumol 2002).

The dynamic efficiency of markets is so important that it may trump static efficiency concerns. Suppose, for example, that a market is dominated by a few large firms. In this market, prices will be somewhat higher than they would be in a more competitive market. But if those large firms invest more in research and development than smaller firms would, it might not be long before the resulting innovation would make consumers better off.

16.2 Market Failure

Despite their many virtues, markets do not always perform well. We will now consider the main reasons markets fail:

1. Externalities
2. Public goods
3. Imperfect competition
4. Imperfect information
5. Natural monopoly
6. Income redistribution

16.2.1 Externalities

Production or consumption of some products may directly affect others. These side effects are called **externalities**. When the side effects benefit others, they are called **external benefits**. When the side effects harm others, they are called **external costs**. When these side effects are not considered in market exchanges, the resulting equilibrium may entail volumes that are too high or too low.

For example, immunization confers external benefits on people who have not been immunized. If you are immunized, my risk of becoming ill decreases. In return for this benefit, I might be willing to pay a part of the cost of your immunization and part of the cost of others' immunizations. As a practical matter, though, providing subsidies to the thousands of people I want to help would be difficult. I'd be able to subsidize only a small number of immunizations, which defeats the purpose of my offer.

Exhibit 16.1 illustrates this concept. The private demand curve, which ignores the product's external benefits, is D_p. The social demand curve, which incorporates these benefits, is D_s. The market equilibrium, which ignores the external benefits of immunization, results in a volume of Q_p. An equilibrium that takes the external benefits into account would result in the larger volume of Q_s. In short, the market equilibrium is not fully efficient.

Externality
A benefit or cost imposed on someone who is not a party to the transaction that causes it

External benefit
A positive impact of a transaction for a consumer or producer not involved in the transaction

External cost
A negative impact of a transaction for a consumer or producer not involved in the transaction

EXHIBIT 16.1
Market
Equilibrium
with External
Benefits

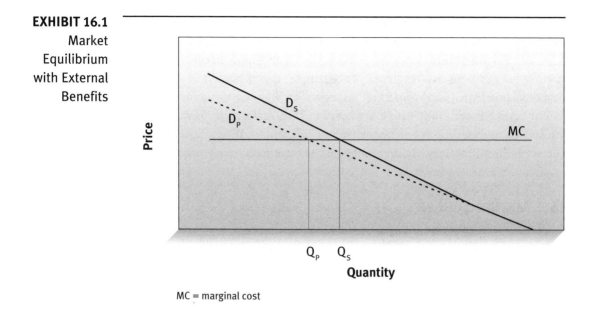

MC = marginal cost

Externalities need not be positive. If I let my untreated sewage contaminate your well, I am imposing external costs on you to have the sewage treated. I am considering the amount I would have to spend on water to get rid of wastes, but I am not considering your costs. If the society includes just the two of us, you could pay me to produce less sewage. If the society includes 100 people like me, and our sewage affects 500 or 5,000 people, these private payments will become complex, and problems are likely to ensue. External benefits and costs that affect large numbers of people are characteristic of *public goods* (see Section 16.2.2).

Tragedy of the commons
Over- or underuse of a resource that occurs when ownership of the resource is unclear and users produce externalities

A classic example of an externality is the **tragedy of the commons**. If everyone in a village can graze livestock on a common pasture, each person has an individual incentive to overuse the resource. The overgrazing may become so severe that all of the livestock starve and the village collapses. In other words, each person's livestock consume resources that imperil everyone else's livestock. More contemporary examples include vehicle congestion in cities, in which each driver ignores the costs imposed on others; overuse of the Ogallala aquifer in the central United States, in which each farmer's pumping increases costs for others; and excessive production of greenhouse gases by one country that causes a climate change affecting all countries.

The use of antibiotics in healthcare is another example of the tragedy of the commons. Patients benefit from the liberal use of antibiotics, but society suffers because overuse speeds the development of antibiotic-resistant strains.

Network externality
The effect each additional user of a product or service has on the value of that product or service to existing users

The flip side of the tragedy of the commons is a **network external-ity**—a value each additional user adds for existing users. Communications equipment of all sorts promotes network externalities. Electronic health record systems are a good example. An electronic health record system is valuable to a hospital. It transmits records quickly throughout the hospital, and any physician can instantly access a patient's record. If the other hospitals in town adopt compatible systems, the value of that electronic health record system increases. Its value increases further if all providers in the country adopt compatible systems. The hospital will be able to offer more appropriate treatment to an emergency department patient from another town because it will have access to that patient's past treatments, test results, and vital signs.

Standards also promote network externalities. For example, one reason that healthcare costs are high in the United States is the absence of widely accepted standards for billing. Insurers have their own systems, and providers must submit bills in a wide range of formats to be paid in a timely fashion. If two insurers adopt a common standard, they will save some money, but hospitals and clinics (which are not parties to the decision to standardize) will save even more. The value of this standardization increases as more and more insurers join.

16.2.2 Public Goods

A **public good** is an extreme example of externalities. A pure public good has two unusual characteristics: Consumption by one person does not prevent consumption by another, and exclusion is difficult. One person's use of a pure public good does not interfere with another's use of it, so its use is **nonrival consumption**: The marginal cost of letting one more person use the public good is zero. For instance, my enjoyment of clean air in the country does not limit your enjoyment of it. Alternatively, I can use the new research you are using. In addition, preventing people from using pure public goods is difficult, so their use is **nonexcludable consumption**, meaning that everyone has access to them.

A radio broadcast illustrates the difference between these two concepts. When a program is broadcast, anyone in the reception area can get the signal. Adding another listener does not affect current listeners, so consumption of the broadcast is clearly nonrival. In contrast, a radio broadcast may or may not be excludable. Most commercial radio in the United States does not exclude any potential listeners, but Sirius Satellite Radio is only available to subscribers, so exclusion is possible. Because exclusion is possible, radio broadcasts are not public goods.

In contrast, a reduction in levels of sulfur dioxide in the air is a public good. One person's enjoyment of better air quality does not prevent another person from enjoying it too, so consumption of improved air quality is nonrival. In addition, preventing anyone from taking advantage of cleaner air would be hard to imagine, so consumption is nonexcludable.

Public good
A good whose consumption is nonrival and nonexcludable

Nonrival consumption
Consumption by one person that does not prevent simultaneous consumption by another person

Nonexcludable consumption
When preventing consumption by someone who did not pay for a product is infeasible

Markets are not likely to result in the right amounts of public goods being consumed. If market transactions lead to any consumption of public goods, the quantities are likely to be too small.

Because everyone can simultaneously enjoy a public good, the marginal benefit of a public good equals the sum of the marginal benefits for everyone in society. So, if a 1 percent reduction in sulfur dioxide (SO_2) in the atmosphere is worth $1 to Jordan, $2 to Kim, and $4 to Logan, it will be worth $7 to the three of them. The marginal benefit to society is the sum of the marginal benefits to the members of society, and the members of this three-person society should be seeking an outcome in which the marginal benefit to society equals the marginal cost.

Exhibit 16.2 illustrates this situation. If the three members of society act independently, only Logan will pay for sulfur dioxide reduction and the level chosen will be 1 percent. In this example, Logan's marginal benefit equals $4.25 minus 25 times the reduction in sulfur dioxide, which amounts to $4 for a 1 percent reduction. (A marginal benefit schedule like this one is simply a recasting of a demand curve in terms of value at each level of consumption.) The marginal cost is $3.60 plus 40 times the reduction in sulfur dioxide, so the marginal cost also equals $4 for a 1 percent reduction.

At this cost Jordan and Kim will be unwilling to pay for any reduction in sulfur dioxide, although they will benefit from Logan's spending. In this example, Jordan's marginal benefit schedule is 1.4 minus 40 times the extent of sulfur dioxide reduction, and Kim's marginal benefit schedule is 2.24 minus 25 times the extent of sulfur dioxide reduction. Jordan would only be willing to spend $1 for a 1 percent reduction, and Kim would be willing to

EXHIBIT 16.2
Demand for a
Public Good

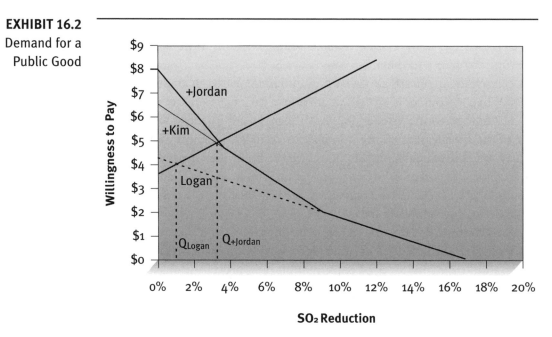

pay $2. However, they will be willing to pay for a much larger reduction in sulfur dioxide if they recognize that reducing sulfur dioxide levels is a public good and pool their resources. In this example they will be willing to pay for a 3.306 percent reduction in sulfur dioxide, with Logan paying $3.42, Kim paying $1.42, and Jordan paying $0.08. The sum of these marginal benefits is $4.92, which is equal to the marginal cost. This level of reduction, which equates the marginal benefit and marginal cost, would be optimal for this three-person society.

Cooperation could therefore lead to an optimal result. The difficulty is that Jordan would be even better off if Kim and Logan paid for the reduction in sulfur dioxide. After all, Jordan will benefit whether he pays or not. This situation is called the **free rider** problem. In a three-person society everyone could probably be persuaded to pay, but cooperation is less likely to be possible in a society of 3 million or 300 million people.

Free rider
Someone who benefits from a public good without bearing its cost

---

CASE 16.2	**To Vaccinate or Not**

"Look, the chicken pox vaccine comes with some risks. The chicken pox vaccine is a live attenuated vaccine. It can cause a mild case of chicken pox or shingles. Plus, it's not necessary. As long as everyone else at work has had chicken pox or has been vaccinated, I don't need to be vaccinated. And I don't like needles or doctors," said Sam.

"But, Sam," replied Dakota, "what if everyone or even just a third of the population followed your example? Then there would be no herd immunity. Everyone who had not been vaccinated would be at risk. In addition, chicken pox is a different disease in adults. The rash is usually more widespread, the fever lasts longer, and complications are more common. And if a pregnant woman gets chicken pox, a lot of really nasty things can happen to her baby. I know it takes two shots, I know you don't want to spend the money, and I know you hate shots. But you really ought to get vaccinated, for yourself and for the other people here at work."

Discussion questions:
- What are the external effects of a vaccine?
- Would too few people be vaccinated if it were not mandatory? What evidence supports your conclusion?
- What steps do governments take to increase vaccination rates?
- What steps do private companies take to increase vaccination rates? Why?

16.2.3 Imperfect Competition

At equilibrium in a perfectly competitive market, price equals marginal cost. Producing more volume than that produced at equilibrium would be inefficient because the value of the additional output would be less than its cost. In an imperfectly competitive market, however, every producer has some market power, so producers will set prices to make marginal revenue equal marginal cost.

Exhibit 16.3 illustrates an imperfectly competitive market. Marginal cost (MC) is $60. To maximize profits, the producer sets a price of $80, which yields marginal revenue (MR) of $60. As a result, some customers who would be willing to pay more than marginal cost, but not $80, would not buy this product. In a perfectly competitive market, the price would be $60 and volume would be twice as large.

16.2.4 Imperfect Information and Incomplete Markets

The efficiency of market outcomes rests on the assumption that buyers and sellers have perfect information, which is seldom the case in healthcare. As Arrow (1963) argued, the purpose of a visit to a physician is often the reduction of uncertainty; people seek care because they need more complete information. If patients are unsure about the benefit they will gain from a physician visit, they may decide to forgo the visit, which can lead to less-than-optimal market outcomes.

Exhibit 16.4 illustrates three possible outcomes for the scenario above. D_1, D_2, and D_3 describe different consumers' willingness to pay for care. D_1 represents the willingness of a consumer who correctly understands the value of a physician visit. Given the marginal cost of producing this information,

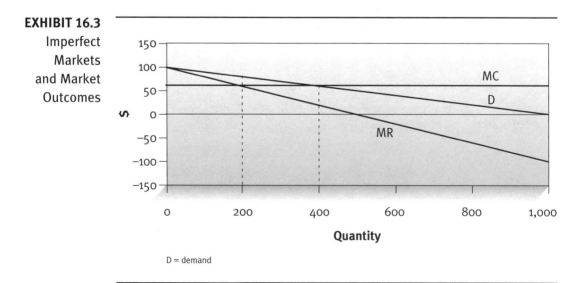

EXHIBIT 16.3
Imperfect
Markets
and Market
Outcomes

D = demand

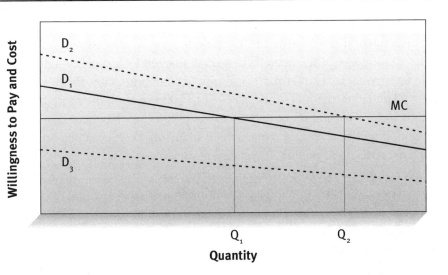

EXHIBIT 16.4
Market
Outcomes
with Imperfect
Information

the consumer will buy Q_1. D_2 describes the willingness of a consumer who overstates the value of a physician visit. This consumer will buy Q_2, which is substantially larger than Q_1. More important, the true value of the visit at Q_2 is well below marginal cost. (The true value lies on the D_1 demand curve.) This individual would be better off reallocating spending to other products. Finally, D_3 describes the willingness of a consumer who understates the value of a physician visit. In this example, the consumer makes no visits and forgoes all the benefits those visits might have provided. This consumer would be better off reallocating spending from other areas to physician visits. In short, we cannot be sure that the market outcome will be optimal if information is imperfect.

The situation is even more complex than Exhibit 16.4 suggests. Physicians and other experts may have discretion in recommending services. Even after a service has been provided, the consumer may have difficulty ascertaining whether the expert made the best recommendation, especially if the expert reaps large profits from the recommended service. Insurance further complicates matters. Insurers have difficulty tracking the true costs of services, and the conventional wisdom is that slow adjustments in insurance fees distort the profitability of some services. For example, the cost of MRI equipment has dropped sharply even as the quality of images has increased and the time needed to obtain an image has gone down. As a result, the cost of producing a scan dropped, but prices for scans went down only slowly. As a result, MRI scans became so profitable that many individual physicians began installing them in their offices, and use of MRI scans increased rapidly through 2006 (Lee and Levy 2012). Growth has slowed considerably since 2006, as coverage has become more restrictive and patients have faced higher copayments.

16.2.5 Natural Monopoly

If fixed costs are so high that only one firm can survive in the long run, that firm is a **natural monopoly**. Monopolies develop relative to the structure of costs and the size of the market. In a small market, only one hospital may be able to survive. In a larger market, multiple competitors can thrive.

The larger the investment needed to set up a firm, the more likely the firm is to be a natural monopoly. If an imaging center has fixed costs of $20 million, it will be a natural monopoly in many markets. If an imaging center has fixed costs of $2 million, it will be a natural monopoly only in the smallest markets. Like any monopoly, natural monopolies tend to sell their products and services at overly high prices, resulting in low sales.

CASE 16.3   **Diagnosing Chest Pains**

One evening during the summer of 2012, a Connecticut woman experienced chest pain (Brill 2013). She took an ambulance to a local not-for-profit hospital. After several hours in the emergency room, she was sent home with a diagnosis of indigestion.

Shortly thereafter, she received a bill of $995 for the ambulance, $3,000 for physicians' services, and $17,000 for the hospital. A major part of the hospital bill was a $7,998 charge for a CT scan with contrast. (The Medicare rate is $554.) The alternative to the CT scan would have been a stress test using an electrocardiograph. Its list price was $1,200 and the Medicare rate was $96. Unfortunately for the patient, she was not offered this option, was uninsured, and was a year too young to be eligible for Medicare.

When questioned about the bill, a hospital representative said, "I've told you I don't think a bill like this is relevant. Very few people actually pay those rates." Nonetheless, the patient was asked to pay it. A medical billing advocate was able to negotiate a $10,000 discount but made it clear that she thought even this amount was excessive.

Discussion questions:
- After reading this case, would you be more or less willing to have a CT scan done if an emergency room physician recommended it? How confident would you be that your choice was a good one?
- Had the woman asked her physicians what the alternatives were, they probably would have discussed a stress test. Would you expect a patient who fears that she is having a heart attack to ask for alternatives? Explain your logic.

(continued)

CASE 16.3
(continued)

- Emergency department staff are unlikely to know the list prices or allowed fees for a CT scan. How can consumers make good choices without information about price?
- Do you think hospitals should be required to provide an estimate of the cost of procedures before a patient chooses to have one done? Explain your logic.
- Do you think information about prices would have influenced the patient's decision or the physicians' recommendations?

16.2.6 Income Redistribution

A substantial part of government spending can be described as insurance or redistribution. Medicaid and Social Security Disability Insurance are examples. Taxes are levied on the healthy and wealthy to provide medical care and income to those less fortunate.

Redistribution is usually rationalized in one of two ways. One views redistribution as a public good. We all have some sympathy for the unfortunate, and we all benefit if someone offers them aid. Individual gains are small, however, and we may be tempted to let others provide our share of the redistribution. People who obtain a benefit at another's expense or without the usual cost or effort are free riders. Free riding results in underprovision of the public good.

A related approach introduced by John Rawls (1971) argues that if we were ignorant of our circumstances, we would want a society that allowed for some redistribution. In this approach, we would decide on how much redistribution was appropriate behind a "veil of ignorance," meaning that we would not know whether we were healthy or unhealthy, wealthy or poor.

16.3 Remedies

The remainder of this chapter explores possible remedies for market failure. Remember that doing nothing is always an option. Government intervention will not necessarily improve the situation. Governments also fail, and intervention could even worsen the situation.

16.3.1 Assignment of Property Rights

Many externalities result from ambiguities about the ownership of property rights. For example, does a downstream city have a right to clean water, or does an upstream city have a right to use a river as a sewer? Often the first step in solving externality problems is defining who has the right to use an asset. Once users are defined, asset sales, private agreements, regulations, or taxes can be used to produce efficient outcomes.

An influential analysis by Coase (1960) pointed out that ambiguity about property rights underlies many externality problems. As long as the costs of reaching and enforcing an agreement are small, the people involved in an externality case can reach agreements that solve the problem. For example, if the upstream city has the right to pollute, the downstream city can pay it to refrain from polluting the river. If the downstream city has the right to pure water, the upstream city will have to pay for the right to pollute (and will usually find it can pay less if it limits its pollution). Either way, the property owners can reach an efficient solution. With unclear property rights, who should pay whom is unclear, and too much of the externality is likely to be produced. If it is not clear that the upstream city has to pay for the right to pollute or it is not clear that the downstream city has to pay to prevent pollution, the upstream city is likely to underestimate the cost of pollution as a way of disposing of waste and dump too much waste into the water.

If an externality affects many people or is caused by many people, the costs of reaching and enforcing an agreement will be high. As a result, workable private agreements will be hard to reach. For example, pollution of Chesapeake Bay is caused by millions of people and affects millions of people. In such cases, governments typically claim property rights and use a variety of tools to improve outcomes.

In recent years, governments have taken steps to create markets for pollutants. First, the government asserts its ownership of the property right affected by pollution. Then, firms or jurisdictions are issued permits to pollute. These permits are worth more to firms or jurisdictions that have difficulty reducing pollution and are worth less to firms that reduce pollution more easily. Trades among potential polluters establish a price per unit of pollution and push potential polluters to equalize the costs of pollution reduction. Firms that incur low costs to reduce pollution have an incentive to do more to clean up than do firms that incur high costs to reduce pollution; the latter buy permits so that they can limit their cleanup efforts.

The 1990 Clean Air Act amendments set national caps for emission of sulfur dioxide by power plants, issued permits equal to this cap to plants, and allowed plants to trade permits. This program significantly reduced emissions of sulfur dioxide, and most observers consider it a success. The price of compliance was low, so compliance was high, and firms were encouraged to innovate to reduce emissions.

16.3.2 Taxes and Subsidies

If a product generates significant external benefits, a subsidy can be used to make the market outcome more efficient. Whether the subsidy goes to producers or consumers does not matter. Either way, the market price will fall and consumption will rise.

Exhibit 16.5 illustrates the effects of a subsidy. The demand curve D_1 describes the willingness of consumers to pay for a product. Because it yields external benefits, the market outcome will be Q_1, which is inefficiently small. Giving consumers a subsidy (S) will expand consumption to Q_2, which will be the efficient level if the right subsidy has been chosen. Alternatively, one could subsidize producers, thereby reducing the marginal cost by S. This subsidy will also cause consumption to increase to Q_2.

If this product generated external costs, a tax could be imposed to reduce consumption. The challenge with the tax or subsidy is determining the appropriate rate. Changing tax or subsidy rates is not an easy political process, and the market will not always make the appropriate rate evident.

16.3.3 Public Production

Public provision of products is another approach to market failure. Public provision is especially useful for pure public goods. When significant externalities are present and excluding certain potential customers is difficult or inefficient, public provision may be the best response. Even if private firms can profitably produce some of the output consumers seek, using prices (as private firms must) to pay for such products is undesirable. For example, private research firms might be able to profitably conduct some public health research by disseminating the results only to organizations that pay to get access to it. But this approach is inefficient because too few people will get access to the research. The cost of sharing the results with additional

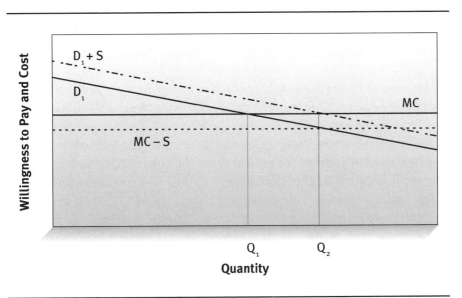

EXHIBIT 16.5
Market Outcomes with a Subsidy

organizations is very small, and the value of the research is not reduced if it is more widely shared.

If redistribution is a goal, using prices to affect product consumption may also be undesirable. For example, prices that are high enough to allow a clinic to survive may also be high enough to prevent low-income citizens from using the clinic.

Public provision does not necessarily mean public production. For example, medical research has many of the attributes of public goods. Although government employees perform medical research, a large share of research is performed by scholars who are not government employees, but private researchers competing for tax-supported research funds. In another example of public provision with private production, medical care for the poor is usually provided to improve the health of our least fortunate citizens, meaning that the goal is largely redistribution. In some cases, this care is provided by government hospitals and clinics. More commonly, though, care is provided by private hospitals and clinics but funded by tax-supported programs like Medicaid.

16.3.4 Regulation

The next chapter examines regulation. Regulation is an important form of government intervention in markets, especially in healthcare. Markets need rules to work, so regulation is not an alternative to markets. Some regulations cause markets to work well; other regulations have the opposite effect.

16.4 Conclusion

Markets have many virtues, not the least of which is the ability to reveal information about cost and value. Many forms of government intervention falter because key information about cost and value is lacking. In addition, the impulse to innovate inherent in markets is important for improved health and well-being. A long-standing criticism of governments is their bias toward inaction and the status quo.

A key question about government intervention is hard to answer: Will intervention improve the well-being of the public? Intervention will not necessarily improve an imperfect market. Effective interventions are hard to design and even harder to implement. In the rough-and-tumble of political life, good intentions do not always translate into good effects, and proposals backed by advocates are not always good ideas. Furthermore, government interventions can improve the well-being of individuals or groups even if the interventions do not improve overall well-being.

This critique should not be pushed too far. Government support for research has problems, but the strong consensus seems to be that the overall benefits are considerable and that government action is necessary. The government's public health activities also have problems, but there is no consensus that ending these activities would make our citizens better off. On the other hand, some interventions should be ended. The challenge is to determine what new programs to start and which existing programs to expand, contract, or terminate.

Exercises

16.1 Global warming is a classic example of a public good. Analyze this comment and explain your answer.

16.2 The existence of market failure does not signal what should be done in response. Analyze this comment and explain your answer.

16.3 Imperfect competition is the norm, so healthcare markets cannot work. Analyze this comment and explain your answer.

16.4 Markets work; governments do not. Analyze this comment and explain your answer.

16.5 Are market forces strong enough to deliver efficient healthcare? Please explain your answer.

16.6 For each scenario, assess whether an externality is present.
   a. Vaccinating children against influenza reduces its incidence among the elderly.
   b. Newly graduated nurses flock to teaching hospitals for training. After working for a year, many leave to work for competitors.
   c. A couple who planned to move to Florida to retire find that the plummeting housing market has wiped out their equity.
   d. Physicians complain that they spend a third of their time explaining to patients why television advertisements about medications for their conditions do not apply to them.

16.7 The supply of measles vaccine is given by $Q = 450 \times P$. The demand for measles vaccine is given by $Q = 20,000 - 50 \times P$.
   a. What is the market equilibrium price and quantity?
   b. The demand curve implies that private willingness to pay is $P = 400 - Q/50$. However, external benefits are associated with each measles vaccination, so the social demand curve is $Q = 20,000 - 50 \times (P - 5)$. What are the equilibrium price and quantity if these external benefits are considered?
   c. Propose an intervention that will result in this equilibrium volume.

16.8 The supply of an antibiotic is $Q = 30 \times P - 200$. The demand for it is $Q = 8,800 - 20 \times P$.

a. What is the market equilibrium price and quantity?

b. Use of the antibiotic creates $20 in external costs due to water pollution. Would the market outcome be different if a $20 tax were levied on producers instead?

16.9 Vaccination schedules are predictable, meaning that insurance coverage for vaccinations does not protect consumers against risks. Insurance coverage for vaccinations drives up costs because more people get vaccinated if coverage is available and because insurers have overhead costs. Does insurance coverage for vaccines do anything useful? Explain your answer.

16.10 About two-thirds of funding for substance abuse treatment comes from taxpayers. Does substance abuse treatment have external benefits that warrant this level of public funding?

16.11 Provide examples of the following types of government intervention in healthcare:

a. Government production

b. Subsidies for products

c. Taxes on products

d. Price regulation

e. Quality regulation

f. Inaction

16.12 Provide healthcare examples of the following types of market failure:

a. External benefits

b. External costs

c. Public goods

d. Imperfect competition

e. Imperfect information

16.13 Private foundations support medical research. Doesn't their support prove that tax funding of medical research is unnecessary? Please explain.

16.14 Public health information can be broadcast at a cost of $100. Public health information is a pure public good, in that many people can use the information simultaneously and preventing people from using the information is very difficult. One group of residents has a demand curve for public health information of the form $Q = 50 - P$. Here Q is the number of public health broadcasts per month and P is the price per broadcast. Another group has a demand curve of $Q = 140 - P$.

    a. At a price of $100 per broadcast, how many broadcasts per month will be demanded? (Add the quantities demanded by each group.)

    b. What is the total willingness to pay for 85 broadcasts? (Recast the demand curve to reveal willingness to pay and add the amounts for the two groups. For one group, willingness to pay equals $50 - Q$. For the other, it equals $140 - Q$. For both groups the minimum is $0.)

    c. At what level of output does willingness to pay equal $100?

    d. What do these results imply?

16.15 Every 1 percent reduction in the level of particulates in the air costs $200,000. Low-income residents in a region have a demand for particulate reduction of $R = 10 - P$ (R is the level of particulate reduction and P is the price per 1 percent reduction). High-income residents have a demand for particulate reduction of $R = 40 - 2P$.

    a. Is reduction of the level of particulates a public or private good?

    b. What will the market demand for particulate reduction be?

    c. What is the optimal level of particulate reduction?

16.16 Few orthopedic surgeons publish data describing their surgical volumes, infection rates, mortality rates, functional gain rates, or customer satisfaction rates.

    a. How much would a regulation requiring publication of such data cost?

    b. Would such a regulation improve the workings of the market?

    c. Would such regulation be an appropriate government activity?

    d. Do we need a regulation requiring publication of data for surgeons if private physician rating firms already exist?

References

Arrow, K. J. 1963. "Uncertainty and the Welfare Economics of Medical Care." *American Economic Review* 53 (5): 941–73.

Baumol, W. J. 2002. *The Free-Market Innovation Machine: Analyzing the Growth Miracle of Capital.* Princeton, NJ: Princeton University Press.

Blum, J. 2013. "Cure for Affordable Medical Devices." *Politico.* Published June 23. www.politico.com/story/2013/06/affordable-medical-devices-medicare-bidding-program-93204.html.

Brill, S. 2013. "Bitter Pill: Why Medical Bills Are Killing Us." *Time.* Published April 4. http://time.com/198/bitter-pill-why-medical-bills-are-killing-us/.

Coase, R. 1960. "The Problem of Social Cost." *Journal of Law and Economics* 3: 1–44.

Debreu, G. 1959. *Theory of Value*. New York: Wiley.

Japsen, B. 2013. "Obama Administration Not Budging on Medicare Competitive Bidding." *Forbes*. Published June 29. www.forbes.com/sites/bruce japsen/2013/06/29/obama-administration-not-budging-on-medicare-competitive-bidding/.

Lee, D. W., and F. Levy. 2012. "The Sharp Slowdown in Growth of Medical Imaging: An Early Analysis Suggests Combination of Policies Was the Cause." *Health Affairs* 31 (8): 1876–84.

Leonhardt, D. 2008. "High Medicare Costs, Courtesy of Congress." *New York Times*. Published June 25. www.nytimes.com/2008/06/25/business/25leonhardt. html.

Rawls, J. 1971. *A Theory of Justice*. Cambridge, MA: Harvard University Press.

US Government Accountability Office. 2012. *Review of the First Year of CMS's Durable Medical Equipment Competitive Bidding Program's Round 1 Rebid*. Published May. www.gao.gov/assets/600/590712.pdf.

CHAPTER

17

REGULATION

Learning Objectives

After reading this chapter, students will be able to

- describe the importance of regulation for managers;
- explain the interest group model of regulation;
- analyze the effects of regulations on firms, rivals, and consumers; and
- discuss alternative approaches to market failure.

Key Concepts

- Healthcare is extensively regulated.
- Regulation can make or break an organization (or its competitors).
- The objective of regulation is consumer protection.
- The rationale for consumer protection regulations is consumer ignorance.
- Legislation and regulation reflect interest group politics.
- When markets are imperfect, regulation cannot always improve outcomes.
- Providers are likely to "capture" the regulatory process.
- Market responses to consumer ignorance can limit the need for regulation.

17.1 Introduction

Healthcare is extensively regulated, and new regulations are constantly under consideration. Regulation is important to managers for five reasons:

1. Changes to regulations can make or break an organization. For example, in 2013 some health insurers withdrew from the market and others jumped in. Many of those who withdrew concluded that

the benefits required by the Affordable Care Act (ACA) meant that they would no longer be competitive. Those who entered the market concluded that the emergence of public and private exchanges would allow them to compete effectively (Olberding 2013).

2. In some circumstances, firms can use regulations to gain a competitive edge, especially when the regulations can be used to prevent entry by a potential rival. For example, Armstrong County Memorial Hospital was able to use the Pennsylvania **certificate of need law** to prevent the construction of a competing ambulatory surgery center (US Department of Justice 2000). Claims of regulatory violations by competitors can delay or derail projects, even if the claims are ultimately dismissed. For these reasons, managers must understand the impact of regulations on their organizations, react effectively to changes to regulations, and know when political action is necessary.

Certificate of need law
A law requiring state approval of healthcare construction projects

3. Managers need to understand the impetus behind healthcare regulation. Regulations are politically acceptable because the complexity of healthcare makes consumers feel vulnerable. Healthcare organizations must address these feelings of vulnerability because failure to do so invites additional regulation or loss of business.

4. Managers need to understand that legislating and regulating are continuing political contests. Most organizations have little to gain and much to lose in these risky contests. Few organizations can command enough political power to win lasting advantages through the political process, but all organizations need to be aware of the threats these contests pose.

5. Some regulations work poorly because they conflict with powerful financial incentives. Many of the same incentives that reinforce or undermine regulations also affect private contracts. Managers must know when regulations or contracts will work and when incentives will undermine them.

As noted in Chapter 16, markets and regulation are inseparable. Markets function badly with poorly designed rules, and regulations work badly when they conflict with market incentives. How well a healthcare market functions depends crucially on its regulatory structure.

17.2 Market Imperfections

Objections to regulation often stress that unfettered markets serve consumers well. This assertion may be true for perfectly competitive markets, but most healthcare markets fall far short of this ideal. At the heart of these imperfections lies "rational ignorance," or consumers' inability to make good choices. Before we discuss this important issue in healthcare regulation, let's look at the three other main imperfections that beset healthcare markets: insurance, market power, and **externalities**.

Externality
A benefit or cost imposed on someone who is not a party to the transaction that causes it

17.2.1 Insurance

By distorting consumers' incentives, insurance reduces the likelihood that healthcare markets will function ideally. Patients are shielded from the true costs of healthcare, and even the most ethical provider will feel comfortable recommending goods and services that the patient would be unwilling to buy if he or she faced the full cost. Moreover, the healthcare system in the United States limits the role of consumers in choosing insurance plans. Because patients are insulated from the true costs of care, their healthcare choices are unlikely to fully reflect their values. This lack of connection between what consumers value and what healthcare products cost is an important market imperfection.

17.2.2 Market Power

Most healthcare providers have some market power, which means prices will exceed marginal cost. To guarantee that markets will allocate resources at least as well as any other system, prices need to reflect the opportunity cost of using a good or service. By driving a wedge between the costs and prices of products, market power compounds the distortions introduced by insurance and may cause markets to function poorly. Moreover, in markets with firms that have market power, price controls can be useful tools. In a perfectly competitive market, price controls can be irrelevant (when market prices fall below regulated levels) or harmful (when market prices rise above regulated levels). When organizations have significant market power, a third outcome is possible: Price controls can result in lower prices and higher output. Price controls are not guaranteed to work in such markets, however; they can still be irrelevant or harmful. But price controls can be beneficial if the distortions they create are smaller than the distortions they remove.

17.2.3 Externalities

Some healthcare issues involve significant externalities. As noted in Chapter 16, an externality is a benefit received by, or a cost imposed on, someone who is not a party to a transaction. For example, installation of a catalytic converter in a car in Los Angeles will make the air cleaner not only for the owner of the car but also for others who live there and across the country. Markets tend not to work well when externalities are significant. Consumers and producers generally focus on the private benefits of transactions, which results in underconsumption of products that generate external benefits and overconsumption of products that generate external costs. Not surprisingly, the regulatory role of government tends to be substantial in these instances. For example, consider three activities that generate externalities: the search for new knowledge, the control of communicable diseases, and the maintenance of the environment. Patent and copyright laws restrict use of new knowledge, so producers are able to profit from selling it and thus are motivated to produce it. Public health regulations can mandate immunizations or require treatment of those infected with communicable diseases. Environmental regulations may restrict how resources are used or effectively change ownership rights. The details of these regulations can be controversial, but few societies leave resource allocation in such areas entirely to market forces.

17.3 Rational Consumer Ignorance

Healthcare regulations serve multiple purposes, but the ostensible objective of most regulations has long been consumer protection. The argument is that consumers need protection because they are rationally ignorant about the healthcare choices they must make.

At some point, everyone has difficulty making healthcare choices. In many cases decision makers have to rely on ambiguous or incomplete information. Although the scientific aura of modern medicine may suggest otherwise, many therapies lack a firm scientific basis. Even when the scientific evidence is good (in cases where investigators have carried out controlled clinical trials), decision makers may have a hard time applying it. Moreover, the results of controlled trials do not always translate to the uncontrolled environment of community practice. Even valid evidence involves probabilities, and most people (including most healthcare providers) have difficulty using this sort of information well. We tend to see patterns where none exist, place too much emphasis on cases that are memorable or recent, and ignore the rules of probability.

Patients face additional problems. They often must make decisions when they do not feel well and are experiencing a great deal of stress. They typically lack the experience, information, and skills they need to make healthcare choices. Even after they have chosen a course of action, consumers may have difficulty assessing whether they were diagnosed correctly, whether they were prescribed the right therapy, and whether that therapy was executed properly.

The ignorance of most patients is explainable. Few of us know the healthcare choices we will have to make or when we will have to make them. We don't want to invest the time to inform ourselves because we might not ever use the information. We'd rather have somebody else do the research. Of course, rational ignorance is not universal. Patients with chronic illnesses often are well informed about their care because they expect to make ongoing decisions and are motivated to become knowledgeable.

Consumers' struggle with medical decisions makes them vulnerable in a number of ways. Consumers often do not know when to seek care. They can have difficulty evaluating the recommendations of healthcare professionals, the quality of care, or the price of that care. They may be unable to differentiate care that is worth more from care that costs more. To reduce their vulnerability, consumers may turn to medical professionals for advice.

Unfortunately, securing provider recommendations does not render consumers unassailable. Providers often have incentives to be imperfect agents. A provider may sell a product because he or she is being paid by the producer to sell it, or may recommend a therapy because it is more profitable than another treatment. Patients may wind up undergoing treatment that is ineffective or harmful, or taking the advice of incompetent or unethical providers. In short, relying on providers for advice can reduce, but not necessarily efface, consumers' vulnerability.

For these reasons, providers have an interest in reducing consumers' concerns about their vulnerability. Consumers who cannot distinguish good advice from bad may ignore all of it. Consumers who cannot distinguish reliable from unreliable healthcare professionals may decide to forgo care. Regulations serve provider interests by signaling quality to consumers. As long as competent, trustworthy professionals find it easier to live with the regulations than incompetent, untrustworthy professionals do, regulations can be useful for both consumers and providers. Indeed, for this reason, much of the demand for regulation comes from the groups to be regulated, and many groups engage in self-regulation. For example, a group of physicians with a particular specialty may decide to create its own regulations that it expects will keep lesser-qualified physicians out of the specialty. This approach would help the group's own market share and help the public.

Rational ignorance and distortions induced by insurance, market power, and externalities will continue to make healthcare markets imperfect. Remember, however, that market regulation of such influences does not guarantee improved outcomes. Regulations are usually imperfectly designed and imperfectly implemented. In addition, the consumer protection rationale of regulations may be just that: a rationale. Regulations can be used to gain a competitive advantage and may harm, not help, consumers.

17.4 The Interest Group Model of Regulation

Legislation need not serve the public interest. Given that groups can use regulations to expand their markets and gain market power, the **interest group**

Interest group model of regulation
Model that views regulations as attempts to further the interests of affected groups, usually producer groups

model of regulation argues that legislatures are similar to markets, in that individuals and groups seek regulations to further their interests. Regulatory barriers to competition are often better than other competitive advantages because they are often harder for competitors to breach (especially for new firms or firms from outside an area, which have little or no political influence). Product features can be duplicated and marketing plans can be copied by even the most insignificant start-up firm, but large, well-established firms have significant political advantage.

17.4.1 Limiting Competition

One of the best ways to gain market power is to limit competition. Regulation is an effective way of limiting competition. For example, when confronted by the development of freestanding ambulatory surgical centers, the American Hospital Association sought to use state certificate of need laws to restrict their expansion (National Conference of State Legislatures 2013). Similarly, dental societies have long supported state laws prohibiting persons not licensed as dentists to fit and dispense dentures. Although lobbying the legislature to pass laws to prevent competition is legal, working together to prevent competition is illegal. In addition, the industry being regulated is likely to control the regulatory process, so consumer protection legislation may represent "existing firm protection" and not protect the consumer. Managers cannot ignore politics; doing so can put an organization at risk.

17.4.2 Licensure

Licensure is professional control of the regulatory process. A profession can be regulated in many ways. Professional regulation often protects the economic interests of the regulated group far better than it protects the health and safety interests of the public. States generally regulate health professionals via licensure, certification, and registration. Licensure prohibits people from performing the duties of a profession without meeting requirements set by the state. Certification prohibits those who do not meet requirements set by the state from using a title, but not from practicing. Registration requires practitioners to file their names, addresses, and relevant qualifications.

Licensure is the most restrictive form of regulation. It can prohibit practice by individuals without the right qualifications or require that they practice under the supervision of another professional. Its use is often justified by concerns about safety. While recognizing that certification considerably reduces consumer ignorance, advocates of licensure contend that it prevents unwary consumers from making unsafe choices. In some cases, however, licensure can prevent consumers from making choices that might make sense for them. Furthermore, it forces consumers to use highly trained, expensive personnel even when viable alternatives may be available.

CASE 17.1   Monks, Caskets, and the Supreme Court

The Louisiana State Board of Embalmers and Funeral Directors was formed in 1914 to regulate embalmers, funeral homes, and funeral directors and to handle consumer complaints. The board has one consumer representative. The other members all work in funeral homes (Louisiana State Board of Embalmers and Funeral Directors 2014).

Louisiana does not require burials in caskets, nor does it set any standards for caskets. Buying a casket online is legal. Nonetheless, Louisiana deemed it a crime to sell "funeral merchandise" without a funeral director's license (Institute for Justice 2014b).

The monks of Louisiana's Saint Joseph Abbey have to work to support it. After receiving inquiries from consumers, they decided to sell the cypress caskets in which Saint Joseph Abbey has long buried its dead. A funeral director filed a complaint arguing that "illegal third-party casket sales place funeral homes in an unfavorable position with families" (Institute for Justice 2014a). The Louisiana State Board of Embalmers and Funeral Directors moved to prevent the monks from selling caskets. To meet the board's standards, each monk would have to earn 30 hours of college credit and apprentice for a year at a licensed funeral home. None of the skills thus gained would be related to coffin building.

After opposition from the funeral industry prevented it from getting the law changed, the Abbey sued the board. The Abbey won in the district court in 2011 and in the Fifth US Circuit Court of Appeals in 2013. In its unanimous decision, the Circuit Court said, "The great deference due state economic regulation does not demand judicial blindness to the history of a challenged rule or the context of its adoption nor does it require courts to accept nonsensical explanations for regulation" (Institute for Justice 2014b). The US Supreme Court rejected the board's petition for review, so the Circuit Court's ruling stands (Institute for Justice 2014b).

Discussion questions:
- Why were funeral directors so opposed to the monks making caskets?
- Why would licensing casket makers be a good idea?
- In medicine, licensure and certification coexist. Is this true in any other fields?
- How do licensure and certification differ in their protections for ill-informed consumers?

17.4.3 Regulation as a Competitive Strategy

Regulations that affect the structure or process of an organization's operations typically increase its costs and reduce its flexibility. Naturally, firms resist regulation (even if their business plans are consistent with the goals of the regulation). For these reasons, imposing regulations on rivals (but not on oneself) can be an effective competitive strategy. Most regulation of the health professions has been a result of this strategy because existing professionals have been grandfathered in and regulations apply only to newly licensed practitioners.

17.5 Regulatory Imperfections

Capture
Takeover of the regulatory process by a special interest

When markets are not perfect, regulation can improve outcomes. For three reasons, however, regulation is likely to be equally imperfect: the need for decentralized decision making, conflicts between regulatory and financial incentives, and **capture** by regulated firms. Therefore, although new regulations can improve outcomes, this result is not guaranteed.

Regulations work best when decision making is centralized and when "one size fits all." Healthcare does not fit these criteria. Patients' healthcare needs, preferences, and circumstances vary considerably, so decision making needs to be decentralized and individualized. In addition, regulatory and financial incentives need to be aligned to work well. When they are not, regulations are likely to be ignored or circumvented. For example, we know that healthcare organizations respond to financial incentives. If physicians find that treating patients in the hospital is more convenient than treating them in their offices, and the physicians receive no financial incentives to encourage outpatient care, utilization review (an analysis of patterns of care by an employer or insurer) is unlikely to reduce hospitalization rates.

Furthermore, the groups being regulated are likely to capture the process, even if it is based on the noblest of intentions. Capture occurs when a group gains control of the administration of the regulations. Capture matters because the way the laws are implemented and enforced is as important as the laws themselves, and sooner or later the groups being regulated are likely to take control of the enforcement process. They have better information than consumers, pay more attention to the regulatory process than consumers, and have a more intense interest in the regulatory process than consumers. Regulation does not eliminate consumers' rational ignorance (although regulations about disclosing information may reduce it). As a result, regulators are likely to be members of the regulated group or are likely to rely on members of the regulated group for advice. Compounding this dependence is the regulated group's ongoing interest in the regulations. Consumers and their advocates, in contrast, are likely to lose interest once the problems that led to the regulations have eased. Finally, the group being regulated typically has an intense interest in the outcome of the process, and most consumers do not. This disparity further increases the odds of capture because in the political arena, a small group with an intense interest is likely to prevail over a larger group with more diffuse interests. As a result, regulation can best be described as "for the profession" rather than "of the profession."

CASE 17.2   Self-Regulation

"State pharmacy boards are too lax in their enforcement of the laws, too slow in innovating, and too prone to favor the interests of pharmacists. The public is often not represented on boards, and pharmacists are a majority of the board in every state," Avery said. "This situation is regulation for pharmacists, by pharmacists. If the safety of the public and the financial interests of the profession clash, the public will lose. Board members are almost always drawn from a list submitted by the state association of pharmacists. This approach is just another example of a profession using licensure to prevent competition, while talking about safety. For example, most pharmacists are opposed to periodic competency examinations. Concerns that some pharmacists might lose their licenses appear to outweigh concerns that incompetent practitioners might be at work."

Discussion questions:
- Who sits on your state's board that regulates pharmacy, medicine, and dentistry? Does the board include any consumer representatives? Are members of the regulated profession a majority of the board?
- Could such boards function without representatives of the profession? Realistically, could a licensing board not be dominated by the profession in question?
- How would consumers be hurt if your state stopped licensing pharmacists and started certifying them instead? How would these two systems differ? Is this scenario an example of a result of regulatory capture? Can you suggest a strategy that would ensure that the licensing board would serve the public interest?
- Suppose your state stopped licensing pharmacists. Would hospitals replace high-paid pharmacists with untrained or minimally trained personnel? Would retail pharmacies replace high-paid pharmacists with untrained or minimally trained personnel? Explain your answers.

17.6 Market Responses to Market Imperfections

Market responses to consumer ignorance can limit the need for regulation. Even imperfectly functioning markets incorporate incentives to serve consumers well. For most providers, repeat sales and customers are essential, so the incentives to meet customers' expectations are strong. Even when repeat customers are not major contributors to the business (as with a nursing home or plastic surgeon), the provider's reputation is one of its most important assets. Customers may not detect even profound agency problems. (See Chapter 13 for a fuller discussion of asymmetric information and agency.) Aware of their ineptitude for assessing poor performance, they often are willing to pay for information about quality and turn to consumer organizations (such as AARP) or information services (such as the National Committee for Quality Assurance) to aid them.

17.6.1 Tort Law and Contract Law

Tort law, which addresses compensation for a broad array of injuries, and contract law, which addresses breaches of agreement, can also remediate the shortcomings of healthcare markets. These legal remedies have powerful advantages. First, the threat of action is often enough to ensure compliance with explicit or implicit norms. If the probability of detecting noncompliance is high enough and the penalties are large enough, the threat of legal action will keep firms' behavior in check. Second, an agent's financial liability for nonperformance of a treatment usually exceeds the expected costs of the treatment, so tort law and contract law create incentives for providers to perform. Aside from prompting legal costs, fines, and penalties, liability can damage the agent's reputation. Third, legal liability is outcome oriented. Historically, regulation has focused on whether the structure of care and the processes of care comply with unverified norms, so its utility in matters of law is limited. Fourth, the legal system is more difficult to capture than most regulatory systems, especially when plaintiffs can take their cases to juries. Because consumers can initiate legal action themselves and because some lawyers are willing to accept the financial risks of failed suits by accepting contingency fees, access to legal remedies is more difficult to restrict than access to regulatory remedies.

Despite the power of tort law and contract law, their use also has disadvantages. To begin, legal remedies are costly to apply. Because of the costs of bringing suit, consumers may face barriers when accessing the legal system. Second, consumer ignorance may compromise the effectiveness of legal remedies. If consumers do not realize that their bad outcome resulted from a breach of duty on the part of their provider, they will not bring suit.

Alternatively, ignorant consumers may file suits when undesired outcomes resulted from bad luck, not negligence.

Absent a credible threat of being sued, incompetent or unscrupulous providers can continue unchecked. Even worse, the incentive for competent, scrupulous providers to invest resources in improving the quality of care may become diluted.

17.6.2 Information Dissemination

The legal system is both powerful and limited. First, it limits physicians to areas in which they are competent, doing so more effectively than state licensing boards. Medical licenses do not recognize differences in the skills of physicians. Were licenses the only guide, family practitioners would be able to perform neurosurgery. In fear of liability claims, hospitals also limit physicians to specific practices. Physicians, too, restrict their practices.

Second, studies of medical malpractice have shown that the majority of consumers who have suffered serious injuries as a result of negligence do not sue and receive no compensation. In addition, a high proportion of malpractice suits do not appear to involve provider negligence (Weiler et al. 1993). As a result, the malpractice system does not provide useful information on quality, and malpractice litigation's effect on the quality of care is not clear. In principle, publication of providers' malpractice histories should help consumers choose. Publication of risk-adjusted outcomes data would be better because it would put pressure on organizations to improve quality and could reduce consumer ignorance.

17.6.3 Contracts

Contracts are a private regulatory system (albeit one that does not work when collective mechanisms for enforcing contracts do not function effectively). As with public regulations, contracts work best when financial and regulatory incentives are aligned. A contract that pays more for better performance will usually produce more satisfactory results than a contract that stipulates minimum performance requirements.

For example, modification of physicians' practice patterns is a challenge for physician organizations seeking to become medical homes or accountable care organizations. Edwards and colleagues (2014) note that these new organizations will need new payment systems to align incentives for physicians. These new contracts with physicians may blend capitation, pay for performance, gainsharing, and fee-for-service payment. For example, a primary care physician might receive a base capitation payment, share a bonus if the practice meets patient satisfaction targets, and share another bonus if the practice meets cost targets. These contracts seek to change practice patterns by aligning the organization's and physicians' incentives.

CASE 17.3   Changing Consumer Information

"Quality report cards are everywhere," said Kai.

"Some of the early efforts were real clunkers, but most look pretty sensible now. It makes sense to offer consumers information instead of protecting them from the consequences of their ignorance. A lot of the report cards emphasize clinical issues, but some look at courtesy and customer service. The advantages of report cards are immense. Physicians and patients get systematic information that helps them choose specialists and hospitals. Providers have an incentive to improve performance in areas they might have overlooked, and those who cannot compete are likely to drop out of the market. Quality report cards have no downside. Setting up elaborate pay-for-performance schemes may not even be necessary. Fear of the fickle consumer may be incentive enough."

"While I like the idea of report cards," replied Leslie, "researchers have found little evidence that they have a significant impact. In principle, report cards may push out low quality firms, induce entry by high quality firms, or encourage existing firms to improve quality, but the evidence is far from compelling, as Dranove and Jin argued in 2010. Epstein noted in 2010 that study after study has found that report cards seem to have modest impacts on referrals and market share, probably because referring physicians already steer patients to higher quality providers. I like the idea of public reporting of price and quality data, but it's hard to make the case that report cards have had much of an effect."

"Whoa," replied Kai. "I think you are getting confused. Most doctors and hospitals provide comparable levels of service. Only a few fall short of the mark. The goal is to improve population outcomes by steering patients away from those providers or getting the providers to improve. A few patient switches are enough to move market share, and even if we can't show clearly that report cards work, everyone is improving. Where we have report cards, we see better performance. That's enough for me."

Discussion questions:
- What evidence can you find that report cards have improved quality?
- By what mechanisms could report cards improve reported market outcomes?

(continued)

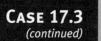

CASE 17.3
(continued)

- Does the scarcity of scientific evidence on the effectiveness of report cards matter?
- Could publication of performance data be advantageous to hospitals or physicians?
- How do report cards address information asymmetries? Would reducing information asymmetries guarantee better markets?
- Does it matter whether report cards are produced by governments or private organizations?
- Why are a few patient switches enough to influence market outcomes?

17.7 Implications for Managers

Markets and regulations complement each other because badly regulated markets will perform poorly. The usual reaction of managers is that less regulation is better than more, but this view is not always true. For example, the regulations that governed the market for individual health insurance before the passage of the ACA appear to have driven up costs, made coverage difficult to buy, and reduced the value of policies for potential customers. Buying health insurance in the individual market was a "nightmare" (Metcalf 2013). But regulatory changes have revitalized the individual market and transformed it into a growing sector (Keckley, Copeland, and Scott 2013).

Healthcare managers must understand the importance of regulations for their organizations and incorporate the effects of regulations into their decision making. Losses in the legislative or bureaucratic arenas may instigate regulations that put an organization at a significant disadvantage. Although managers may be tempted to see regulations as competitive tools, in practice their value is usually limited in competing with rivals in the same sector. Although zoning laws and certificate of need laws are notable exceptions, regulations usually apply the same rules for all the competitors in a sector.

Even when regulations could afford them a competitive advantage (perhaps by suppressing competition from rivals from other sectors), few organizations have the political strength and staying power to secure a long-lasting competitive advantage through political action. The exceptions tend to be large organizations that have a well-defined goal shared by all members, are well funded, have a positive reputation, and advocate policies that benefit the public (although less influential interest groups often have the capacity to shape laws and subsequent regulations when the stakes are small for other groups). For most organizations the challenge will be to resist the creation of laws and administrative rulings that threaten to put them at a disadvantage. Fortunately, preventing change usually takes much less influence than does causing it.

The interests of healthcare providers appear to require more regulation than governments can be induced to develop. Nongovernmental regulation is widespread in healthcare. For example, certification of health plans and physicians grew out of the need to give customers more detailed information about quality than regulatory bodies could provide. This trend is likely to continue. Managers need to prepare their organizations to compete in environments in which competitive pressures force the release of detailed, audited information about costs and outcomes. Organizations that don't perform well, and are thus unable to attract well-informed customers, will fail.

17.8 Conclusion

Markets need a sound regulatory underpinning to secure property rights, define liability, create a mechanism for enforcing contracts, and constrain or sanction forms of competition. For example, Enthoven and Singer (1997) point out that for an insurance market to function effectively, it must have a mechanism for deciding when care is medically necessary. Such a mechanism benefits both insurers and patients. An insurer will lose sales if its contracts are too ambiguous because consumers will perceive the contracts' terms as meaningless. On the other hand, simple, rigid interpretations of medically necessary care would not take into account the diverse circumstances consumers face. Designing effective regulations is not easy. Even well-intentioned regulations can stifle innovation, and regulations do not guarantee to improve outcomes.

Exercises

17.1 Why are many consumers apt to be rationally ignorant about their options?

17.2 Why would insurance coverage tend to increase rational ignorance?

17.3 A proposal has been advanced to limit advertising of pharmaceutical prices to prevent unfair pricing by national chains. You estimate that limits on price advertising will change the price elasticity of demand from –5.63 to –4.43. The marginal cost of a typical prescription is $40. A typical small pharmacy fills 25 prescriptions per day. A typical consumer fills 20 prescriptions per year. What economic effects will the limit have on consumers and on pharmacists? Which group is likely to be the more effective advocate for its position?

17.4 Prices for a medical procedure average $1,000 and range from $800 to $1,200. How much could a consumer paying full price save by getting the best price? Suppose that insurance is responsible for 75 percent of the consumer's spending and that out-of-pocket spending is limited to $250. How much could the consumer save by getting the best price?

17.5 Why are many economists opposed to licensure of medical facilities and personnel?

17.6 Identify circumstances in which both public and private regulation are present. Which serves consumers better? Why?

17.7 Find out who is on the board of the licensing agency for one of the health professions for your state. Does the board include more members of the profession being regulated or more consumers?

17.8 To reduce the costs of resolving insurance disputes, insurers have required that customers use arbitration. Arbitrators are required to be knowledgeable about medicine and insurance contracts. Why might you anticipate that the arbitration mechanism would wind up favoring the interests of the insurers?

17.9 How might the Food and Drug Administration be subject to capture? Who would be likely to capture the agency?

17.10 Hospital privileges usually restrict what physicians can do. Medical licenses do not. What drives this difference?

17.11 Consumers Union, the Leapfrog Group, and the Department of Health and Human Services have websites that provide consumer information about hospitals. Why are multiple sources of information available? Which of these sources did you find the most interesting?

17.12 Give an example of a healthcare product that is financed by the government but produced by private firms. Can you explain why this arrangement exists?

References

Dranove, D., and G. Z. Jin. 2010. "Quality Disclosure and Certification: Theory and Practice." *Journal of Economic Literature* 48 (4): 935–63.

Edwards, S. T., M. K. Abrams, R. J. Baron, R. A. Berenson, E. C. Rich, G. E. Rosenthal, M. B. Rosenthal, and B. E. Landon. 2014. "Structuring Payment to Medical Homes After the Affordable Care Act." *Journal of General Internal Medicine.* Published online April 1. doi:10.1007/s11606-014-2848-3.

Enthoven, A. C., and S. J. Singer. 1997. "Markets and Collective Action in Regulating Managed Care." *Health Affairs* 16 (6): 26–32.

Epstein, A. J. 2010. "Effects of Report Cards on Referral Patterns to Cardiac Surgeons." *Journal of Health Economics* 29 (5): 718–31.

Institute for Justice. 2014a. "Free the Monks and Free Enterprise: Challenging Louisiana's Casket Cartel." Accessed April 21. www.ij.org/louisiana-caskets-background-2.

———. 2014b. "Saint Joseph Abbey, et al. v. Castille, et al.: Challenging Louisiana's Casket Cartel." Accessed April 15. www.ij.org/saint-joseph-abbey-et-al-v-castille-et-al.

Keckley, P., B. Copeland, and G. Scott. 2013. "The Future of Health Care Insurance: What's Ahead?" *Deloitte Review* 13: 117–31.

Louisiana State Board of Embalmers and Funeral Directors. 2014. "Members." Accessed April 15. http://lsbefd.state.la.us/members.html.

Metcalf, N. 2013. "Remember Health Insurance Before the Affordable Care Act?" *ConsumerReports.org*. Published November 18. www.consumerreports.org/cro/news/2013/11/health-insurance-before-obamacare/index.htm.

National Conference of State Legislatures. 2013. "Certificate of Need: State Health Laws and Programs." Modified November. www.ncsl.org/research/health/con-certificate-of-need-state-laws.aspx.

Olberding, M. 2013. "Some Small Insurers Dropping Health Policies in Nebraska." *Lincoln Journal Star*. Published October 11. http://journalstar.com/business/local/some-small-insurers-dropping-health-policies-in-nebraska/article_eda9bbd9-dc93-5135-abe7-aadaef579ba6.html.

US Department of Justice. 2000. "Brief for the United States and the Federal Trade Commission as Amici Curiae." Accessed February 3, 2009. www.usdoj.gov/atr/cases/f230700/230741.htm.

Weiler, P. C., H. H. Hiatt, J. P. Newhouse, W. G. Johnson, T. A. Brennan, and L. L. Leape. 1993. *A Measure of Malpractice: Medical Injury, Malpractice Litigation, and Patient Compensation*. Cambridge, MA: Harvard University Press.

18

BEHAVIORAL ECONOMICS

After reading this chapter, students will be able to

- explain why rational decision making has its limits,
- describe some ways that bounded rationality affects decision making, and
- identify several ways to use behavioral economics to improve decision making.

Key Concepts

- Brainpower and time are scarce resources, so shortcuts in decision making make sense.
- Some shortcuts result in poor decisions.
- Some decisions appear to reveal inconsistent preferences.
- Status quo bias means that some people tend to avoid even beneficial changes.
- Overconfidence often leads to poor decisions.
- Problematic shortcuts include availability, anchoring, confirmation, and hindsight bias.
- Awareness of framing bias is especially important in management.
- Changes in how choices are set up can improve decision making.

18.1 Introduction

Standard economic models start with assumptions that are not really true. These assumptions include the notions that decision makers are always rational, have unlimited willpower, and are concerned only about themselves. These assumptions were previously viewed as harmless simplifications, but researchers have demonstrated that being more realistic could be important in management and policy. For example, cash bonuses may reduce work effort (especially if the work is intrinsically interesting or important), but symbolic payments (such as praise) tend to increase work effort (Gneezy, Meier, and Rey-Biel 2011). For a purely rational worker, that finding would not make sense. Surely praise coupled with cash would be a more powerful motivator than praise alone. Economics that drops the assumptions of complete rationality, complete willpower, and complete selfishness is called **behavioral economics**.

Behavioral economics
A scholarly discipline that integrates psychology and economics

Behavioral economics addresses the choices that individuals make when they use shortcuts and rules of thumb in decision making. Our brainpower and our time are scarce resources, so it makes sense to use rules of thumb in making decisions. Unfortunately, these shortcuts sometimes result in poor decisions.

Children's Health Insurance

Nearly two-thirds of the millions of children without health insurance appear to be eligible for Medicaid or the Children's Health Insurance Program (Kenney et al. 2011). For many of these children, health insurance would be free. Not accepting free health insurance makes sense in standard economics only if you believe that the hassles of signing up for these programs outweigh their considerable benefits, but behavioral economics notes several reasons for this pattern. First, parents may focus on the up-front hassles and give much less emphasis to the future benefits. That is, the parents may heavily discount the future benefits. Second, the well-known problem of procrastination means that tomorrow or next week are always better times than today to go to the trouble of enrolling a child. (We will discuss procrastination more in Section 18.2.) Third, we know that many decision makers have trouble with probabilities, meaning that the parents of these uninsured children make poor assessments of the chance that their child will become seriously ill or that better access to medical care will be important (Kahneman and Tversky 1979).

To boost enrollment of eligible children after the reauthorization of the Children's Health Insurance Program in 2009, the Department of Health and Human Services authorized bonus payments to states that made enrollment in the program easier and increased enrollment more than a formula would predict. Eighteen states applied for the bonuses and fifteen got them. As a result of this program, more than 800,000 children gained coverage. Alabama added 133,000 children to its Medicaid rolls and got the largest bonus, just over $55 million. To simplify

(continued)

(continued)

enrollment, Alabama removed asset tests for children, stopped requirements for an in-person interview, made eligibility last for a full year, and simplified the application process in other ways (Kenney et al. 2011).

Both the Alabama program and the national program incorporate ideas from behavioral economics. The Alabama program focused on making enrollment easier, rather than emphasizing traditional outreach strategies. The national program was voluntary and let states choose how to try to increase enrollment (with some broad limits). These features limited resistance to the program and focused resources on states that wanted to expand enrollment. Unfortunately, many children who are eligible for health insurance subsidies remain uninsured, and adults are likely to face a similar problem under the Affordable Care Act (ACA).

18.2 Inconsistent Preferences

A standard assumption in economics is that consumers make reasonable forecasts about what they will do in the future and make plans on that basis. Behavioral economics notes, to the contrary, that many people appear to have inconsistent preferences. A classic example is the tendency to procrastinate. For example, we may conclude that the cost of exercising is more than offset by its benefits, especially if we commit to starting exercising next week. But when next week arrives, we don't want to work out; we want to put it off for another week. Last week the costs were in the future; this week they will be realized right now. Decisions that I make today may conflict with decisions that I make next week, even though nothing has changed.

This inconsistency appears to involve rather odd patterns of **discounting** future benefits and costs (Frederick, Loewenstein, and O'Donoghue 2002). For example, if you regard being paid $988 today as being just as good as being paid $1,000 in three months, your personal discount rate is less than 5 percent per year.[1] Would you prefer getting $790 now to getting $1,000 in three months? If so, you are acting as though your discount rate is more than 150 percent per year. A discount rate of more than 150 percent per year seems pretty high, but the real anomaly is that people sometimes use 5 percent and sometimes use 150 percent or more for seemingly similar transactions.

A standard assumption is that people will use the same discount rate for short-term financial gains, long-term financial gains, short-term financial

Discounting
Adjusting the value of future costs and benefits to reflect the willingness of consumers to trade current consumption for future consumption

costs, and long-term financial costs because someone could make money by exploiting discount rate variations. But many people discount the future very heavily and treat short delays much differently from longer delays. For example, would you be willing to pay an annual rate of more than 300 percent for a $200 three-week loan? More than 18 million taxpayers thought this proposition was a good deal in 2011, when they signed up for refund anticipation checks that allowed them to pay their tax preparation fees out of their tax refunds (Wu, Fox, and Feltner 2013). The fee for this privilege was typically $30 or more. Most people who agreed to refund anticipation checks had very low incomes (so coming up with $200 to pay a tax preparation fee would be a problem) and probably were not financially sophisticated (given that a number of ways to have a simple return filled out cost much less than $200).

Paying Not to Go to the Gym

People who are cash strapped are not the only ones who act inconsistently. Health club members make some odd choices too.

Most health clubs offer several payment plans. You can pay by the visit, buy a monthly membership (which lets you cancel at the end of every month), or buy an annual membership. If you are not sure how much you'll go or whether you will stick with this particular gym, paying by the visit makes sense. Choosing a monthly contract makes sense for members who plan to use the gym a lot but may want to quit after a couple of months.

However, the plans that people buy often don't match how they use the gym. For example, people who bought a monthly membership averaged 4.3 sessions per month (DellaVigna and Malmendier 2006). That means they paid more than $17 per session, even though they could have averaged only $10 if they bought a ten-visit pass or $12 if they simply paid for each visit. The difference is not trivial. Making this poor choice increased club fees by more than $600 per year.

The second oddity is that members who chose a monthly contract were 17 percent more likely to be enrolled for more than a year than members who chose an annual contract. Compared to a monthly contract, an annual contract offers the equivalent of one or two months free, which suggests that neither group was good at predicting what they would do. At least some members who chose annual contracts should have chosen monthly contracts, and some members who chose monthly contracts should have chosen annual ones.

(continued)

(continued)

Why do people overestimate how much they will work out? They heavily discount the psychic cost of doing so when they sign the contract. (If you like working out, obviously this statement does not apply.) If you discount the pain of exercising by enough, tomorrow will be a much better day to work out than today. Unfortunately, if you apply that logic for 365 days, you never go to the gym.

A service called Gym Pact promises to help. It charges you if you go to the gym less than you intended to. (Your smart phone GPS knows if you've been to the gym or not.) Gym Pact uses the money from slackers to pay people who actually met their exercise targets (Gym Pact 2014). The idea is that creating an immediate financial reward for working out will offset the pain of doing so. The company founders got the idea after taking a class in behavioral economics (Bernard 2012).

18.3 Risk Preferences

Why do people smoke or drive without seat belts? That these behaviors are risky is not exactly news. One could argue that many smokers are addicted, but that argument just pushes the question back a step. Why do people start smoking if they know that cigarettes are addictive and that smoking is dangerous? One possibility is that people who make risky choices like risk. Another is that they misunderstand the risks they are taking. For example, many people appear to underestimate health risks, and this underestimation is a factor in their decision not to buy insurance. Another way to describe underestimation of risk is to say that people are overconfident (as we discuss further in Section 18.4). This observation is not entirely new. In *An Inquiry into the Nature and Causes of the Wealth of Nations* ([1776] 1904), Adam Smith observed that many people did not buy insurance on their homes because of their "presumptuous contempt of the risk." Whether we should treat this choice as the result of overconfidence (as Smith did), bad information about risk, or difficulty in understanding the meaning of risks does not matter too much. Any of these will lead to poor decisions.

Some evidence links risk preferences to risky behavior. (Recall from Chapter 4 that risk seekers seek more variable outcomes and risk-averse people seek less variable outcomes. Risk seekers seldom buy insurance. Risk-averse people will buy insurance if the premium is not too much larger than the expected loss.) For example, Anderson and Mellor (2008) found that people who did not use seat belts very often were more likely to be smokers as well. They also found that people who were risk seekers (less than 15 percent of their sample) were more likely to smoke, drink heavily, be obese, not use seat belts, and drive fast.

Misunderstanding the dangers of risky behavior and the likelihood of those dangers is a major problem for younger people. Aversion to risk typically increases with age. Few children are risk averse, a slightly larger share of adolescents are risk averse, and most adults are risk averse (Paulsen et al. 2012). Recall that being risk averse means being willing to accept somewhat lower average rewards (financial or other) in exchange for a reduction in the variability of those rewards. Most people who buy health insurance are risk averse because the expected benefits are less than the premium. Typically, someone who is risk averse tends to discount the future less than someone who is risk seeking, so these two tendencies reinforce each other (Jusot and Khlat 2013).

Not surprisingly, most people who become addicted to cigarettes did so as adolescents (Sloan and Wang 2008). Their willingness to accept risk was high, their concern about the future was low, and their ability to imagine the consequences of becoming addicted was limited.

Employer-Sponsored Health Insurance and Behavioral Economics

Among Americans who are not eligible for Medicare, a majority get their health insurance through their employer. Because it allows insurers to reduce marketing and underwriting costs, employer-sponsored health insurance typically costs less than comparable individual coverage. Employer-sponsored health insurance also benefits from tax subsidies because employer contributions are not treated as taxable income and many employees can pay their premiums with pretax dollars.

Employer-sponsored insurance also has some features that are likely to boost enrollment. First, it limits the number of choices. Too many choices may lead to no decision, so a limited number of choices is likely to increase enrollment. Second, the employee's share shows up as a deduction from gross pay. Apparently a deduction feels like less of a burden than writing a check even though they are financially identical.

The ACA also allows employers to make health insurance enrollment the default option. Because employees are free to disenroll or switch plans, this enrollment does not affect their freedom of choice.

(continued)

(continued)

Evidence suggests, however, that such a seemingly trivial change could have dramatic effects. Evidence about the effects of default enrollment on health insurance decisions is modest, but multiple studies show dramatic increases in pension plan enrollment when enrollment becomes the default option (Carroll et al. 2009). Consumers often find complex choices difficult to make, and some will respond by not choosing.

18.4 Incorrect Beliefs

In Lake Wobegon all the children are above average. That's mathematically possible, but over 90 percent of American students reported that their driving skills were above average—something that tells us more about our capacity for self-delusion than about our driving abilities or our ability to do math (White, Cunningham, and Titchener 2011). Oddly, others don't share this assessment, and nearly two-thirds of young drivers admit to texting and other unsafe behaviors while driving (Allstate 2011). But does this overconfidence or "Lake Wobegon effect" matter?

It does because overconfident decision makers are likely to make bad choices. They are likely to overestimate their chances of success and apt to attribute failures to bad luck (hence not learning from them). For example, the fact that companies often lose money when they buy other companies is common knowledge. Acquiring a company requires a bid above its current market valuation, and its current market valuation is as likely to be too high as to be too low. So, it takes a very confident management team—one convinced of their skill and of unrecognized synergies—to buy another company. In many cases this confidence amounts to overconfidence and the acquisition is unprofitable (Armstrong and Huck 2010). Overconfident CEOs often make money-losing acquisitions.

Several cognitive traps feed into overconfidence:

- Availability bias
- Anchoring bias
- Confirmation bias
- Hindsight bias

We will discuss each of these in turn.

Availability bias can occur because certain outcomes are overly easy to imagine or overly hard to imagine. For example, if you run a public health

Availability bias
A cognitive trap that occurs when some facts are overly easy or overly hard to recall

agency, which threat to life should be your top priority, tornadoes or asthma? If you were asked this question right after hearing about the Oklahoma City tornadoes, you might have said tornadoes. The news reports made them easy to remember. In fact, the two threats are not even close. Between 2010 and 2012, tornadoes killed an average of 222 people each year (National Oceanic and Atmospheric Administration 2014). Nearly 3,500 people die from asthma each year, and quite a few of these deaths are preventable. If you have never known anyone who died as a result of asthma, you might have a difficult time imagining asthma as a cause of death and may pay too little attention to it.

Anchoring bias
A cognitive trap that occurs when an irrelevant fact influences a decision

Anchoring bias occurs when some initial estimate, even if it is not based on evidence or is simply wrong, affects future discussions. In a strategy discussion about whether to add a long-term care facility to a system, one of the board members says, "I hope the return on equity is better than the 5 percent that home health care firms earn." That comment is not really relevant because long-term care and home health care are fairly distinct markets. True or not, the comment is likely to influence the subsequent discussion.

Irrelevant information can influence decision making. If a job candidate starts by mentioning a desired salary of $150,000, the candidate will probably get a higher offer than if he or she started by mentioning a current salary of $85,000. Neither of these numbers may fall within the pay range for the job in question, but mentioning the $150,000 tends to anchor the discussion.

Even experienced professionals can be affected by anchoring. Two groups of Scandinavian financial advisers were asked to forecast returns for European stock markets (Kaustia, Alho, and Puttonen 2008). One group was told that the historical average was a return of 4.5 percent and forecast returns of 4.6 percent. The other group was not given any information and forecast returns of 8.1 percent. In another experiment the financial advisers were prompted with irrelevant data about very high returns in Sweden or very low returns in Japan. Those given the Swedish data gave much higher forecasts. The good news is that financial professionals were less subject to anchoring effects than students. Students given the Swedish data forecast rates of return more than twice as high as students given the Japanese data.

Confirmation bias
The tendency to focus on information that supports one's beliefs

Confirmation bias occurs when we filter evidence to prove that our conclusions are right. How did you react when a political candidate that you support said something stupid? Most of us will offer an example of the opponent's failings rather than switch candidates.

A management example of confirmation bias can be found in the hiring process. Suppose you interview several people, and Ms. Jones seems to stand out. You are confident that she is the best choice. You call several references, they say mostly good things about the candidate, and those are the comments that you include in your notes. Ms. Jones turns out to be a disaster. You used the interview to support your positive impression, not to look for warning signs. You didn't follow up when a reference said, "Well, she wasn't here that long," and another said, "She was only in my unit for about three months."

Hindsight bias occurs when you feel that you "knew it all along," that is, when you believe that you made a prediction that you did not. This bias creates two decision traps. First, your overconfidence may grow. Second, you have no incentive to explore why your predictions were faulty. Neither of these bodes well for future decisions.

> **Hindsight bias**
> The tendency to overstate how predictable an outcome was beforehand

Hindsight bias is widespread, having been documented in diverse situations including labor disputes, medical diagnoses, managerial decisions, and public policy (Roese and Vohs 2012). Hindsight bias has serious consequences because it impairs performance. For example, researchers have found that investment bankers who earned the least had the largest hindsight bias (Biais and Weber 2009). Hindsight bias also makes effective investigations of accidents and near misses difficult, leaving future patients at risk because no fundamental changes are made (Hugh and Dekker 2009).

18.5 Representativeness and the Law of Small Numbers

To assess a possible merger with another practice, you interview six CEOs from practices that went through mergers. After you complete the interviews, you notice that the three CEOs from the successful mergers were accountants and the three CEOs from the failed mergers were physicians. What should you infer from that?

You should infer nothing. Your sample is too small and may be biased. If you looked at a larger, more representative sample, you might find any pattern. For example, you might find that merged practices led by accountants were more likely to fail. Nonetheless, you may be tempted to think that having an accountant as the CEO is important.

Several factors are at work here. First, humans are prone to see patterns even if no pattern exists. We are apt to think that our experience with a small number of people will be typical of the whole group. This tendency is called **representativeness bias** (Tversky and Kahneman 1971). We are also apt to forget that statistics based on small numbers can be very misleading. This tendency is the **law of small numbers bias**.

> **Representativeness bias**
> The tendency to overstate how typical a small sample is
>
> **Law of small numbers bias**
> Generalizations based on small samples

The problem is greatest when our own experience suggests a conclusion. We easily dismiss colleagues' stories as being mere anecdotes. Our stories seem different. They feel meaningful to us. We have no trouble saying, "The plural of *anecdote* is not *evidence*," unless the anecdote is ours. Our stories seem compelling.

18.6 Inconsistent Decision Making: Framing

Real-life choices appear to be affected by how they are presented. In fact, framing appears to be one of the strongest decision-making biases. Framing is especially relevant to health decisions because the stakes are high and because older adults (who are more likely to have to make health decisions) appear more likely to use shortcuts that cause **framing bias** (Perneger and Agoritsas 2011).

Framing bias
The effects of presenting the same data in different ways

A standard way of illustrating framing bias is via a treatment choice problem. Treatment 1 is guaranteed to save 200 of 1,000 people with a fatal disease. Treatment 2 offers a 20 percent chance of saving 1,000 lives and an 80 percent chance of saving no one. Which do you prefer? Most people prefer treatment 1 because it seems less risky.

Now consider another scenario. If you choose treatment 3, 800 of 1,000 people with a fatal disease will die. With treatment 4, you have an 80 percent chance that everyone will die and a 20 percent chance that no one will die. Which do you prefer? Most people choose treatment 4.

The only difference between these two scenarios is that the first is framed in terms of how many people live and the second is framed in terms of how many die. They are otherwise identical, yet choices typically differ. By changing the emotional context of a decision, framing can change choices.

Framing can take several forms. It can describe the attributes of choices in different ways, describe the outcomes of choices in different ways, and describe the risks of choices in different ways. For example, people tend to prefer a choice when its attributes are presented in positive terms (Mishra, Gregson, and Lalumiere 2012). Thus, consumers are more apt to choose a hospital that stresses its high patient satisfaction (a positive attribute frame) rather than its low mortality rates (a negative attribute frame). An example of goal framing would be to describe the effect of a new strategy as a gain in market share (a positive goal frame) or as avoiding stagnation (a negative goal frame). Most people are influenced by **loss aversion**, meaning they worry more about avoiding losses than they do about realizing gains. As a result, people may respond more to negative goal frames. The treatment choice example given earlier in this section illustrates risk framing. The same problem can be presented in terms of lives saved (a positive risk frame) or in terms of deaths prevented (a negative risk frame). People tend to be more willing to accept risk to avoid negative outcomes than they are to gain positive outcomes.

Loss aversion
A focus on avoiding losses rather than maximizing gains

The importance of framing appears to vary. Some decision makers appear to be immune to framing, with decision makers with the best mathematics skills the least likely to be affected. In addition, goal framing appears to have smaller effects than attribute or risk framing (Armstrong and Huck 2010). The challenge for managers is determining when framing will matter and when it will not.

Framing Insurance Choices to Improve Consumer Decision Making

A number of countries rely on consumer demand to limit medical costs. An important mechanism is the willingness of consumers to switch to less expensive health insurance plans, which pressures insurers to offer low-cost plans and pressures providers to reduce what they charge for care. However, consumers often find insurance choices daunting, which may result in reluctance to switch plans. This reluctance dilutes the effects of competition on costs. For example, in Switzerland (which has an insurance system similar to the ACA) rates of switching between insurers have been very low, even though prices varied among comparable plans. Annual switching rates in 2004 were around 3 percent, even though the monthly premium for the most expensive plan averaged 140 Swiss francs more than the least expensive plan (Frank and Lamiraud 2009).

Why were switching rates so low? Behavioral economics offers several reasons. First, a significant **status quo bias** is at work. Consumers are often reluctant to make changes if they do not have to. Second, too many choices can stop consumers from making any choice. This problem is called **decision overload**. Because the average Swiss consumer had 56 plans to choose from in 2004, decision overload appears to have been relevant. Third, consumers tend to worry about making what turns out to be a bad choice. One way to avoid regret about a choice is to avoid making a choice. Fourth, consumers appear to give more weight to avoiding losses than to realizing gains. This response is loss aversion. Loss aversion is a powerful emotional response to the potential for losses in health or income. Loss aversion tends to inhibit making changes.

Status quo bias
The tendency not to change, even when it would be advantageous to do so

Decision overload
Poorer decision making that occurs as choices become more complex

18.7 Conclusion

People use shortcuts when they make hard or emotionally charged decisions. In other words, patients, clinicians, and managers use shortcuts when they buy insurance, when they make medical decisions, when they make strategic decisions at work, and when they hire and fire employees. Shortcuts are common.

Sometimes, unfortunately, shortcuts lead to poor choices. Patients may choose insurance plans that expose them to significant financial risks. Clinicians may recommend problematic treatment plans. And managers may make business decisions that harm patients or their organizations. The stakes can be high.

What can managers do to limit bad decision making due to shortcuts? Fortunately, a number of strategies are available.

- Look hard for evidence that you are wrong.
- Appoint someone to tear apart your analyses.
- Reward those who express honest disagreement.
- Seek out the opinions of people who disagree with you, and listen carefully.
- Try to reframe problems to view them from different perspectives.
- Talk about your feelings to see if they are leading you astray.
- Postpone committing to strategies as long as you can.
- Make sure that a review process and an exit strategy are part of decision making.
- Be aware that your decision making can lead to mistakes.

These steps will not shield you from making errors. They may help you make fewer mistakes, though.

Exercises

18.1 You will receive a $10,000 insurance payment in two months. If you are willing to pay for expedited handling, you can be paid in one month. Would you be willing to pay $50? $100? $200? More?

18.2 You will receive a $20,000 insurance payment in 12 months. If you are willing to accept a reduced payment, you can be paid in 11 months. Would you be willing to accept $19,800? $19,500? $19,000? Less?

18.3 What annual interest rate is implied by your answer to Exercise 18.1? You calculate this by dividing $10,000 by the difference of $10,000 and the amount you are willing to pay for expedited handling, then taking the result to the 12th power and subtracting 1. For example, if you were willing to pay $100, the result would be $(\$10,000/\$9,900)^{12} - 1 = 0.1281781$, or 12 percent.

18.4 What annual interest rate is implied by your answer to Exercise 18.2? Is it the same as the rate in Exercise 18.3? Why would this comparison matter?

18.5 How are Exercises 18.1 and 18.2 different? How are your answers to them different?

18.6 How could you use behavioral economics to increase the number of insured employees in your firm?

18.7 How likely is someone aged 25 to 44 to have an emergency department visit? What is the probability of having two visits? What is a typical charge for an emergency department visit? On the basis of your answers, would someone aged 25 to 44 be willing to buy coverage for emergency department care (with a $50 copayment) if it cost $250 per year?

18.8 What was your forecast of emergency department spending in Exercise 18.7? Your forecast should equal the probability of one emergency department visit times the typical charge plus the probability of two visits times the typical charge.

18.9 A town has two hospitals. One averages 30 births per day; the other averages 15. Overall, half of the babies are boys, but some days more than 60 percent of the babies are boys. Is either hospital likely to have a greater number of days with a high proportion of boys?

18.10 Eighty percent of the participants at a meeting are physicians. The rest are nurse practitioners. Your neighbor Amy is there. She is 40, married, and highly motivated. Colleagues have told you that Amy is extremely capable and promises to be very successful. What is the probability that Amy is a physician?

18.11 Will you be in the top half of your class or the bottom? What proportion of your classmates will forecast that they will be in the top half? What implications does this scenario have for decision making?

18.12 You have finished interviewing candidates for an assistant director position. One of them stands out as the best candidate to you. You know that this view sets you up for confirmation bias as you check references. What steps can you take to prevent this bias?

18.13 Your vice president is an accountant and believes that accountants make the best practice managers. One of the three finalists for a practice management has an accounting background. Everyone on the search team has ranked this candidate lowest of the finalists. You fear that your vice president will tend to selectively read the team's recommendations and lean toward hiring this person. What can you do to offset this potential confirmation bias?

18.14 Thirty-four percent of the employees in your health system are obese, and 16 percent of their children are obese as well. Obese employees are less productive, have higher medical costs, and miss more work. Employees with obese children also miss more work, so persuading employees and their families to lose weight looks like a good investment for the system. In fact, effective, clearly cost-effective interventions are available to reduce obesity, and you offer them to your employees and their families. You have recently begun to make weight loss interventions available for free, but only 1 percent of your employees have signed up for them. What behavioral economics tools can you use to help your employees lose weight?

Note

1. If getting $988 is as good as getting $1,000 in three months, your discount rate is 4.95 percent per year. Dividing $1,000 by $988 gives a three-month discount factor of 1.012145749. Taking this result to the fourth power (to convert it to an annual rate) gives 1.04948. It is customary to subtract 1.00 from this discount factor and express the results in percentage terms. Doing so gives 4.95 percent.

References

Allstate. 2011. "New Allstate Survey Shows Americans Think They Are Great Drivers—Habits Tell a Different Story." Published August 2. www.prnewswire.com/news-releases/new-allstate-survey-shows-americans-think-they-are-great-drivers---habits-tell-a-different-story-126563103.html.

Anderson, L. R., and J. M. Mellor. 2008. "Predicting Health Behaviors with an Experimental Measure of Risk Preference." *Journal of Health Economics* 27 (5): 1260–74.

Armstrong, M., and S. Huck. 2010. "Behavioral Economics as Applied to Firms: A Primer." *Competition Policy International* 6 (1): 3–45.

Bernard, T. S. 2012. "Gym-Pact Fines You for Not Exercising." *New York Times.* Published January 2. http://bucks.blogs.nytimes.com/2012/01/02/gym-pact-fines-you-for-not-exercising/.

Biais, B., and M. Weber. 2009. "Hindsight Bias, Risk Perception, and Investment Performance." *Management Science* 55 (6): 1018–29.

Carroll, G. D., J. J. Choi, D. Laibson, B. C. Madrian, and A. Metrick. 2009. "Optimal Defaults and Active Decisions." *Quarterly Journal of Economics* 124 (4): 1639–74.

DellaVigna, S., and U. Malmendier. 2006. "Paying Not to Go to the Gym." *American Economic Review* 96 (3): 694–719.

Frank, R. G., and K. Lamiraud. 2009. "Choice, Price Competition and Complexity in Markets for Health Insurance." *Journal of Economic Behavior & Organization* 71 (2): 550–62.

Frederick, S., G. Loewenstein, and T. O'Donoghue. 2002. "Time Discounting and Time Preference: A Critical Review." *Journal of Economic Literature* 40 (2): 351–401.

Gneezy, U., S. Meier, and P. Rey-Biel. 2011. "When and Why Incentives (Don't) Work to Modify Behavior." *Journal of Economic Perspectives* 25 (4): 191–209.

Gym Pact. 2014. "Pact Creates Powerful Incentives for Health." Accessed April 18. www.gym-pact.com.

Hugh, T. B., and S. W. Dekker. 2009. "Hindsight Bias and Outcome Bias in the Social Construction of Medical Negligence: A Review." *Journal of Law and Medicine* 16 (5): 846–57.

Jusot, F., and M. Khlat. 2013. "The Role of Time and Risk Preferences in Smoking Inequalities: A Population-Based Study." *Addictive Behaviors* 38 (5): 2167–73.

Kahneman, D., and A. Tversky. 1979. "Prospect Theory: An Analysis of Decision Under Risk." *Econometrica* 47 (2): 263–92.

Kaustia, M., E. Alho, and V. Puttonen. 2008. "How Much Does Expertise Reduce Behavioral Biases? The Case of Anchoring Effects in Stock Return Estimates." *Financial Management* 37 (3): 391–412.

Kenney, G. M., V. Lynch, J. M. Haley, M. Huntress, D. Resnick, and C. Coyer. 2011. *Gains for Children: Increased Participation in Medicaid and CHIP in 2009.* Washington, DC: Urban Institute.

Mishra, S., M. Gregson, and M. L. Lalumiere. 2012. "Framing Effects and Risk-Sensitive Decision Making." *British Journal of Psychology* 103 (1): 83–97.

National Oceanic and Atmospheric Administration. 2014. "Monthly and Annual U.S. Tornado Summaries." Accessed April 23. www.spc.noaa.gov/climo/online/monthly/newm.html.

Paulsen, D. J., M. L. Platt, S. A. Huettel, and E. M. Brannon. 2012. "From Risk-Seeking to Risk-Averse: The Development of Economic Risk Preference from Childhood to Adulthood." *Frontiers in Psychology* 3: 313.

Perneger, V., and T. Agoritsas. 2011. "Doctors and Patients' Susceptibility to Framing Bias: A Randomized Trial." *Journal of General Internal Medicine* 26 (12): 1411–17.

Roese, N. J., and K. D. Vohs. 2012. "Hindsight Bias." *Perspectives on Psychological Science* 7 (5): 411–26.

Sloan, F. A., and Y. Wang. 2008. "Economic Theory and Evidence on Smoking Behavior of Adults." *Addiction* 103 (11): 1777–85.

Smith, A. [1776] 1904. *An Inquiry into the Nature and Causes of the Wealth of Nations.* London: Methuen.

Tversky, A., and D. Kahneman. 1971. "Belief in the Law of Small Numbers." *Psychological Bulletin* 76 (2): 105–10.

White, M. J., L. C. Cunningham, and K. Titchener. 2011. "Young Drivers' Optimism Bias for Accident Risk and Driving Skill: Accountability and Insight Experience Manipulations." *Accident Analysis and Prevention* 43 (4): 1309–15.

Wu, C. C., J. A. Fox, and T. Feltner. 2013. *Something Old, Something New in Tax-Time Financial Products: Refund Anticipation Checks and the Next Wave of Quickie Tax Loans.* Boston: National Consumer Law Center.

GLOSSARY

A

Accountable care organization. A provider organization that contracts to be paid based on the cost and quality metrics of a patient population

Adverse selection. High-risk consumers' willingness to pay more for insurance than low-risk consumers (Organizations that have difficulty distinguishing high-risk from low-risk consumers are unlikely to be profitable.)

Agency. An arrangement in which one person (the agent) takes actions on behalf of another (the principal)

Agent. A person who takes actions on behalf of another person (the principal)

Anchoring bias. A cognitive trap that occurs when an irrelevant fact influences a decision

Arc elasticity. A ratio of percentage changes that is calculated using the average of two points (For example, a percentage change in price between $8 and $2 would be calculated by subtracting $2 from $8 and then dividing the result by $5, the average of the two values.)

Asymmetric information. Information known to one party in a transaction but not another

Attribute-based differentiation. Making customers aware of differences among products

Availability bias. A cognitive trap that occurs when some facts are overly easy or overly hard to recall

Average cost. Total cost divided by total output

B

Behavioral economics. A scholarly discipline that integrates psychology and economics

Bundled payment. A single payment, also called a *bundled episode payment*, that covers all services delivered during a given episode of care (Examples of an episode of care include hip replacement, a year of diabetes care, or pregnancy.)

C

Capitated. Payment is per person (The payment does not depend on the services provided.)

Capitation. Payment per person (The payment does not depend on the services provided.)

Capture. Takeover of the regulatory process by a special interest

Case-based payment. A single payment for an episode of care (The payment does not change if fewer services or more services are provided.)

Certificate of need law. A law requiring state approval of healthcare construction projects

Coinsurance. A form of cost sharing in which a patient pays a share of the bill rather than a set fee

Collusion. A secret agreement between parties for a fraudulent, illegal, or deceitful purpose

Complement. A product used in conjunction with another product

Concentrated market. A market with few competitors or dominant firms

Confirmation bias. The tendency to focus on information that supports one's beliefs

Copayment. A fee the patient must pay in addition to the amount paid by insurance

Cost. The value of a resource in its next best use

Cost–benefit analysis. An analysis that compares the value of an innovation with its costs (Value is measured as willingness to pay for the innovation or willingness to accept compensation to allow it to be implemented.)

Cost-effectiveness analysis. An analysis that measures the cost of an innovation per unit of change in a single outcome

Cost-minimization analysis. An analysis that measures the cost of two or more innovations with the same patient outcomes

Cost sharing. The general term for direct payments to providers by insurance beneficiaries (Deductibles, copayments, and coinsurance are forms of cost sharing.)

Cost shifting. The hypothesis that price differences are due to efforts by providers to make up for losses in some lines of business by charging higher prices in other lines of business

Cost–utility analysis. An analysis that measures the cost of an innovation per quality-adjusted life year

Cross-price elasticity. The percentage change in the quantity demanded associated with a 1 percent change in the price of a related product

D

Decision overload. Poorer decision making that occurs as choices become more complex

Decision tree. A visual decision support tool that depicts the values and probabilities of the outcomes of a choice

Deductible. Amount a consumer must pay before insurance covers any healthcare costs

Demand. The amounts of a good or service that will be purchased at different prices when all other factors are held constant

Demand curve. A graphic depiction of how much consumers are willing to buy at different prices

Demand shift. A shift that occurs when a factor other than the price of the product itself (e.g., consumer incomes) changes

Diagnosis-related groups (DRGs). Case groups that underlie Medicare's case-based payment system for hospitals

Discounting. Adjusting the value of future costs and benefits to reflect the willingness of consumers to trade current consumption for future consumption

E

Economies of scale. When larger organizations have lower average costs

Economies of scope. When multiproduct organizations have lower average costs

Efficient. Producing the most valuable output possible, given the inputs used (Viewed differently, an efficient organization uses the least expensive inputs possible, given the quality and quantity of output it produces.)

Elastic. A term used to describe demand when the quantity demanded falls by more than 1 percent when the price rises by 1 percent (This term is usually applied only to price elasticities of demand.)

Elasticity. The percentage change in a dependent variable associated with a 1 percent change in an independent variable

Equilibrium price. Price at which the quantity demanded equals the quantity supplied (There is no shortage or surplus.)

Expected value. The sum of the probability of each possible outcome multiplied by the value of the outcome

External benefit. A positive impact of a transaction for a consumer or producer not involved in the transaction

External cost. A negative impact of a transaction for a consumer or producer not involved in the transaction

Externality. A benefit or cost imposed on someone who is not a party to the transaction that causes it

F

Favorable risk selection. When an insurance plan attracts customers who use fewer services than average and therefore has lower costs

Fee-for-service. A reimbursement model that pays providers on the basis of their charges for services

Fixed costs. Costs that do not vary according to output

Framing bias. The effects of presenting the same data in different ways

Free rider. Someone who benefits from a public good without bearing its cost

G

Gainsharing. A strategy for rewarding those who contribute to an organization's success

Group model HMO. HMO that contracts with a physician group to provide services

H

Hindsight bias. The tendency to overstate how predictable an outcome was beforehand

HMO (health maintenance organization). A firm that provides comprehensive healthcare benefits to enrollees in exchange for a premium (Originally, HMOs were distinct from other insurance firms because providers were not paid on a fee-for-service basis and because enrollees faced no cost-sharing requirements.)

I

Income effects. Effects of income shifts on amounts demanded or supplied (Shifts may be due to changes in income or due to changes in purchasing power caused by price changes.)

Income elasticity of demand. The percentage change in the quantity demanded associated with a 1 percent increase in income

Increase or decrease in demand. A shift in the entire price-quantity schedule (a new demand curve, not a movement along an existing curve)

Incremental. Involving a small change from the current situation

Independent practice association (IPA) HMO. HMO that contracts with an independent practice association, which in turn contracts with physician groups

Inelastic. A term used to describe demand when the quantity demanded falls by less than 1 percent when the price rises by 1 percent (This term is usually applied only to price elasticities of demand.)

Information asymmetry. When one party in a transaction has less information than another

Information-based differentiation. Making customers aware of a product's popularity, reputation, or other signals that suggest high value

Input. Goods and services used in production

Interest group model of regulation. Model that views regulations as attempts to further the interests of affected groups, usually producer groups

L

Law of small numbers bias. Generalizations based on small samples

Life year. One additional year of life (A life year can equal one added year of life for an individual or an average of $1/n$th of a year of life for n people.)

Limit pricing. Setting prices low enough to discourage entry into a market

Loss aversion. A focus on avoiding losses rather than maximizing gains

M

Managed care. A loosely defined term that includes all plans except open-ended fee-for-service, sometimes used to describe the techniques insurance companies use

Marginal. Involving a small change from the current situation

Marginal analysis. The assessment of the effects of small changes in a decision variable (such as price or volume of output) on outcomes (such as costs, profits, or probability of recovery)

Marginal cost pricing. Using information about marginal costs and the price elasticity of demand to set profit-maximizing prices

Marginal or **incremental cost.** The cost of producing an additional unit of output

Marginal or **incremental revenue.** The revenue from selling an additional unit of output

Market system. A system that uses prices to ration goods and services

Mean absolute deviation. The average absolute difference between a forecast and the actual value (It is absolute because it converts both 9 and –9 to 9. The Excel function *ABS()* performs this conversion.)

Medicaid. A collection of state-run programs that meet standards set by the Centers for Medicare & Medicaid Services (Medicaid serves those with incomes low enough to qualify for their state's program.)

Medical home. A primary care model, often called a *patient-centered medical home*, that emphasizes being patient centered, comprehensive, team based, coordinated, accessible, and committed to quality and safety (A medical home devotes resources to coordinating care, improving communication, and making care available after office hours.)

Medicare. An insurance program for the elderly and disabled that is run by the Centers for Medicare & Medicaid Services

Medicare Part A. Coverage for inpatient hospital, skilled nursing, hospice, and home health care services

Medicare Part B. Coverage for outpatient services and medical equipment

Monopolist. A firm with no rivals

Monopolistic competitor. A competitor with multiple rivals whose products are imperfect substitutes

Moral hazard. The incentive to use additional care that having insurance creates

Moving average. The unweighted mean of the previous n data points

N

Narrow network. A limited group of providers who have contracted with an insurance company (Patients will usually pay more if they get care from a provider not in the network. The network is usually restricted to providers with good quality who will accept low payments.)

Natural monopoly. A market that can be most efficiently served by a single firm

Network externality. The effect each additional user of a product or service has on the value of that product or service to existing users

Network HMO. HMO that has a variety of contracts (including contracts with physician groups, IPAs, and individual physicians)

Nonexcludable consumption. When preventing consumption by someone who did not pay for a product is infeasible

Nonrival consumption. Consumption by one person that does not prevent simultaneous consumption by another person

Normative economics. Using values to identify the best options

O

Objective probability. An estimate of probability based on observed frequencies

Oligopolist. A firm with only a few rivals or a firm with only a few large rivals

Opportunism. Taking advantage of a situation without regard for the interests of others

Opportunity cost. The value of a resource in its next best use (The opportunity cost of a product consists of the other goods and services we cannot have because we have chosen to produce the product in question.)

Out-of-pocket payment. Total amount that a consumer spends directly for healthcare

Out-of-pocket price. The amount of money a consumer pays for a good or service

Output. Goods and services produced by an organization

Overuse of care. When the harms of services exceed the benefits

P

Pareto optimal. An allocation of resources in which no reallocation of resources is possible that will improve the well-being of one person without worsening the well-being of another

Percentage adjustment. Percentage adjustment of the past n periods of historic demand (The adjustment is essentially a best guess of what is expected to happen in the next year.)

Point-of-service (POS) plan. Plan that allows members to see any physician but increases cost sharing for physicians outside the plan's network (This arrangement has become so common that POS plans may not be labeled as such.)

Positive economics. Using objective analysis and evidence to answer questions about individuals, organizations, and societies

PPO (preferred provider organization). An insurance plan that contracts with a network of providers (Network providers may be chosen for a variety of reasons, but a willingness to discount fees is usually required.)

Preemption. Building excess capacity in a market to discourage potential entrants

Price discrimination. Selling similar products to different individuals at different prices

Price elasticity of demand. The percentage change in sales volume associated with a 1 percent change in a product's price

Principal. The organization or individual represented by an agent

Producing to order. Setting prices and then filling customers' orders

Producing to stock. Producing output and then adjusting prices to sell what has been produced

Product differentiation. The process of distinguishing a product from others

Profits. Total revenue minus total cost

Public good. A good whose consumption is nonrival and nonexcludable

Q

Quantity demanded. The amount of a good or service that will be purchased at a specific price when all other factors are held constant

R

Range. The difference between the largest and smallest values of a variable

Rational decision making. Choosing the course of action that gives you the best outcomes, given the constraints you face

Reference pricing. A system in which an insurer's allowed fee has an upper limit (A customer who chooses a provider with a price above the limit will pay the difference between the limit and the price.)

Representativeness bias. The tendency to overstate how typical a small sample is

Return on equity. Profits divided by shareholder equity

Risk adjustment. Payments (or insurance premiums) that vary to reflect patient characteristics, especially age, sex, other demographic characteristics, and health status

Risk aversion. The reluctance of a decision maker to accept an outcome with an uncertain payoff rather than a smaller, more certain outcome (A risk-averse person would prefer getting $5 for sure to a gamble with a 50 percent chance of getting nothing and a 50 percent chance of getting $10.)

Risk neutral. Indifferent to risk in decision making (A risk-neutral person would think that getting $5 for sure is as good as a gamble with a 50 percent chance of getting nothing and a 50 percent chance of getting $10.)

Risk seeker. A decision maker who prefers more risk to less (A risk seeker would prefer a gamble with a 50 percent chance of getting nothing and a 50 percent chance of getting $10 to getting $5 for sure.)

S

Salary. Fixed compensation paid per period

Scarce resources. Anything useful in consumption or production that has alternative uses

Seasonalized regression analysis. A least squares regression that includes variables that identify subperiods (e.g., weeks) that historically have had above- or below-trend sales

Sensitivity analysis. The process of varying the assumptions in an analysis over a reasonable range and observing how the outcome changes

Shortage. Situation in which the quantity demanded at the prevailing price exceeds the quantity supplied (The best indication of a shortage is that prices are rising.)

Signaling. Sending messages that reveal information another party does not observe

Societal perspective. A perspective that takes account of all costs and benefits, no matter to whom they accrue

Staff model HMO. HMO that directly employs staff physicians to provide services

Standard deviation. The square root of a variance

Status quo bias. The tendency not to change, even when it would be advantageous to do so

Subjective probability. An individual's judgment about how likely a particular event is to occur

Substitute. A product used instead of another product

Sunk costs. Costs that have been incurred and cannot be recouped

Supply curve. A graphic depiction of how much producers are willing to sell at different prices

Supply shift. Shift that occurs when a factor (e.g., an input price) other than the price of the product changes

Surplus. Situation in which the quantity supplied at the prevailing price exceeds the quantity demanded (The best indication of a surplus is that prices are falling.)

T

Tragedy of the commons. Over- or underuse of a resource that occurs when ownership of the resource is unclear and users produce externalities

U

Underwriting. The process of assessing the risks associated with an insurance policy and setting the premium accordingly

V

Variable costs. Costs that change as output changes

Variance. The squared deviation of a random variable from its expected value (If a variable takes the value 3 with a probability of 0.2, the value 6 with a probability of 0.3, and the value 9 with a probability of 0.5, its expected value is 6.9. Its variance is 5.49, which is $0.2 \times [3 - 6.9]^2 + 0.3 \times [6 - 6.9]^2 + 0.5 \times [9 - 6.9]^2$.)

INDEX

Note: Italicized page locators refer to figures or tables in exhibits.